&Nursing
midwifery
research

METHODS AND APPRAISAL FOR EVIDENCE-BASED PRACTICE **3rd** edition

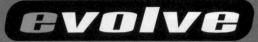

The Latest *Evolution* in Learning

Evolve provides online access to free learning resources and activities designed specifically for the textbook you are using in your class.

The resources will enhance your learning of the material covered in the book and much more.

Visit the website listed below to start your learning evolution today!

Think outside the book... evolve.

&Nursing midwifery
research

METHODS AND APPRAISAL FOR EVIDENCE-BASED PRACTICE 3rd edition

ZEVIA SCHNEIDER
DEAN WHITEHEAD
DOUG ELLIOTT
GERI LOBIONDO-WOOD
JUDITH HABER

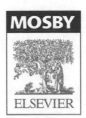

MOSBY

ELSEVIER

Sydney   Edinburgh   London   New York   Philadelphia   St Louis   Toronto

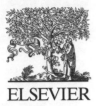

ELSEVIER

Mosby
is an imprint of Elsevier

Elsevier Australia
(a division of Reed International Books Australia Pty Ltd)
30–52 Smidmore Street, Marrickville, NSW 2204
ACN 001 002 357

National Library of Australia Cataloguing-in-Publication Data

Schneider, Zevia.
Nursing & midwifery research : methods and appraisal for
evidence-based practice.

3rd ed.
Bibliography.
Includes index.
ISBN 978 0 7295 3791 9 (pbk.).

1. Nursing - Research. 2. Midwifery - Research. I. Whitehead, Dean.
II. Elliott, Doug. III. Title. IV. Title : Nursing and midwifery research.
610.73072

Publisher: Debbie Lee
Developmental Editor: Mae-wha Boadle
Publishing Services Manager: Helena Klijn
Edited, project managed and indexed by Forsyth Publishing Services
Proofread by Pam Dunne
Typesetting, cover and internal design by DiZign
Printed in Australia by Southwood Press

Printed on paper manufactured from sustainable forests.

Foreword

It is with pleasure that I introduce this third edition of *Nursing and midwifery research: methods and appraisal for evidence-based practice*. This edition has a fresh new look, with numerous features that aid in understanding. As each of the authors contend, today's research agenda is complex and multi-dimensional, reflecting the professional worlds of nursing and midwifery. They have succeeded in writing a text that deconstructs some of this complexity and gives the reader an appreciative view of the power of research in celebrating, changing and improving practice. The central tenet of this work is outlined with remarkable clarity in the introductory chapter: scientific investigation promotes accountability, one of the hallmarks of a profession. This theme is picked up throughout subsequent chapters with illustrations from contemporary research studies. A second theme is cogently argued within the various methodological explanations; namely that to advance the professions of nursing and midwifery we have unprecedented need for accurate measurement, appropriate modes of enquiry, evidence-based decision making and innovative management and leadership. Appreciation of research is a further thread running through the text, and it is underlined with prolific examples of research studies of particular relevance to an Australasian readership.

Each of the chapters is written with an eye on developing the skills, knowledge and attitudes needed by both novice researchers and experienced professionals seeking to update their knowledge. Several features make this text an excellent educational resource for both of these groups. Chapter 3, on searching the literature, breaks down the skills required to search efficiently into small, strategic steps. It adds current information on web-searching and where to find the resources to expedite the research process. This sets the stage for the inclusion of other web resources in each subsequent chapter. Each chapter contains at least one distinctive feature in moving from the philosophical roots of various methodologies to the design features necessary for successful implementation. The emphasis on translational research is important, as are the arguments for an eclectic approach to interpretive research to make research findings relevant to practice settings. In each chapter there is a balanced discussion of pros and cons of each method, culminating in an insightful discussion of mixed methods in Chapter 15. Chapter 16, on critical evaluation, is outstanding. It will be helpful to students completing assignments, but equally as important, it provides a solid foundation of knowledge for aspiring journal referees. Chapters 19 and 20 are also excellent resources for researchers, especially in providing essential information for grant proposals, generating plausible budgets, and addressing the challenges of managing research projects and teams.

Students and teachers will appreciate the *tutorial triggers*, the many *research in brief* accounts, and the *evidence-based practice tips*. These features and the excellent figures and tables illustrating the various methodological approaches make the book highly readable and readily understood. The writers set out to foster an appreciation of nursing and midwifery research and to provide a roadmap for success. They have succeeded in both. I am extremely pleased to commend it to you, and congratulate this team of researchers and their new recruits to a third edition. I trust you will enjoy it as much as I have.

Professor Anne McMurray
Peel Health Campus Chair in Nursing
Murdoch University
February, 2007

Preface

In the five years since the 2nd edition of this book appeared, nurses and midwives, as conductors and consumers of research, have continued to champion the need for critical reading and evaluation of research reports. This edition is different from previous editions in many respects. The difference was initiated mainly by our dynamic response to market events and feedback from the Australasian region. Market events include the continuing impetus of basing practice on research evidence, and the importance of including all nurses and midwives in the research process — either through the conduct of research or the implementation of findings into practice. Events also include the recognition of midwifery as a discipline in itself. This said, research methods, be they quantitative or qualitative approaches, are generic to both nursing and midwifery. That is why midwifery commands distinct recognition in this research textbook.

Knowledge about research process, design, data collection and data analysis is essential in today's healthcare settings, and all nurses and midwives need to understand what the findings mean and their implications for changing practice. This book, then, is directed in the first instance to those health professionals, the consumers of research, who base their clinical decisions on how and when to utilise research findings to change practice. Clinical researchers will also find the content important for their beginning and continuing development in research methods applied to clinical practice. The revision of the text was guided by constructive comments from our students, colleagues and friends in allied health professions. We gratefully acknowledge their contribution in making this edition more inclusive and broader in scope, while maintaining a detailed account of the variety of common research approaches.

This edition has been restructured into three sections and 21 chapters. Section 1 *Research awareness* sets the scene for the importance of nursing and midwifery research and provides an overview of research theory and its underpinning processes. Chapters on searching for and reviewing the literature provide detailed advice for undergraduates and facilitates online access of research articles. Ethical and legal issues focussing on Australia and New Zealand are also discussed. Section 2 *Research appreciation and application* provides a detailed discussion of qualitative, quantitative and mixed-methods research approaches with many useful examples from the clinical area. Chapters are devoted to critical evaluation, implementation, sampling, collecting and analysing data in qualitative and quantitative approaches. Evidence-based practice, practice development and changing practice through research are also discussed in the latter chapters of this section.

Section 3 *Conducting primary research* is a new section and is designed to enhance the previous two sections by supporting both undergraduate and postgraduate students in their original research endeavours. Writing research proposals may be a requirement for undergraduates in their research program and postgraduates will find the information useful for developing an ethics proposal or applying for university or external funding. Research project management and useful advice on how to present research and the publishing process are detailed in the final two chapters.

We hope that you enjoy using the third edition of this text and that it stimulates and encourages you to read and think about research and its place in your professional practice. We also hope it assists in the development of your skills and confidence in critically appraising the research literature. Most importantly, we hope that you will share your information about research with your colleagues and use research findings to inform the care that you deliver to your patients. The delivery of quality nursing and midwifery care is a challenge in our dynamic health care environment. Used appropriately, this text will be a valuable tool to assist you in that process.

Zevia Schneider, Dean Whitehead
and Doug Elliott
April 2007

Contents

Section three
Conducting primary research   337

Editors

Zevia Schneider, RN, RM, PhD, MEd, MAppSc, BEd, BA FRCNA

Consultant, Formerly Associate Professor, Research, Faculty of Nursing, RMIT University, Melbourne, Vic

Dean Whitehead, MSc (Hlth Ed), BEd, PGDip (Hlth), PGCert (Hlth Ed), RN, PhD candidature

Senior Lecturer, School of Health Sciences — Nursing, Massey University, Palmerston North, NZ

Doug Elliott, RN, PhD, MAppSc (Nurs), BAppSc (Nurs), ICCert

Professor of Nursing, Director of Research, Faculty of Nursing, Midwifery and Health, University of Technology, Sydney, NSW

Contributors

Leanne M Aitken, PhD, BHSc (Nurs) (Hons), GDipScMed (ClinEpi), GCertMgt, ICCert RN FRCNA

Professor of Critical Care Nursing, Research Centre for Clinical Practice Innovation, Griffith University and Princess Alexandra Hospital, Brisbane, Qld

Merilyn Annells, PhD, MNS, BN (Ed), DipAppSc (NS), RN

Professor of Community Nursing, School of Nursing & Midwifery, Faculty of Health Sciences, La Trobe University, Bundoora, Vic

Paul Arbon AM, PhD, Med (Studies), Grad Dip Health Ed, DipEd, BSc, RN

Professor of Nursing (Population Health), Flinders University, Adelaide, SA; Adjunct Professor of Nursing and Nursing Research, University of Canberra, Canberra, ACT

Anne Coup, MPhil, BA, Dip Grad, ADN, RGON

Senior Lecturer, School of Nursing, Otago Polytechnic, Dunedin, NZ; Member College of Nurses of Aotearoa, NZ; Member New Zealand Institute for Research on Ageing

Murray J Fisher, ITcert, DipAppSc, BHSc, MHPEd, RN

Senior Lecturer, Associate Dean (Academic) (Acting), Faculty of Nursing and Midwifery, University of Sydney, NSW

Bridie Kent, PhD BSc (Hons), RN, FCNA

Associate Professor, Director of Clinical Nursing Research, University of Auckland and Auckland District Health Board, NZ; Director of the Centre for Evidence Based Nursing Aotearoa, NZ

Brendan McCormack, D.Phil (Oxon), BSc (Hons), PGCEA, RNT, RMN, RGN

Director of Nursing Research and Practice Development, Royal Group of Hospitals, Belfast and University of Ulster at Jordanstown, UK
Adjunct Professor, Faculty of Medicine, Nursing & Health Sciences, Monash University, Melbourne, Vic

David R Thompson, RN BSC MA PhD MBA FRCN FESC

Professor of Nursing & Director, The Nethersole School of Nursing, The Chinese University of Hong Kong, Hong Kong

Reviewers

Shirin Caldwell, MEd, BA, PGCert
(Public Health), RN

Lecturer, School of Health Science,
UNITEC Institute of Technology,
Te Whare Wananga o Wairaka, NZ

Glenn W Doolan, MNA, BAppSc Adv Nur
(Admin), RN, FRCNA, AFACHSE

Honorary Senior Lecturer, School of
Nursing and Midwifery, Gippsland
Campus, Monash University; DPH
Scholar, Dept Epidemiology and
Preventive Medicine, Faculty of Medicine,
Nursing and Health Sciences, Monash
University, Burnett Tower, Alfred
Hospital, Melbourne, Vic

Trudy Dwyer, RN, ICU Cert, BHlthScn
(Nurs), MClinEd, PhD

Senior Lecturer, Nursing and Health
Studies, Faculty of Science, Engineering
and Health, Central Queensland
University; RN, Rockhampton Hospital,
Qld

Susan Gallagher, RN, RPN, RMRN, BEd,
MA (Ed), MRCNA, MANZCMHN

Senior Lecturer, School of Nursing (NSW
& ACT), Faculty of Health Sciences,
Australian Catholic University, NSW

Pauline Glover, EdD, MNSt, BEd, Dip T
(Nurse Ed) RM, FACM

Associate Professor, Nursing and
Midwifery, Associate Dean Academic
Programs School of Nursing and
Midwifery, Flinders University,
Adelaide, SA

Gavin D Leslie, RN, IC Cert, PhD, BAppSc,
Post Grad Dip (Clin Nurs) FRCNA

Associate Professor, Critical Care
Nursing, Edith Cowan University and
Royal Perth Hospital; Coordinator
Master of Clinical Nursing Course, Edith
Cowan University; Head Postgraduate
Nursing Studies, Royal Perth Hospital,
WA; Editor, *Australian Critical Care*

Nita Purcal, MEd (Hons), Grad Dip Admin,
BA, Paed Cert, RM, RN

Head of Program, Midwifery, School of
Nursing, University of Western Sydney,
NSW

Frances Ward, MPH (Hons), BHSc (Nsg),
ADN, RN

Lecturer School of Health Science,
UNITEC Institute of Technology,
Te Whare Wananga o Wairaka, NZ

Donna L Waters, PhD, MPH, BA, RN

Manager, Research and Projects, The
College of Nursing; Honorary Associate,
Faculty of Nursing, Midwifery and
Health, University of Technology, Sydney,
NSW

Acknowledgments

The title and content of this third edition have been updated to reflect the ever-changing and widening scope of nursing and midwifery research, especially in relation to how we seek to develop and improve clinical practice on the basis of systematic and rigorous research. We gratefully acknowledge the strong base provided by our editors from the United States, from which the first and second Australasian editions were adapted. Our appreciation is extended to all of our contributors for their collegiality and support and also to each other for creating a friendly, supportive and cooperative environment in which to achieve our aims.

The production of this edition was facilitated by the Elsevier Australia publishing team with their assistance and support throughout the writing and production process: Vaughn Curtis, Regional Director, for his continuing support of Australasian authors; Debbie Lee, Publisher, for her insightful guidance, encouragement and management of the text's development; Amanda Simons, Editorial Coordinator, and Mae-wha Boadle and Suzanne Hall, Developmental Editors. We also thank the manuscript reviewers, colleagues and students who collectively provided feedback, suggestions and ideas to make this text more relevant, useful and meaningful to nurses and midwives.

We gratefully acknowledge the copyright holders for allowing us to reproduce their works in the text.

Most importantly we are indebted to our families who enthusiastically provided encouragement and support and were with us all the way. Zevia thanks Saul, Cheryl and Brenda for their continuing love, encouragement and support. Dean would like to express his heartfelt gratitude to Katie, Thomas and James for their unstinting love and support. Doug thanks Maureen, Kate, Nick and Josh for their love, understanding and commitment during this project.

Zevia Schneider, *Dean Whitehead* and *Doug Elliott*

Evolve ancillary authors

Elsevier Australia would like to thank the editors for their additional contribution to the Evolve website that accompanies the third edition of *Nursing and midwifery research*. In addition, Elsevier Australia would like to thank the following authors who specifically prepared the instructors' PowerPoint slides:

Glenn W Doolan MNA, BAppSc AdvNur (Admin), RN, FRCNA, AFACHSE

Honorary Senior Lecturer, School of Nursing and Midwifery, Gippsland Campus, Monash University; DPH Scholar, Dept Epidemiology and Preventive Medicine, Faculty of Medicine, Nursing and Health Sciences, Monash University, Burnett Tower, Alfred Hospital, Melbourne, Vic

Donna L Waters PhD, MPH, BA, RN

Manager, Research and Projects, The College of Nursing; Honorary Associate, Faculty of Nursing, Midwifery and Health, University of Technology, Sydney, NSW

Research
awareness

The significance of nursing research

ZEVIA SCHNEIDER AND DEAN WHITEHEAD

Learning outcomes

After reading this chapter, you should be able to:

- state the significance of research to the practice of nursing and midwifery
- discuss the major developments of international nursing research over the last 100 years
- describe the major events in the history of nursing and midwifery in Australia
- describe Australasian perspectives of the relationships between research, education and practice
- identify the place of the consumer of nursing and midwifery research
- evaluate the nurse's and midwife's role in the research process as it relates to their level of educational preparation through research units
- recognise the relationship of research to evidence-based practice (EBP) and practice development (PD)
- identify future trends in nursing and midwifery research.

Introduction

The recent proliferation of nursing and midwifery-related textbooks and journal articles on differing research issues are evidence of a heightened interest and activity in research overall. Many nurses and midwives share the belief that a knowledge of and involvement in research can have a significant effect on the depth and breadth of their professional practice. Much of this interest and belief has been generated through the advent of evidence-based practice (EBP), also referred to as evidence-based nursing (EBN), an increasing emphasis on professional accountability, and through drives to provide quality clinical outcomes.

The purpose of this opening chapter is to help develop an appreciation of the significance of research in nursing and midwifery and their research roles through historical and futuristic views. This chapter explores the relationships between research, practice and professional development, including a brief examination of developments in nursing and midwifery, particularly in terms of professional organisations and journals. It seeks to explore these issues, as does the rest of this book, while grounded in and through a particular emphasis on the Australasian perspective.

Background of evidence-based nursing and evidence-based midwifery

EBN and EBM have their roots in the evidence-based medicine movement that grew from clinicians' concerns about the proliferation of clinical trials without attempts to integrate research findings into medical practice. Similarly, definitions of evidence-based practice emphasise the principle of integration of the best available evidence with the practitioner's clinical expertise, together with patient preferences within a context of limited resources. EBN and EBM have brought about a change in emphasis from 'doing' research to 'understanding' research (see Chapters 17 and 18), which reflects a move from 'research generation' towards 'research utilisation' in practice. A strong policy emphasis on clinical effectiveness means that nurses and midwives are increasingly called upon to justify their clinical decisions and outcomes — to peers, colleagues, commissioners and consumers of healthcare (French 2005). There is clear direction in the Australian Nursing and Midwifery Council (ANMC) National Competency Standards (2005) for the graduate midwife to use research to inform practice.

Health professionals are cognisant that they are accountable and responsible for providing the best possible standard of patient care. It is well accepted that effective research activity, aligned with evidence-based practice, is the best way to ensure quality healthcare provision.

Nursing and midwifery are diverse disciplines in an epistemological sense — that is, the philosophical examination of human knowledge in terms of its origins, nature, methods and limits (see Chapter 2). As such, research in both disciplines encompasses the full range of philosophical and methodological pursuits — from studying an 'n of one' (an in-depth study of one participant) through to large epidemiological studies (large-scale surveys); from in-depth understanding of unique personal experiences through to broad survey findings. Nursing and midwifery have 'unique' places in the world of research endeavour by the nature of their role and function (Leslie & McAllister 2002). This said, they do not always effectively conduct or make good use of research findings and often find themselves criticised for this. Many nursing studies highlight why this is the case; mostly suggesting that nurses find it difficult to translate the findings of published research into practice (Edwards et al. 2002; Olade 2003; Veeramah 2004).

One of the aims of this book is to assist nurses, midwives and other health professionals in developing critical appraisal skills and research consumer expertise, as well as to provide some beginning skills in conducting research. This book then acts as an organiser for learning in conjunction with formal research courses undertaken primarily at the undergraduate level. There are three sections: Section 1 examines the key aspects of research awareness, research process, critical reading and appraisal skills (searching and reviewing literature), formulating research questions and ethical issues. Section 2 incorporates chapters on common qualitative and quantitative approaches and processes, mixed method research, critical evaluation of research, evidence-based practice and practice development, and changing practice through research. Section 3 provides practical information about writing research proposals and grant applications, managing a research project and presenting and publishing conducted research.

Research awareness and consumerism — how this book accommodates these

Many nurses and midwives who are not committed to conducting research do at least recognise the necessity of having the knowledge to critically read research reports, because it is on the basis of understanding the report that decisions about practice change can be made. This is often the first step that health professionals take in their quest to become familiar with research and the process of research; that is the critical searching and review of the research literature (see Chapters 4 and 5). It is also the first step towards 'research awareness' — the intention of the first section of this book. Many students of nursing and midwifery acknowledge the importance and need of research units in their undergraduate programs where, again, this often represents their introduction to the research process. This text is designed in such a way that it introduces the reader gradually to the nuances of the research process and allows them to progress, or access at will, from 'research awareness', to 'research consumerism', through to 'research application'.

There is now a focus on research awareness and consumerism and an acknowledgment that nursing is not presently a 'purely research-driven' profession (Koziol-McLain et al. 2002 p 364). This applies to midwifery also. In essence, both disciplines rely not just on 'hard research-driven data' for evidencing

practice and change of practice, but other forms of evidence apply as well; that is, tacit knowledge, professional experience, patients' needs and values, conceptual/theoretical knowledge etc. Research then must be critically read and evaluated, as well as aligned with other forms of professional evidence, before it can be implemented and practice changed. The internet has provided quick and easy access to current research articles concurrent with declarations from federal, state and territory governments, stakeholders, hospital administration, and not least the public, who want to be assured that the community is receiving the best possible care. Accessing the information from the internet also requires knowledge of information technology (Pravikoff et al. 2005). As the ability to appraise research studies develops, the complexity of practice and the associated critical-thinking skills will become more appreciated. This, in turn, will help to refine clinical judgment and decision-making skills. The ultimate beneficiaries will be the recipients of quality care.

● **Evidence-based practice tip**
Patient needs and values, together with the RNs', or RMs', clinical expertise and critical analysis of research findings, must also be considered when implementing practice change.

A short history of international and Australasian nursing research

A good place to start an appreciation of nursing research is to explore its historical roots and origins. The development of nursing, and therefore nursing research, has a long and interesting history which has included many theories, models and innovations. The groundwork for what has blossomed into an international research-based discipline was laid in the late nineteenth century and the first half of the twentieth century, and is intimately related to the development of clinical practice, education and disciplinary knowledge.

Post-1850

In the mid-nineteenth century, nursing as a formal discipline began evolving with the ideas and practices of Florence Nightingale. Her concepts are congruent with the present priorities of nursing research, particularly epidemiological methods. Nightingale believed that the systematic collection and exploration of data were necessary for nursing. Her collection and analysis of data on the health status of British soldiers during the Crimean War led to a variety of reforms in healthcare (Palmer 1977). Nightingale also noted the need for measuring outcomes of nursing and medical care.

Other than Nightingale's work, there appears to have been little documented research during the early years of the development of nursing, perhaps in part because schools of nursing had just begun to be established internationally and nursing leadership was beginning to develop independently of medicine. Lucy Osborn introduced the Nightingale model of nurse training to Australia in 1868 (Godden & Forsyth 2000). This was a formalised apprenticeship where student nurses provided the majority of direct nursing care in hospitals while undertaking the course (Russell 1990). The Japanese Red Cross established a similar model in 1890 (Hisama 2001), as did other countries in the Western Pacific region.

1900–1950 Regulation and journals

The Australasian Trained Nurses Association was formed at the turn of the century, but it was not until the 1920s that nursing training and practice began to be regulated and standardised within the states and territories of Australia (Russell 1990). In the case of Midwifery, the *Midwives Act* of 1901 was the mechanism through which formal regulation was introduced and, with the exception of the Australian Capital Territory and Northern Territory, all Australian states were registering midwives (Bogossian 1998). Although nursing and midwifery in Australia are considered discrete occupations, midwifery has been subordinated because of the absence of strong leadership to fight for independent status and practice (ACMI 1990), and lack of protection through government policy and legislation (Bogossian 1998). Also, legislation regulating the practice of midwives varies across states and territories.

1950–2006

In Australia, by the 1960s, there were six separate areas of nursing: general, psychiatric, geriatric, mental retardation, midwifery and mothercraft (Russell 1990). The 1970s saw the enrolled nurse (EN) role introduced and, while not the cause of introducing ENs, poor wages for registered nurses (RNs) and the strict regulations requiring trainees to live-in impacted on the supply of student nurses and registered nurses. A period of industrial and professional changes coincided with changes in societal factors (including the role of women and increased general education). This ultimately resulted in undergraduate nursing education transferring from hospital-based certificate programs into higher education diploma programs (1985–1993): postgraduate programs in research and speciality coursework developed from the late 1980s. Doctoral studies in nursing were possible following implementation of the unified national tertiary education system in 1993. Prior to this time, nurse academics had qualifications predominantly from education, arts and social sciences.

In Australia, the debate regarding 'direct entry' midwifery involved issues about whether midwives should also be nurses, how recognition of prior learning would impact on nurses wishing to enter the program, and whether 'direct entry' should become a mainstream option (Leap 1999).

Issues were resolved and by 2003 a direct entry midwifery (DEM) three-year degree had been introduced into some Australian universities.

A comprehensive examination of the development of nursing research globally and the works of so many excellent researchers, especially in the 1980s and 1990s, is beyond the scope of this chapter, but is discussed elsewhere from Australian (Russell 1990; Wiles & Daffurn 2002), New Zealand (New Zealand Nurses Organisation, NZNO; http://www.NZNO.org.nz), British (Crookes & Davies 1998) and United States (US National Institute for Nursing Research, NINR; http://www.nih.gov/ninr/amission.html) perspectives. As the profession developed during the 1990s, a number of peer-reviewed Australian and New Zealand nursing research journals commenced publication (see Table 1.1). Both the Royal College of Nursing, Australia (RCNA) and the College of Nursing were producing professional journals, and the development of clinical chairs (professorships) in Australia and New Zealand created effective links between the healthcare sector and tertiary education sectors. The role of clinical professors has traditionally included research, education and politics. Research centres developed to support the professors and provided guidance for research efforts in the clinical environment (Dunn & Yates 2000).

The East Asian Forum of Nursing Scholars was formed for cross-national support of academic nursing. Currently both national-based and state/territory-based nursing professional groups and organisations are developing priorities for nursing research and strategies for promoting evidence-based nursing (EBN) practice in Australasia (see Chapters 17 & 18). In New Zealand, for instance, the Nursing Council of New Zealand (NCNZ) has, through its *Health Practitioners Competence Assurance Act* (2003 — www.nursingcouncil. org.nz), legislated for nurse registration against 'recertification' (professional competence and development audit). The requirement for all nurses to maintain a required standard of continuing competence clearly identifies the place of research and evidence-based practice, as an integral part of this process.

A re-ordering of research priorities and a targeting of practice-oriented research occurred in the 1960s in the US. Studies on nurses and nursing continued, but at the same time the pioneers in the development of nursing theories and models, such as Orlando (1961), Peplau (1952) and Wiedenbach (1964), called for the development of nursing practice based on theory. However, even with support from major nursing organisations, research did not flourish. Where research education did exist, nurses had not yet developed sufficient expertise in research design and methodology to teach their own research courses and were, until recently, dependent on others from related disciplines such as psychology, education and sociology to teach these courses. Today this is not usually the case; units in research methods are being taught by nurses throughout the undergraduate program.

The 1970s also saw extended growth among US graduate programs in nursing, especially at the doctoral level. Many nurses from Australia went to the United States to complete higher degree programs as none were available locally at the time. These programs, along with the American Nurses Association (ANA) and Sigma Theta Tau (the international honour society for nurses — see http://www.nursingsociety.org), clearly supported nurses learning the research process as well as producing research that could be used to enhance care quality. Sigma Theta Tau has over 400 chapters throughout the world, including Australia, New Zealand, Hong Kong, Korea, Taiwan and Pakistan. Alliances with this and other international organisations committed to the goal of health for all will create natural research partnerships. The International Council of Nurses (ICN), to which the RCNA and New Zealand Nursing Organisation (NZNO) are affiliated, and groups such as the American Academy of Nursing (http://www.nursingworld.org/aan), and other organisations are examples of international nursing research forums designed to inform nurses of the global breadth of health issues.

Additional journals, such as *Advances in Nursing Sciences*, *Nurse Researcher*, *Journal of Advanced Nursing*, *Research in Nursing and Health*, *Western Journal of Nursing Research*, and *Journal of Nursing Scholarship*, were established in the 1970s and continue to promote the generation of nursing theory and research. Since then, other successful journals — such as the highly regarded *Journal of Clinical Nursing* — have been established to further this cause. Of course, a number of textbooks (including this one), exclusively devoted to nursing and midwifery-related research, have been successfully developed and published over the last few decades, to add to the research literature of both disciplines.

The efforts in the last 20 years have been aimed at the refinement and development of research and the utilisation of research findings in clinical practice in Western healthcare delivery. Adoption of research findings to practice is often based on findings from a systematic review of a series of method-related studies. There are now many resources available to assist clinicians to provide best practice. The Joanna Briggs Institute for Evidence Based Nursing and Midwifery (http://www.joannabriggs.edu.au) was formed to examine the literature in relation to practice and has established collaborating centres — such as an active centre based at the University of Auckland in New Zealand. Elsewhere, the EBP movement remains to the fore (e.g. Cochrane Collaboration, York Centre for Evidence-Based Nursing).

Journal publications

The *Australian Nurses Journal* (ANJ) was first published in 1903 and the *Australian Journal of Advanced Nursing* commenced publication in 1983.

The first midwifery journal, the *College of Midwives Journal*, was published in 1988 and reflected the growing stature of the profession. In 2006 the name changed to *Women & Birth* and became an international journal. Research studies, articles, and theoretical and philosophical papers are invited from midwives, health professionals, consumers and scholars from other disciplines that focus on all matters that affect women and birth. *Kai Tiaki Nursing New Zealand*, under a variety of titles, has been published since 1908, and details similarly occurring events and processes as those detailed in the Australian history of nursing throughout the 1900s. *Nursing Praxis in New Zealand* was first published in 1985.

In the United States, development and documentation of nursing research focused mainly on nursing education, but some patient- and technique-oriented research was evident. That is, nurses, not patients, were predominantly the subjects of study. This was later reflected in initial nursing research in Australia. The pioneering works of some US nurses (e.g. Dock 1900; Wald 1915; Goodrich 1932), were for the purpose of reforming education in nursing and establishing it as a viable profession in the US. Some clinical research emerged in the US in the early half of the twentieth century and centred mainly on the morbidity and mortality rates associated with such problems as pneumonia and contaminated milk (Carnegie 1976).

Social change and World War II affected all aspects of nursing, including research.

Military needs created a shortage of nursing personnel. After the war, nursing, like the rest of the world, began to reassess itself and its goals. A number of reports from the US demonstrated the need for nursing to enter the university setting and to update the description of nursing practices. A number of studies on nursing roles and needs followed (Simmons & Henderson 1964).

The significance of research in nursing and midwifery

Nursing and midwifery are practised in a complex and structured environment with many competing demands — hence practitioners need to work effectively within the clinical environment. Increasingly, healthcare environments evolve at an unprecedented pace, forcing nurses to challenge and expand their 'comfort zone' through considering creative approaches to old and new health problems (Davidson & Elliott 2001). The complexity of maintaining and improving the quality of care and increasing government and consumer questioning of the quality and increasing costs of healthcare has invited the query 'How do nurses or midwives make a difference?' Using research findings from rigorous, high quality studies to justify practice is an appropriate way to address this question and its associated challenges.

Points to ponder
▶ Consider some of the ways in which nurses and midwives can become involved in using research findings in the clinical area.
▶ Consumers of research will have as much say about implementing findings into practice as those who conduct research.

There is general consensus that the research role for nursing and midwifery graduates, from both Bachelor of Nursing and Bachelor of Midwifery programs, calls for the skills of critical appraisal. That is, nurses and midwives must be knowledgeable research consumers, able to critique and evaluate research findings to determine their merit for utilisation in clinical practice.

Nursing and midwifery research provides a specialised scientific knowledge base that empowers both professions to participate actively in constantly shifting clinical-care related challenges and to maintain their place and role in society. While this has occurred throughout the world, a significant number of professional organisations have concurrently emerged from within the Australasian and Asia–Pacific region. Table 1.1 lists examples of professional nursing organisations that have formed and journals that have been developed to advance the professions through various activities, including research and publishing. The listing is for illustrative purposes only, and does not encompass all organisations or journals associated with nursing or midwifery in Australasia.

There are also many other intradisciplinary and interdisciplinary professional groups promoting education, research and practice development throughout the Asia–Pacific region and elsewhere; for example, Australian Cardiac Rehabilitation Association (http://www.acra.net.au); Renal Society of Australasia (http://www.renalsociety.org).

The Australian Nursing and Midwifery Council Incorporated (ANMC) and the Nursing Council of New Zealand (NCNZ) developed a set of national competencies and domains for registered nurses and midwives in both countries, and identified research as a core competency of the registered professional nurse and midwife role. The elements relating to these competencies state that an RN acknowledges the importance of research in improving nursing outcomes; incorporates research findings into nursing practice; and contributes to the process of nursing research. The National Competency Standards for the Midwife regarding research directs a midwife to incorporate research evidence into practice. While there is no directive to conduct research, the midwife must show evidence of being a knowledgeable research consumer who uses analytic skills to evaluate evidence and inform practice. The Royal College of Nursing Australia (RCNA) (http://www.rcna.org.au) statement on nursing research reiterated this view. The statement noted that scientific investigation promotes accountability, which is one of the hallmarks of a profession. The

RCNA also has a research network to support members interested in research. Similarly, the New Zealand Nurses Organisation (NZNO), through its nursing research section (NRS), promotes and fosters research as an integral component of nursing practice (www.nzno.org.nz).

Point to ponder

▶ Commitment to the research process is required of all nurses and midwives in Australia and New Zealand: this commitment involves the critical analysis of research and the will to implement research findings into practice.

Speciality nursing groups also highlight the importance of research in their practice settings. For example, the Australian College of Critical Care Nurses (ACCCN) developed a set of competencies for specialist critical care nurses. These included participating in collaborative research within the multidisciplinary team, and incorporating research findings into nursing practice (ACCCN 2002). The College also has a research advisory panel to support members and advise the National Executive. Other professional colleges have similar statements relating to the importance of research in their practice. The Australian and New Zealand College of Mental Health Nurses Incorporated has a research board to support professional practice development. The Australian College of Midwives Incorporated (ACMI) recognises that midwifery practice, as an independent discipline, requires demonstration of evidence-based knowledge (ACMI 1998). The New Zealand Nurses Organisation continues to promote research as an integral component of nursing practice, and helps develop organisational research through their nursing research section (NRS) and affiliated nurse speciality groups. Similarly, the East Asian Forum of Nurse Scholars (EAFONS) convened in 1997 to promote research and scholarship among its university members from Hong Kong, South Korea, Taiwan, Thailand and the Philippines — particularly in terms of doctoral education and support.

TABLE 1.1 Sample of professional nursing organisations and journals in Australasia

Nursing organisation	Affiliated journal	Further details — website
New Zealand Nursing Organisation (NZNO)	*Kai Tiaki Nursing New Zealand*	http://www.nzno.org.nz
College of Nurses — Aotearoa (NZ)	*Te Puawai*	http://www.nurse.org.nz
Association for Australian Rural Nurses	newsletter	http://www.aarn.asn.au
Australasian Neuroscience Nurses' Association	*Australian Journal of Neuroscience*	http://www.users.bigpond/com/annaexecutive
Australian and New Zealand College of Mental Health Nurses	*Australian and New Zealand Journal of Mental Health Nursing*	http://healthsci.utas.edu.au/nursing/college/index
Australian College of Critical Care Nurses	*Australian Critical Care*	http://www.acccn.com.au
Australian Confederation of Operating Room Nurses	*ACORN: the Journal of Perioperative Nursing in Australia*	http://www.acornjournalcjb.net.au
Australian College of Midwives Incorporated	*Women & Birth*	http://acmi.org.au
Australian Nursing Federation	*Australian Journal of Advanced Nursing*	http://www.anf.org.au
Congress of Aboriginal and Torres Strait Islander Nurses	newsletter	http://www.indiginet.com.au/catsin
Joanna Briggs Institute for Evidence Based Nursing and Midwifery	*Changing Practice information sheets*	http://www.joannabriggs.edu.au
Royal College of Nursing, Australia	*Collegian*	http://www.rcna.org.au
New South Wales College of Nursing	*Nursing.Aust*	http://www.nursing.aust.edu.au
South East Asian Forum of Nursing Scholars	*Asian Journal of Nursing Studies*	http://nhs.polyu.edu.hk/nhs/schacht/schact-asian
Transplant Nurses Association	*Transplant Nurses Journal*	http://www.tna.asn.au
Independent and other professional publications		
New Zealand Nursing Review — www.nursingreview.co.nz *Australian Journal of Rural Health* *Australian Journal of Advanced Nursing* *Contemporary Nurse* *Hong Kong Nursing Journal* *International Journal of Nursing Practice* *Journal of Korean Academy of Nursing* *Nursing Inquiry* *Singapore Nursing Journal*		

Linking theory, education and practice to nursing research

Research links theory, education and practice. Theory supported by research findings becomes the foundation of theory-based practice in nursing. The educational setting provides an environment in which students can learn about the research process. In this setting, they can also explore different theories and begin to evaluate them in light of research findings. All primary research adheres to a set of principles and guidelines regarding the ethical conduct of research — see, for example, the Australian Vice-Chancellors Committee and National Health and Medical Research Council guidelines (http://www.avcc.edu.au/news/publications). These issues are also discussed in more detail in Chapter 6.

Three examples of linking research to practice are outlined below, and discussed further throughout this book.

1. Campbell and Torrance (2005) explored self-reported changes in coronary risk factors by patients three to nine months following coronary artery angioplasty. It appeared that many patients did not understand that they still had coronary artery disease and that the angioplasty was not a cure. Despite the seriousness of chest pain, few patients reported this information to their doctor. As a result of these findings pre-procedure education programs were recommended.

2. Jirojwong et al. (2005) assessed health outcomes of home follow up visits after postpartum discharge. While a positive relationship between the number of home visits and a woman's confidence to perform maternal roles was found, there was no positive correlation between number of home visits and the Edinburgh postpartum depression scale. The researchers acknowledged their inability to control for extraneous variables and recommended further investigation.

3. In a study exploring medication knowledge and self-management practices of people with type 2 diabetes who regularly attended the diabetic outpatient clinic, Dunning and Manias (2005) found that patients' medication knowledge and self-management were inadequate. They recommended that asking about

complementary and self-initiated medicine use should be standard nursing practice.

The three research studies above highlight the importance of examining one's clinical practice. The recommendations do much to enhance patient care.

At this point it could be asked how education in nursing and midwifery research links theory and practice. The answer is twofold. First, knowledge about research methods provides an appreciation and an understanding of the research process to encourage participation in research activities. Second, it should enable students to become intelligent research consumers. A research consumer uses and applies research to practice in an active and systematic manner. To be knowledgeable consumers, nurses and midwives must have knowledge about the relevant research process, the ability to evaluate information logically and the skills to apply the knowledge gained. It is not necessary to undertake research studies to be able to critically evaluate research projects and make decisions about the usefulness of the findings in practice.

Research in brief

Alexander et al. (2003) evaluated a newly created breastfeeding support group run by a breastfeeding counsellor and a midwife in a socioeconomically disadvantaged housing estate in the UK. 'Bosom Buddies' were trained to assist with the weekly drop-in group. Fifty three women attended and consented to complete an anonymous questionnaire six weeks after their first attendance. The response rate was 87%. Findings indicated that the group was highly successful in supporting women to continue to breastfeed for at least six weeks following their first attendance. There also appeared to be psychosocial benefits.

Educational preparation for conducting research

A Bachelor of Nursing or Bachelor of Midwifery qualification prepares the graduate to use research findings to inform their clinical practice. This also occurs at the postgraduate level — depending on the level of research experience that students have already been exposed to. The *ability* to conduct research is nowadays generally learnt at a bachelor honours or graduate research level. In particular, nurses and midwives are educationally prepared at the research master's and doctoral levels to conduct independent primary research. At the master's level, nurses and midwives are prepared to be active members of research teams. They are able to assume the role of clinical expert, collaborating with an experienced researcher in proposal development, data collection, data analysis and interpretation. Master's-prepared nurses enhance the quality and relevance of nursing research by providing clinical expertise about problems and by providing knowledge about the way the clinical services are delivered. They facilitate the investigation of clinical problems by providing a conducive climate for research activity and provide leadership by assisting colleagues in applying research-based knowledge to their practice.

Nurses or midwives who have a PhD (Doctor of Philosophy, an advanced higher research degree) have the greatest amount of expertise in appraising, designing and conducting research. They develop theoretical explanations of phenomena relevant to their discipline, methods of scientific inquiry, and use analytical and empirical methods to discover ways to extend the knowledge base of the discipline. In addition to their role as producers of research, doctoral-prepared nurses and midwives act as role models and mentors who guide, stimulate and encourage others who are developing their research skills. They also collaborate with and serve as consultants to social, educational or healthcare institutions or governmental agencies in their research endeavours. Doctoral-prepared nurses and midwives are expected to disseminate their research findings to the scientific community, to clinicians and, as appropriate, to the lay public. Scientific journals, professional conferences and the news media are among the avenues for dissemination (see Chapter 21).

The most important implication of the delineation of research activities according to educational preparation is the necessity of having a collaborative research relationship within the professions. Nursing and midwifery education programs affiliated with universities enable the study of research through to the doctoral level. Nurses and midwives at all educational levels, whether they are consumers or producers of research or both, need to view the research process as something of integral value to their discipline's growing professionalism.

Clinical programs of research

Nurses and midwives who are prepared to direct the conduct of research will head an expanding number of nursing research departments in clinical settings. Nurse and midwife researchers, often clinical professors, who head these centres will increasingly involve clinical nursing staff in generating and conducting research projects, and critically evaluating existing research data to enable improvements in clinical practice. Collaborative centres that link healthcare services and universities in partnership are established focuses for nursing research development in Australasia.

Research training for the scientific role of nurses and midwives will increasingly become an essential component of a research career plan. Programs that support a clinician scientist track, such as with the Canadian Institutes of Health Research (http://www.cihr.ca/funding_opportunities/) or the US National Institute of Nursing Research (NINR; http://www.nih.gov/ninr/research) will develop more widely. Succession planning for clinical chairs will become more sophisticated, and linked to developing programs of research that are supported by public and private funding sources at national and international levels. They will also subscribe to a lifestyle of periodic education and re-training, supported by awards, grants and fellowships. For instance, in Australia the Prime Minister announced, in late 2002, the national research priorities:
- an environmentally sustainable Australia
- promoting and maintaining good health
- frontier technologies for building and transforming Australian industries
- safeguarding Australia.

(http://www.dest.gov.au/sectors/research_sector/policies_issues_reviewers/key_issues/national_research_priorities/default.htm)

There is currently minimal documentation or systematic examination of specific priority areas for nursing research within Australasia although health professionals fit comfortably in *promoting and maintaining good health* and *safeguarding Australia*. Some organisations (e.g. Joanna Briggs Institute for Evidence Based Nursing and Midwifery; NZNO) maintain registers of projects submitted by individual researchers, but in the case of the RCNA, a directory of research ceased publication in 1994. Readers are therefore directed to publications from Australasian professional nursing organisations (listed in Table1.1) and the NHMRC for current or future opportunities for primary research in priority areas.

In the US, research priorities are much more established as a result of the National Institute of Health's infrastructure and significant funding: the 2002 priority areas include management of chronic pain; cachexia; biobehavioural management and quality of life; informal care giving; infrastructure development in nursing research training and career development; and training opportunities in clinical genetics research (http://www.nih.gov/ninr/research/dea).

Promoting nursing and midwifery research

There are a number of ways of promoting research studies in nursing and midwifery. For example, clinical consortia — that is, a number of clinical departments from different institutions, formed for a particular purpose (e.g. treatment of venous leg ulcers, factors influencing breastfeeding in first-time mothers) — will help delineate the common aspects of patient care for the various health professions. Cluster studies, multiple site investigations and programs of research will facilitate the accumulation of evidence supporting or refuting an existing theory and thereby contribute to defining the base of practice.

Nursing and midwifery researchers will continue to gain increased methodological expertise across the full range of the paradigm (see Chapter 2), and are increasingly sophisticated regarding the development and application of computer technology to the research process. A greater emphasis will be placed on measurement issues such as the development of valid tools that accurately measure clinical phenomena. The increasing focus on the need to use multiple measures to assess clinical phenomena accurately is also apparent. Related to the need to measure clinical phenomena accurately will be the development of non-invasive methods to measure physiological parameters of interest in high technology settings (e.g. non-invasive, minimally invasive and invasive haemodynamic measurement). Qualitative research methods (see Chapter 7) will continue to evolve as an increasingly important mode of enquiry, contributing to theory development and providing essential descriptive data that provide direction for clinical practice and future research studies. To facilitate involvement in the research process, it would be helpful for nurses and midwives to join their agency's quality improvement (QI) or quality assurance (QA) committees. Here research articles, projects and clinical practice guidelines are often reviewed and evaluated for evidence-based clinical decision-making. A discussion of other factors that may enhance nursing and midwifery research follows.

Other important factors in facilitating effective nursing and midwifery research

Research roles

There are many roles for nurses, midwives and other health professionals in clinical research (e.g. Dunn & Yates 2000; Ocker & Pawlick Plank 2000). Academic nurses, midwives and senior clinicians are commonly involved as both primary researchers and in the utilisation of research into clinical practice. As noted earlier, all registered nurses and midwives are expected to be proactive consumers of research within the domain of their clinical practice. Thus, the role of the Bachelor of Nursing and the Bachelor of Midwifery graduates in the research process is primarily that of a knowledgeable consumer, a role that promotes the integration of research and clinical practice. Health professionals with direct patient care responsibilities within the healthcare and tertiary sector need skills and experience in critical reading and the determination to work collaboratively. In her study on the changing context of clinical research, McCallin (2006) concluded that experienced nurse researchers should take active roles as interdisciplinary research leaders, innovators and managers. As members of a profession, it is also incumbent on nurses and midwives to share research findings with colleagues, through local education sessions, conference presentations and publications (see Chapter 21).

> ● **Evidence-based practice tip**
> Once a clinical nursing or midwifery issue has been identified, a literature search and review will reveal the extent to which the issue has been researched.

Collaborative research teams

Nurses and midwives also participate in primary or secondary research projects as members of an interdisciplinary or intra-disciplinary research team in one or more phases of such a project. Primary research is where original data are being collected as part of a defined research project. For example, a nurse may work on a clinical research unit where a particular type of nursing care is part of an established research protocol, such as for nurse-initiated analgesia in the emergency department, management of decubitus ulcers (pressure sores), or urinary incontinence. In such a situation, the nurse manages the care according to the format described in the protocol. The protocol may be substantiated by a systematic review developed by the unit staff or available from a data repository (e.g. http://cochrane.hcn.net.au/clib). Nurses and midwives may also be involved in the design of the study, collection and recording of data relevant to patient care delivery, and evaluation of that care, including clients' responses. Secondary research refers to the collection and new synthesis and analysis of findings, as in a review of previous studies. In this case, a collaborative team of multidisciplinary stakeholders may form to establish the best available evidence for a specific clinical practice (e.g. the management of mucositis for individuals with cancer). These activities inform the development of clinical guidelines and other documents to guide clinical practice.

Research in brief

Johnston et al. (2005) recruited thousands of nurses and social workers in a knowledge, attitude and practice cross-sectional survey for training in smoking cessation counselling in Hong Kong. Findings revealed an unmet need in the health professionals working with the elderly regarding smoking cessation. It is recommended that future research should develop and evaluate programs that encourage nurses and social workers to provide cessation interventions — and work collaboratively together in doing so.

Generating relevant research questions

Another important consideration is to match the research question being asked to an appropriate method (see Chapter 5). For example, a question about identifying the most effective clinical intervention needs to be answered using a design and method that will allow comparison of the different interventions or treatments available. Similarly, if the research aim is to gain better understanding of the health problems for a particular population, then a design and method that facilitates exploration of the experiences of individuals with a specific condition are warranted.

Research in brief

A study was designed to explore and describe registered and enrolled nurses' experiences of ethics and human rights issues in nursing practice in Victoria (Johnstone et al. 2004). Frequent and disturbing ethical issues included: safeguarding patients' rights and dignity, possible risk to their own health when providing care, using physical/chemical restraints, working with unethical/impaired colleagues and poor working conditions. From such findings, and linking potentially difficult-to-ask questions against an appropriate method, practice can be improved.

Clinical governance and clinical audit

The concept of 'clinical governance' is integral to the clinicians' goal to provide the most effective and best quality care for their clients. Clinical governance was first described in the United Kingdom as a system designed to ensure that clinical standards are met and that strategies are present to ensure continuous improvement of clinical practice. The major elements of clinical governance are: 'education, clinical audit, clinical effectiveness, risk management, research and development, and openness' (Starey 2001 p 2). Nursing, midwifery and other professional primary healthcare agencies champion the need for continuing education and recognise it as necessary if their goal of providing best quality care to their clients is to be achieved.

'Clinical audit' or measuring clinical performance against a profession's performance indicators has long been a feature of nursing practice. While necessary, clinical experience and expertise are no longer sufficient for ensuring the best care; clinical expertise must be informed by evidence from quality research studies. Ultimately, evidence from research studies should determine clinical practice.

Points to ponder

▶ Nurses and midwives at all levels of education should be invited to participate, and initiated into research projects, in their clinical area.

▶ In addition to research utilisation, it is often nurse clinicians or midwives who generate research ideas or questions, based on hunches, gut feelings, intuition, observations of patients, or nursing care or quality assurance programs in their healthcare environment (see Chapter 5). These ideas are often the seeds of further research investigations or quality improvement projects. For example, Aranda and Pollard (2003) developed a structured process to facilitate practice change from their experience in their mucositis project.

evolve

Future directions for nursing and midwifery research: 2007 and onwards

The future of nursing and midwifery research in the Australasian region looks to be an exciting one in which all will have the opportunity to participate. At the present time, Australian and New Zealand nurses continue to develop a strong and viable research base as evidenced in the many research publications. Research in midwifery has not yet attained the high profile accorded to nursing, however, a sound research profile is emerging and becoming increasingly visible.

Research continues to grow and flourish despite the difficulties being experienced by the profession within the evolving healthcare environment. In Australia, New Zealand and the Western Pacific region there are increasing numbers of doctoral-prepared nurses and higher degree programs are available within most universities. All new nurses graduate with a Bachelor of Nursing degree in Australia and New Zealand, and previously registered nurses are mostly upgrading their qualifications to degree level and above. Development in midwifery as a separate and unique health discipline continues, with direct entry programs being implemented.

It is of paramount importance to define the future direction of nursing and midwifery research and establish research priorities. Equity of access to appropriate healthcare services for all members of society will continue to challenge the collective consciousness of nurses and other stakeholders at the practice and policy-making levels, as well as providing opportunities for research. Also, with the disciplines' emphasis on cultural aspects of care and the influence of such factors on practice, increasing international research is a natural futuristic trend. Access to multiple populations as a function of globalisation allows the generation and testing of healthcare science from many different perspectives. Interaction with colleagues from other countries provides a rich context for the generation and dissemination of research issues (e.g. McKinley et al. 2000; Stewart & Jaasma 2001). Professional speciality organisations will also continue to formalise collaborative networks for mutual benefit, both locally and internationally. For example, in 2001 the World Federation of Critical Care Nurses was formed as an alliance between critical care nursing organisations from Australasia, Europe and North America.

Today, there is a heightened focus on evidence-based practice. To support this, there is the emerging influence of 'Magnet Hospitals' in developing and sustaining an environment where nursing-related evidence-based practice and practice change are more likely to occur. Magnet Hospitals are reviewed, evaluated and judged according to 65 standards developed by the American Nurses Credentialing Centre (ANCC) to meet the highest quality of nursing practice and patient care (http://www.lifespan. org/tmh/services/nursing/magnet.htm). The Magnet Hospital concept is now well developed and its application is strong and increasing in both New Zealand and Australia. More studies are validating the place of Magnet Hospitals in terms of practice change, organisational change and their ability to directly translate and apply appropriate research findings (Baker et al. 2004; Robinson 2006; Caramanica & Small 2006).

To support the evidence-based practice continuum, nursing and midwifery are sure to witness other research reform which will include more outcome-related research and practice-change initiatives. The development and adoption of an increased and diverse range of research methods will fuel this. As a consequence of these improvements, both disciplines will develop growing numbers of diverse research forums, academic and otherwise, to ensure effective dissemination of research findings. Subsequently, nursing and midwifery research will become more apparent and visible, both within and outside the health professions, and enjoy an ever-strengthening presence in the overall research community.

Summary

Nursing and midwifery practice and education cannot be seen to occur by chance or left unscrutinised. All nurses and midwives need to engage, reflect on and evaluate their professional actions and duties. The role of research in facilitating such process is now clearly defined and established for the nursing and midwifery professions. This chapter has aimed to identify the nature and place of nursing research in constructing efficient and effective quality-based practice. In doing so, it is intended that the reader is already beginning to appreciate the integral place of nursing and midwifery research and identify their roles as research consumers. The following chapter leads the reader to an understanding of the actual process of research, alongside its theoretical and philosophical underpinnings.

(K)EY POINTS

- Nursing and midwifery research now has an increasing emphasis on research related to patient outcomes and improving practice. Research, therefore, provides the basis for expanding the body of scientific knowledge that forms the foundation of nursing and midwifery practice. Thus, research links education, theory and practice.

- Nurses and midwives at all levels of educational preparation have a responsibility to participate in the research process. Therefore, as consumers of research, they must have a basic understanding of the research process and critical appraisal skills that provide a standard for evaluating the strengths and weaknesses of research studies before applying them in clinical practice.

- A collaborative research relationship within the nursing and midwifery professions will extend and refine the scientific body of knowledge that provides the grounding for theory and evidence-based practice (EBP). Priority is given to research studies that focus on promoting health, diminishing the negative impact of health problems, ensuring care for the health needs of vulnerable groups and developing cost-effective healthcare systems. Both consumers and producers of research engage in collaborative efforts to further the growth of nursing and midwifery research and accomplish the research objectives of the professions.

Learning activities

1. A research consumer is one who:
   (a) enjoys reading articles
   (b) examines the effects of nursing care on patients
   (c) reads critically and evaluates research findings for implementation into nursing practice
   (d) conducts research in the clinical area.

2. Nurses and midwives do not always conduct or make good use of research findings because:
   (a) they find it difficult to translate findings into practice
   (b) they think that their practice is good enough
   (c) they do not have the time to change their practice
   (d) they find it difficult to conduct research in the clinical area.

3. The Royal College of Nursing Australia and the New Zealand Nurses Organisation:
   (a) want all nurses to conduct research
   (b) do not think that all research is important
   (c) think that all nurses should undertake higher degrees in nursing

   (d) promote research as an integral part of nursing practice.

4. Nurses and midwives, whether consumers or producers of research or both:
   (a) need to recognise the research process as contributing to the professionalism of their discipline
   (b) need to understand that only senior nurses should be involved in research
   (c) want all research findings to be implemented in practice
   (d) want every nurse and midwife to be involved in writing research proposals.

5. Nurses and midwives should work with other health-related departments because:
   (a) it is important to meet other health professionals
   (b) everyone will be conducting the same research
   (c) this will help delineate the common aspects of patient care for the various disciplines
   (d) the hospital administrators will then know how much research is being conducted.

6. Research findings, no matter what the outcome, should be published because:
   (a) everyone wants to know what research has been done
   (b) everyone enjoys reading about the research findings
   (c) all studies are worth publishing
   (d) this is the best way for the nursing and midwifery communities to know what research has been done.

7. Evidence-based nurses ask whether there is a scientific basis for the care they deliver in order to:
   (a) provide the most effective care for their clients
   (b) make certain they can evaluate findings correctly
   (c) convince their colleagues to change practice
   (d) change their practice regularly.

8. Clinical governance was first described as:
   (a) a system designed to ensure research findings are being used
   (b) a system designed to ensure continuing education programs
   (c) a system designed to ensure continuous improvement of clinical practice
   (d) a system designed to ensure the immediate implementation of research findings in clinical practice.

9. In the future nurses and midwives may overcome their funding disadvantage by:
   (a) writing more interesting proposals
   (b) working collaboratively with other health professionals
   (c) working as an independent discipline
   (d) submitting their proposals to a larger number of funding agencies.

10. Nursing and midwifery emphasise cultural aspects of nursing care because:
   (a) Australia and New Zealand are multicultural countries
   (b) equity of access to healthcare for the whole community is a fundamental right
   (c) not all cultures need the same services
   (d) many nurses and midwives come from culturally diverse backgrounds.

References

Alexander J, Anderson T, Grant M, Sanghera J, Jackson D 2003 An evaluation of a support group for breast-feeding women in Salisbury, UK. *Midwifery* 19(3):215–20

Aranda S, Pollard A 2003 Implementing research into practice. In: Schneider Z, Elliott D, LoBiondo-Wood G, Haber J (eds) *Nursing Research: Methods, Critical Appraisal and Utilisation*, 2nd edn. Mosby, Sydney

Australian and New Zealand College of Mental Health Nurses (ANZCMHN). Online. Available: http://www.healthsci.utas.edu.au/nursing/college/ [accessed 22 December 2006]

Australian College of Critical Care Nurses (ACCCN). Online. Available: http://www.acccn.com.au/ [accessed 22 December 2006]

Australian College of Midwives Incorporated (ACMI). Online. Available: http://www.acmi.org.au/ [accessed 22 December 2006]

Australian Nursing and Midwifery Council National Competency Standards. Online. Available: http://www.nursesboard.sa.gov.au/pdf/ANMC.Standards.Sept_2006.pdf/ [accessed 22 December 2006]

Australian Nursing Council (ANC). Online. Available: http://anc.org.au/ [accessed 22 December 2006]

Baker C M, Bingle J M, Hajewski C J, et al. 2004 Advancing the Magnet Recognition Program in master's education through service-learning. *Nursing Outlook* 52:134–41

Bogossian F 1998 A review of midwifery legislation in Australia — history, current state and future directions. *Australian College of Midwives Inc Journal* (March) 24–32

Campbell M, Torrance C 2005 Coronary angioplasty: impact on risk factors and patients' understanding of the severity of their condition. *Australian Journal of Advanced Nursing* 22(4):26–31

Caramanica L, Small D 2006 Seeding the growth of professional nursing practice with the MAGNET Forces. *Nurse Leader* 4:56–61

Carnegie E 1976 Historical perspectives of nursing research and evidence-based practice. *Nurse Researcher* 8(2):55–68

Cochrane Collaboration *Australian Nursing and Midwifery Council Standards*. Online. Available: http://www.cochrane.edu.au [accessed 22 December 2006]

Crookes P, Davies S 1998 *Research into practice: essential skills for reading and applying research in nursing and health care*. Bailliére-Tindall, Edinburgh

Davidson P, Elliott D 2001 Managing approaches to nursing care delivery. In: Chang E, Daly K (eds) *Preparing for professional nursing practice*. MacLennan & Petty, Sydney

Dock L L 1900 What we may expect from the law. *American Journal of Nursing* 1:8–12

Dunn S V, Yates P 2000 The roles of Australian chairs in clinical nursing. *Journal of Advanced Nursing* 31(1):165–71

Dunning T, Manias E 2005 Medication knowledge and self-management by people with type 2 Diabetes. *Australian Journal of Advanced Nursing* 23(1):7–13

East Asian Forum of Nurse Scholars (EAFONS). Online. Available: http://nhs.polu.edu.hk/nhs/schact/schact_eafons.html [accessed 22 December 2006]

Edwards H, Chapman H, Davis L M 2002 Utilization of research evidence by nurses. *Nursing and Health Sciences* 4:89–95

French B 2005 The process of research use in nursing. *Journal of Advanced Nursing* 49:125–34

French P 1999 The development of evidence-based nursing. *Journal of Advanced Nursing* 29(1):72–8

Godden J, Forsyth S 2000 Defining relationships and limiting power: two leaders of Australian nursing, 1868–1904. *Nursing Inquiry* 7(1):10–19

Goodrich A 1932 *The social and ethical significance of nursing: a series of addresses*. Macmillan, New York

Hisama K 2001 Patterns of Japanese clinical nursing: a historical analysis. *Journal of Clinical Nursing* 10(4):451–4

Jirojwong S, Rossi D, Walker S, et al. 2005 What were the outcomes of home follow-up visits after postpartum hospital discharge? *Australian Journal of Advanced Nursing* 23(1):22–9

Joanna Briggs Institute for Evidence Based Nursing and Midwifery. Online. Available: http://www.joannabriggs.edu.au/ [accessed 22 December 2006]

Johnston J M, Chan S S C, Chan S K K et al. 2005 Training nurses and social workers in smoking cessation counselling: a population needs assessment in Hong Kong. *Preventive Medicine* 40:389–406

Johnstone M, Da Costa C D, Turale S 2004 Registered and Enrolled Nurses Experiences of Ethical Issues in Nursing Practice. *Australian Journal of Advanced Nursing* 22(1):24–30

Koziol-McLain J, Drummond J S, Maeve M K, Gunnels M D 2002 Should only nurses do nursing research? *Journal of Emergency Nursing* 28(4):362–4

Leap N 1999 The introduction of 'direct entry' midwifery courses in Australian universities: issues, myths and a need for collaboration. *Australian College of Midwives Inc. Journal* 12(2):11–16

Leslie H, McAllister M 2002 The benefits of being a nurse in critical social research practice. *Qualitative Health Research* 12:700–12

McCallin A M 2006 Interdisciplinary researching: exploring the opportunities and risks of working together. *Nursing and Health Sciences* 8:88–94

McKinley S, Moser D K, Dracup K 2000 Treatment-seeking behavior for acute myocardial infarction symptoms in North America and Australia. *Heart Lung* 29(4):237–47

National Health Service (NHS) Centre for Reviews and Dissemination. Online. Available: http://www.york.ac.uk/inst/crd [accessed 22 December 2006]

National Review of Nursing Education 2006. Online. Available: http://www.dest.gov.au/archive/highered/nuring/pubs/midwifery/1.htm [accessed 22 December 2006]

New Zealand Nurses Organisation (NZNO). Online. Available: http://www.nzno.org.nz/ [accessed 15 January 2007]

Ocker B M, Pawlick Plank D M 2000 The research nurse role in a clinic-based oncology setting. *Cancer Nursing* 23(4):286–91

Olade R A 2003 Attitudes and factors affecting research utilization. *Nursing Forum* 38:5–15

Orlando I J 1961 *The dynamic nurse–patient relationship*. GP Putnam's Sons, New York

Palmer I 1977 Florence Nightingale: reformer, reactionary, researcher. *Nursing Research* 26:84–9

Peplau H E 1952 *Interpersonal relations in nursing: a conceptual frame of reference for psychodynamic nursing*. GP Putnam's Sons, New York

Pravikoff D S, Tanner A B, Pierce S T 2005 Readiness for U.S. Nurses for Evidence-Based Practice. *American Journal of Nursing* 105(9):40–51

Robinson C 2006 From magnet and beyond. *Nurse Leader* 4:23–7

Royal College of Nursing, Australia 1996 *Directory of higher education nursing courses* RCNA, Melbourne

Russell R L 1990 *From Nightingale to now: nurse education in Australia*. Saunders, Sydney

Simmons L W, Henderson V 1964 *Nursing research: a survey and assessment*. Appleton-Century-Crofts, New York

Starey N 2001 What is clinical governance? 'What is…? series' *Evidence-based medicine Bulletin* 1(12):1–7

Stewart S, Jaasma T 2001 Research in cardiovascular nursing in Europe: toward a UNITED approach. *Journal of Cardiovascular Nursing* 16(1):69–72

US National Institute for Nursing Research (NINR). Online. Available: http://www.nih.gov/ninr/amission/html [accessed 15 January 2007]

Veeramah V 2004 Utilization of research findings by graduate nurses and midwives. *Journal of Advanced Nursing* 47:183–91

Wald L D 1915 *House on Henry Street*. Henry Holt & Co, New York

Wiedenbach E 1964 *Clinical nursing: a helping art*. Springer, New York

Wiles V, Daffurn K 2002 *There's a bird in my hand and a bear in the bed, I must be in ICU: the first pivotal years of Australian critical care nursing*. Australian College of Critical Care Nurses, Perth

Answers

Learning activities

1. c	2. a	3. d	4. a
5. c	6. d	7. a	8. c
9. b	10. b		

An overview of research theory and process

DEAN WHITEHEAD

KEY TERMS

critical social theory
epistemology
interpretive
ontology
paradigm tension
paradigms
positivism
qualitative
quantitative
research framework
research process
research theory

Learning outcomes

After reading this chapter, you should be able to:

- identify the theoretical and philosophical positions that underpin research
- explain the existence of a 'paradigm tension' in research
- note broad commonalities and differences between qualitative and quantitative research approaches
- discuss the nature, intention and framework of the research process and research design.

Introduction

Understanding how research works and what methods and processes it adopts is one of the first steps in becoming a knowledgeable research consumer. Research is a systematic and logical process and exists as a mechanism or tool through which knowledge is generated and tested. Generating and testing new knowledge is a vital component in the nursing and midwifery disciplines, because they constantly examine and evaluate their practice. It is anticipated that initial research inquiry equips the individual or group to make those early tentative, and then likely full-scale, attempts at actually conducting and implementing research in a variety of nursing and midwifery environments; for example, clinical, administration, teaching/learning and quality assurance. Without this initial understanding, the research journey rarely flourishes and, instead, confusion and frustration ensue as the research novice struggles to come to terms with the 'language' and instruction of research. It is recommended here then that the novice research consumer adopts a step-by-step approach to understanding research and its different approaches. This chapter offers the initial theoretical and philosophical foundations for understanding research, as well as mapping out the frameworks and processes that stem from such positions.

TT Tutorial trigger 1

How might the absence of knowledge of the underpinning theories and philosophies of research affect nursing and midwifery research?

Research theories, paradigms and frameworks

Kitson (2001), in evaluating the state of nursing research in Australia and New Zealand, believes that there is an explicit need for nurses to understand the underlying theories that underpin research. The same could easily be argued in the case of midwives. The fact that this is not always the case continues to impede the progress of research in these disciplines, in the two countries and beyond. Hutchinson and Johnston (2004), in their Australasian-based study, found that one of the main reasons why nurses fail to utilise research evidence in practice is because they do not know or understand the underpinning theoretical constructs of research. A number of other studies present similar findings for both nursing and midwifery (Edwards et al. 2002; Olade 2003; Veeramah 2004; French 2005; Roxburgh 2006).

Theories are conceptual abstract interpretations of phenomena and their relationships. It is recognised that theory guides practice and that theory, research and practice are inherently linked together (Cody 2003; Marrs & Lowry 2006). According to Graham (2003), research-based theory-building is very appealing, due to its problem-focused nature and its potential to change and improve practice. However, before the novice researcher 'rushes off' to conduct actual research in practice, or use existing research evidence to influence and change practice, it is imperative that they first understand the theoretical and philosophical foundations of research and their associated processes. Fawcett et al. (2001) insist that, as an acknowledgment of diverse forms of 'knowing', any form of evidence has to be both interpreted and critiqued against the consideration of whether or not theory can be applied to practice situations.

It is accepted that we can divide research activities into two broad classifications or 'paradigms' (although multiple paradigms exist within these); that of *qualitative* and *quantitative* research. The philosophical basis of a researcher often stems from a specific paradigm — where a paradigm is a position or view of understanding the world (world-view or view-of-the-world) which encompasses philosophical assumptions that are shared by a community of scholars or scientists. Research paradigms are thus sets of beliefs and practices shared by communities of researchers, which regulate inquiry within disciplines (Weaver & Olson 2006). This research paradigm world-view shapes a researcher's approach to a variety of research-related activities. A paradigm, therefore, guides the direction of conducted research. As to which paradigm position a researcher adopts, depends on a number of factors; such as profession, 'tradition', understanding, and hierarchy. No single theory, paradigm or framework alone can address the disciplines of nursing and midwifery, nor is any superior to another. Therefore, theoretical pluralism exists (Graham 2003; Weaver & Olson 2006).

One of the main aims of this chapter is to introduce the reader to an overview of the different perspectives of quantitative and qualitative research. The basic principles and distinguishing features of both the qualitative and quantitative paradigms are explored within the context of differences and similarities of philosophical origins, terminology and evaluation criteria. The chapters in Section 2 of this book explore different facets of these two paradigms in far more depth than this chapter. Section 2 is purposely divided separately into the paradigms of qualitative and quantitative methods. In Chapter 15, the rapidly evolving phenomenon of 'mixed-methods research' or research triangulation, which looks to 'mix and marry' the processes of both qualitative and quantitative research, are reviewed.

In generating knowledge, researchers can use methods from fundamentally different paradigms. Selection of the paradigm and the resulting research design (plan) is dependent upon the following starting points:

- the purpose of the research and the question/s being asked
- the nature of the issue/s or problem/s being investigated
- what is likely to offer the 'best fit' for process and outcomes
- the knowledge and experience of the researcher
- the need, or not, for generalisability (the application of research findings from a smaller group of research participants to much larger groups).

Regardless of approach, research is conducted to examine and expand current knowledge and understanding of different concepts and phenomena, within a particular philosophical framework. Research is therefore guided by the following concepts (and related questions):

- *Ontology* is the study of existence. It provides the 'world-view' that guides the study (e.g. 'What is the nature of

reality?'; 'What kind of being is the human being?')
- *Epistemology* is the theoretical study of knowledge involved in the search for knowledge and truth. It provides a focus for the study (e.g. what is the relationship between the researcher and the area of study?)
- *Methodology* provides a framework (process) for conducting the study (e.g. how do we know the world, or gain knowledge of it?)

(Parse 2001; Denzin & Lincoln 2005)

Clearly, philosophical ideas such as these are based on values and beliefs — hence there is scope for contention and difference. However, internal consistency and logic are achieved in a study when the links between the three abovementioned concepts are coherent (Parse 2001). Differing views exist regarding these concepts and the ways they interrelate. This difference is to be celebrated because it challenges the premises of what we do and why we do it, and helps us to mould, redefine and manipulate our knowledge base and, subsequently, guide how we conduct our practice.

From a health professional perspective, the study of individuals' responses to disease, treatment and recovery is paramount. Philosophical beliefs about human/environment relationships, and what constitutes knowledge of these areas, are fundamental to such practice (Leddy 2000). Unique experiences or transferable findings form the basis of decision-making for determining whether either a qualitative or quantitative (or both) research method is used. Further delineation is outlined in a common classification of research paradigms. These being:

- *positivist* — reductionist, empirical
- *critical* — emancipatory
- *interpretive* — naturalistic.

Positivist approach

The term positivist or 'positivism' refers to a philosophical position which reflects the traditional scientific approach of objective observation, and prediction and testing of causal relationships (Maggs-Rapport 2001). This paradigm is representative of quantitative research approaches. Positivism (or modernism) is a broad cultural reflection of rationality and known science. The related term 'determinism' adheres to the notion that certain investigated phenomena do not occur by chance, but have predisposing causes that are known to us. This concept is criticised by many though, but especially where supporters adhere to strict and rigid principles, whereby 'pure' positivism is advocated. Labels attached to this paradigm, such as 'proper', 'realist' and 'scientific', have compounded this critique. Consequently, the 'post-positivism' (or post-modernism) movement has developed as a less rigid structure that acknowledges the futility of pursuing 'complete or total objectivity'. Empirical-analytical or logical positivism are equivalent terms used to describe the origins and belief system of the quantitative research paradigm. Another underpinning concept of quantitative research is that of 'deductive reasoning'. This describes a logical thought process whereby research hypotheses (see Chapter 5) are derived from theory — and where reasoning moves from the general to the particular. Chapters 10 through to 14 further add to the understanding of quantitative research.

Critical approach

Critical approaches generally use qualitative methods to examine phenomena of interest. Both critical and interpretive (see next section) approaches are viewed as post-positivist. They developed from researchers wishing to find alternatives to counter and balance out the positivist tradition described above. They are both research methodologies operating within a social-change context, often with a post-modern stance that includes questioning the status quo of social institutions. Consequently, the researcher adopts a position that is free from restraint, especially from the limitations of tradition, and seeks to minimise the 'distance' between the researcher and the study participants.

Critical approaches seek to enable empowerment, emancipation and equality for research participants and to challenge and change social structures. Action research, for instance, is a critical inquiry that describes and interprets social situations and, in doing so, aims to improve social division/inequality through participant involvement. It is essentially a critique of existing social situations, via collaboration and partnership, in order to generate social change (Williamson & Prosser 2002). Chapter 15 expands on the critical process of action research.

Critical approaches are also referred to as emancipatory. In nursing, emancipation has emerged from a longstanding history of social oppression which has been vividly addressed via the means of critical social theory and, in particular, through feminist theory and research (Wittmann-Price 2004; Turris 2005). According to Arslanian-Engoren (2002), feminist research aims to explore underpinning issues that are known to cause discrepancies and inequities in women's healthcare and nursing, preventing them from receiving or delivering comprehensive care and treatment. In doing so, feminist research adopts a 'post-structural' stance by first exposing and then changing power structures that are present within social and political institutions. It is obviously worthwhile to investigate issues that expose any form of marginalisation based purely on gender. It should be noted though that, while a useful approach for investigating such issues in nursing, midwifery and women's healthcare generally, proportionally, feminist research represents a small body of research work in these disciplines overall. For instance, in Edin and Högberg's (2002) midwifery-based study, investigating the incidence of physical and sexual violence encountered by pregnant women, their extensive review of the literature unveiled many survey-based research studies — but uncovered no feminist studies.

Research in brief

Salmon (1999) employed a snowball sampling technique (see Chapter 8), to recruit women into her feminist analysis of women's experiences of perineal trauma, in the immediate post-delivery period. Findings unearthed gender-based anomalies which included the women 'not feeling heard about experienced pain', an alienating doctor–'patient' relationship seemingly based on gender, and a lack of available information or advice. The study concludes that 'listening to women is the key to responsive care' (Salmon 1999 p 247).

For these reasons, this book acknowledges the place of feminist research here, but does not elaborate on it elsewhere. For those that wish to know more about feminist theory and research, they are directed to the references cited immediately above for a theoretical perspective, as well as others that demonstrate actual research examples (i.e. Salmon 1999; Yam 2000; Arslanian-Engoren 2001).

Point to ponder

▶ Some disciplines will lend themselves more to feminist research than others. This would certainly potentially be the case for midwifery, although it is relevant to all those that work with women and on issues of women's health. This said, trawling the midwifery-based research literature, to date, still uncovers scant feminist research examples. The 'Research in brief' box on the previous page is one example.

Interpretive approach

Interpretive approaches to research aim to describe, explore and generate meaning within a social or practice context. The most common post-positivist examples of this approach are phenomenology, grounded theory and ethnography (see Chapter 7). They are also referred to as occurring within a naturalistic or constructivist paradigm. For the interpretive researcher, 'reality' is a fluid entity whereby the phenomenon being investigated exists within contexts that have many different connotations and possibilities. In effect, the reality is not fixed and is constructed according to naturally occurring events and situations. Another related underpinning concept of qualitative research is that of 'inductive reasoning'. This describes a logical thought process whereby generalisations are developed from specific observations — and where reasoning moves from the particular to the general (the opposite to quantitative research). Chapters 7 through to 9, which deal primarily with phenomenology, grounded theory and ethnography, further add to the understanding of interpretive qualitative approaches. Table 2.1 offers a simplified comparative perspective between positivist, critical and interpretive approaches.

Choosing a paradigm

The reasons for selecting a qualitative paradigm position rather than a quantitative one, or vice versa, are based on the research question and the purpose of the study. The formulation of the research problem (research question, problem statement or hypothesis) is an initial and key preliminary step in the process of research, regardless of the method used (see Chapter 5). At this stage, the research consumer examines the consistency between the research problem and the methods used to address that problem. Critical appraisal skills are required to effectively review research studies, and judge whether the findings could be applied to practice or not (see Chapter 4). Recognition of the differences of the characteristics of qualitative research from quantitative research enables the nurse to better interpret the research report findings and identify ways they might be applied. The

TABLE 2.1 A simplified comparison of positivist, critical and interpretive approaches

	Positivist	Critical	Interpretive
Position	Empirico-analytical, reductionist	Post-positive, post-modern, post-structural, emancipatory	Post-positive, post-modern, naturalistic
Methodology	Experimental, quasi-experimental, correlational etc	Feminist research, action research, critical ethnology etc	Phenomenology, grounded theory, ethnography, exploratory/descriptive, case study, historical, Delphi
Data collection	Experiments, closed surveys and interviews	Open observation or interviews, focus groups	Open observation or interviews, focus groups
Researcher position	Distant	Close	Close

TABLE 2.2 A comparison of qualitative and quantitative approaches

Concepts	Qualitative	Quantitative
Origins	Search for meaning; interactive approach	Search for truth in an objective, controlled manner
Beliefs	Complex beings who attribute unique meanings to situations	Biopsychosocial beings with measurable components
Truth	Subjective with multiple realities	Objective reality
Basis of knowing	Meaning, discovery	Cause and effect relationships
Focus	Complex and broad	Concise and narrow
Level	Holistic	Reductionist
Reasoning	Dialectic, inductive	Logistic, deductive
Setting	Occurs in uncontrolled naturalistic (social or human) settings	Investigator seeks experimental control of the setting
Purpose	Develops theory by exploring meaning and describing relationships	Tests hypotheses, theories by control and observation
Sample	People in the sample are referred to as participants, or in ethnographic studies, informants	People in a group are termed the sample, and are referred to as subjects, cases or respondents
Researcher position	An active and interactive participant, immersed in the setting	Uses measuring instruments or tools; e.g. questionnaires
Data elements	Written form (words)	Numerical form (numbers)
Analyses	Interpretive analysis undertaken manually or using software (e.g. NUD*IST, ETHNOGRAPH) that orders and categorises the data	Statistical analysis using software (e.g. SAS, SPSS, Minitab, Statview) to facilitate examination of quantitative data
Outcomes	Are often thematic or conceptual, but not quantifiable	Must be measurable and are reported in numerical terms
Clinical application	Exploration of unique experiences by individuals	Findings able to be generalised to similar groups

origins and belief systems for the qualitative and quantitative paradigms are compared in Table 2.2.

Researchers may sometimes be under the illusion that the differences between qualitative and quantitative paradigms are so wide that one paradigm position is 'incommensurable' with the other (Weaver & Olson 2006). While not intended, the information in Table 2.2 may perpetuate the apparent division between them. It is important, however, to acknowledge their obvious connectedness and inter-relationships. Both approaches are complimentary, not competitive. Broadly speaking, both paradigms are scientific, rigorous and follow very similar process, design and methodology. Neither quantitative

nor qualitative research can occur by chance: both are governed by a systematic adherence to the method and design of the research process (explained later in this chapter).

TT Tutorial trigger 2

Before reading on, from what you or your tutorial group currently understand, which do you believe is the best method to use for conducting nursing or midwifery research — qualitative or quantitative? Can you justify your decision?

The existence of a 'paradigm tension' in research

A 'traditional' paradigm tension has existed for some time within a number of research communities. Essentially, in research terms, the paradigms of qualitative and quantitative research have been (and often still are) viewed as being in direct competition with each other. Conventional/traditional researchers and the research 'communities' they represent, have often initiated and perpetuated this situation. In effect, researchers present the problem, rather than any inherent fault lying with the paradigms themselves. Take, for instance, the fact that medical research is predominantly quantitative in nature, while nursing research is predominantly tipped towards conducting qualitative research. This situation has often resulted in unhelpful, limiting and limited outcomes for healthcare research and created unnecessary division between and within these health professions. Weaver and Olson (2006) suggest that such a state of affairs within nursing and midwifery has, in places, introduced notable confusion, intolerance and competition.

Point to ponder

▶ Medical-based research on women's health issues (e.g. childbirth, osteoporosis) is often criticised for its positivist medicalised orientation, male dominance perspective, and its propensity to reduce all health events (such as childbirth) to a disease state or illness orientation. This said, some midwifery and nursing-specific research has been accused of the same.

The existence of 'hierarchies of research evidence', popularised in the late 1970s in Canada, have contributed (intentionally or not) to the noted paradigm tension. The insinuation of these hierarchies is that some methods of research (especially positivist approaches) are better (or more important) than others. Evans (2003), an Australian nurse, offers a more reasoned interpretation of these hierarchies, in that different research methods are needed to answer different clinical questions — therefore effectiveness, appropriateness and feasibility of method are more important indicators than hierarchy. The Australian Health Advisory Committee (HAC), as part of the National Health and Medical Research Council (NHMRC) has

identified to a certain extent with the above sentiment and, accordingly, developed pilot program guidelines for 2007 (www.nhmrc. gov.au/publications/synopses/cp65syn.htm). Table 2.3 highlights the current proposal for the NHMRC hierarchies of research evidence — although it is important to note that they represent a quantitative hierarchy only.

TABLE 2.3 Designations of levels of evidence according to type of research question

Level	Intervention
1	Systematic reviews of level 2 studies
2	Pseudo-randomised controlled trials (RCTs)
3a	Comparative studies with concurrent controls
3b	Comparative studies without concurrent controls
4	Case series

(Source: NHMRC *Pilot program guidelines for 2007*)

More recent times have seen a more reasoned and enlightened approach to health-related research that now includes research collaboration between all disciplines (including nurses, midwives and doctors), an acknowledgment of the equal and important place of qualitative research, and the advent of 'mixed methods' research (see Chapter 15).

Most researchers are now realising the limitations inherent in championing or rejecting one research paradigm at the expense of another. It is now accepted by many, as both naïve and simplistic, to imply either that one research approach is better than the other, or that they are so different that researchers can only engage in one or the other. It is also acknowledged now that, in many instances, adherence to a single research approach or method might prove inadequate when it comes to answering research questions/ hypotheses — especially with nursing research (see Chapter 15). The key issue really is that the researcher, instead, chooses the most appropriate method for the actual task at hand. Different research methods will always produce different results. One of the main tasks, for the critical reviewer of research, is that they can determine if research studies have adopted the correct method and design for the intended purpose or predicted outcomes.

Theoretical and conceptual frameworks

Research frameworks provide the conceptual underpinnings for research studies. Theoretical research frameworks are underpinned by known and tested theories. There are many 'tried and tested' theories in nursing that researchers can cross-reference against. Therefore, this foundational knowledge serves as a frame of reference from which researchers can either predict or explain their study outcomes. Where studies are unique, however, and are exploring either unknown or previously unexplored domains, it may be that there is no theoretical framework to guide the researcher. This is not a problem, though it would not be recommended for novice researchers to conduct research where this is the case. Conceptual frameworks, on the other hand, relate to single or multiple concepts that are related, but remain untested. They are still useful as a frame of reference but the degree of interpretation is looser and wider than with theoretical frameworks. Verification of an untested nursing theory provides a relatively uncharted area from which research problems can be derived (see the following 'research in brief').

Research in brief

Here we can see that as well as most research possessing a theoretical basis, research can be used to generate new theories. Dalton (2003) extends Kim's theory of collaborative decision-making in nursing practice, in constructing and testing a new theory that moves from Kim's dyadic theory towards a triadic theory — by means of a modified version of Walker and Avant's theory-derivation process.

Evidence-based practice tip

While research theory, philosophy, paradigms, frameworks and concepts can be separately defined, they are interrelated notions and, therefore, it is not uncommon to see the terms used interchangeably. This can cause confusion as to what each one is and how it relates to research overall — and to each other. To avoid such confusion, it is recommended that the reader is conversant with the various nuances of the contexts defined so far in this chapter.

Research process and research design

Research process

If we look at a series of 'typical' research studies, in their entirety and regardless of which paradigm is used, we should note that they all adhere to the same process. By paying attention to this methodological process, critical research consumers can appreciate the integral nature of research method to study development and the relevance of guiding forces on the outcomes of research (Maggs-Rapport 2001). To illuminate the forces, drivers and process of research, this book is designed to take the reader step-by-step on a sequential process-driven research journey — chapter-by-chapter. The order of the chapters therefore, in this book, mostly mirrors the main elements of the 'research process'. The research process then typically adheres to the following structure:

1. identifying the clinical problem/issue
2. critically searching and reviewing the available primary (research-based) and conceptual (theory-based) literature
3. identifying research ideas, questions, statements or hypotheses
4. determining ethical issues and procedures
5. identifying and justifying an appropriate research methodology and method
6. sampling (choosing) appropriate research populations (participants/elements)
7. collecting research data from participants/elements
8. analysing collected research data
9. determining and making sense of research results/findings
10. disseminating (sharing) research findings to wider audiences.

We already note that a number of factors determine the nature and extent of conducted research, which influence the choice of research method or approach. Regardless of research approach though, the process remains constant. This can be seen by looking at the decision path for selecting a research approach as outlined in Figure 2.1.

FIGURE 2.1 Decision path for selecting a research approach

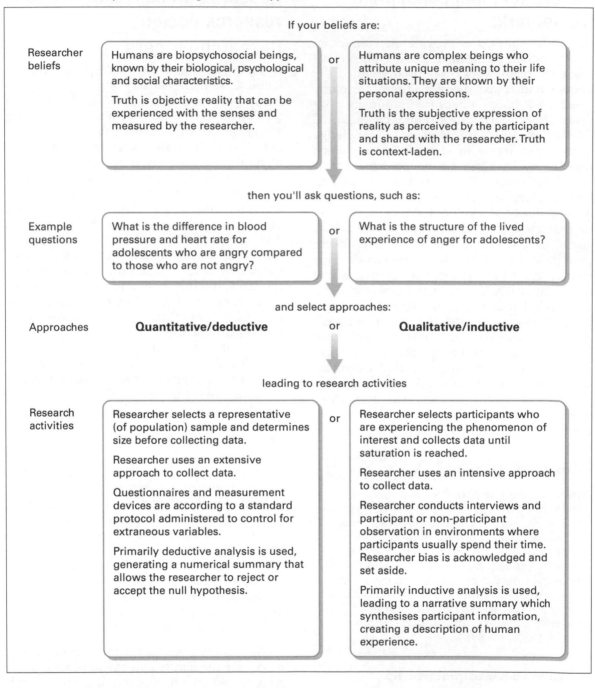

Research design

Research design takes a specific portion of the research process that is more concerned with the actual conducting of the research. This is the part where the researcher plans and designs specific methods for conducting research. These being:

1. the specific methodology and method/methods to be used i.e. qualitative–phenomenology or quantitative–experimental; or potentially both in the case of mixed methods research (see Chapters 7, 10 and 15)
2. ethical consent and approval is sought (see Chapter 6)

3. a sampling framework and technique i.e. the rationale for choosing an appropriate population of research participants or elements to study — such as a random sample of first-year nursing or midwifery students (see Chapters 8 and 11)

4. for quantitative research, variables are operationally defined (see Chapter 12)

5. mostly for quantitative research, measuring instruments are developed or selected and evaluated (see Chapter 13)

6. data collection techniques are employed (see Chapters 8 and 12)

7. the collected data are analysed (see Chapters 9 and 14)

8. results/findings are evaluated (see Chapter 16).

If we look to published research, in academic journals, it will be noted that it too adheres closely to this process in disseminating published research findings — although the format will usually be different for non-research articles. A knowledgeable critical consumer of the nursing and midwifery research literature will likely observe that the research is usually reported in a certain logical fashion. Progressing through Chapters 3, 4, 16 and 21 will help to reinforce this notion. Hudson-Barr (2004) notes the way that nursing- and midwifery-related articles, reported in academic journals, are presented in this very systematic way (an interpretation of likely headings is included in parentheses):

1. the identification of a research problem, idea or issue (introduction)

2. a review of previous research and conceptual work on the identified topic (literature review/background)

3. specification of the research question, statement or hypothesis (aim)

4. a description of how the study was conducted (design, method or approach — to include the possible subheadings of

sampling, ethical procedure, data collection and data analysis)

5. discussion on the results of the research (results/findings)

6. the interpretation of the research findings (discussion — to potentially include limitations, recommendations and conclusion/summary).

> **Evidence-based practice tip**
> The terms research process, design, method, methodology and approach are often used interchangeably. While there are subtle differences between some of them, generally, they are terms used to describe the same thing. For instance, methodology usually refers to the philosophical underpinning that informs what approach is adopted, while method mainly refers to how actual process, i.e. data collection and analysis, are adopted and applied.

Summary

Understanding how research works and what methods and processes it adopts is a part of becoming a knowledgeable research consumer. Without understanding these initial nuances and underpinnings of research, it is unlikely that the research novice is able to progress to become a knowledgeable consumer of research. While some of the theoretical and philosophical terms might initially appear somewhat abstract and unreal, they need to be understood to comprehend the whys and wherefores of conducting research. Following on from this, it is intended that this understanding serves as a springboard to propel the reader towards the first steps of the outlined research process. Much of the available research literature routinely use the terminology and concepts highlighted in this chapter and, to a degree, expects the reader to already be conversant with this material. The next two chapters are devoted to the initial, yet integral, research process steps of critically searching for, retrieving and reviewing the existing research literature.

(K)EY POINTS

- Research stems from, and is underpinned by, a number of theoretical and philosophical positions. These positions create the 'world-view' of the researcher and help determine the research approach that is undertaken.

- The two major paradigms of research are qualitative and quantitative research. Both have their differences and similarities but, ultimately, which paradigm is chosen (if not both) by researchers should be determined on the basis of which approach is the most appropriate for the task at hand and most likely to produce the best possible outcomes for health clients and services.

- Conducted research necessarily conforms to and is conducted in established scientific, systematic and structured frameworks and processes. These must be fully understood before the research consumer can embark on and engage in the application of research findings, or actually conduct research in practice.

Learning activities

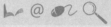

1. The first step in becoming a knowledge-able research consumer involves:
   (a) understanding how to conduct research
   (b) understanding the 'language' of research
   (c) understanding how research works, its underpinning theories and what methods and processes it adopts
   (d) understanding how research impacts on nursing practice.

2. Research is guided by the following concepts (and related questions):
   (a) ontology, epistemology and methodology
   (b) ontology, epistemology and oncology
   (c) ontology, pedagogy and methodology
   (d) ontology, pedagogy and dermatology.

3. Further delineation of qualitative and quantitative research is outlined in a common classification of research paradigms. These being:
   (a) deductive, inductive and productive
   (b) positivist, critical and interpretive
   (c) negativist, uncritical and interpretive
   (d) positivist, critical and productive.

4. The term positivist or 'positivism' refers to:
   (a) philosophical position reflecting the traditional scientific approach of subjective observation and causal relationships

   (b) philosophical position reflecting the traditional scientific approach of objective observation and nursing relationships
   (c) philosophical position reflecting the traditional scientific approach of objective observation and causal relationships
   (d) philosophical position reflecting the traditional scientific approach of subjective observation and nursing relationships.

5. Critical and interpretive research paradigms generally use:
   (a) qualitative methods to examine phenomena of interest
   (b) quantitative methods to examine phenomena of interest
   (c) qualitative methods to examine hypotheses
   (d) quantitative methods to examine hypotheses.

6. The most likely cause for 'paradigm tension' is:
   (a) a researcher feeling anxious about research
   (b) a representation that one research paradigm is more superior over another
   (c) when two different paradigms are used in one study
   (d) when only one paradigm is used.

7. Research frameworks:
   (a) serve as a frame of reference from which researchers can either predict or explain their study methods
   (b) serve as a frame of reference from which researchers can either predict or explain their study designs
   (c) serve as a frame of reference from which researchers can either predict or explain their study inputs
   (d) serve as a frame of reference from which researchers can either predict or explain their study outcomes.

8. The first part of the research process involves:
   (a) identifying the problem/issue
   (b) critically searching and reviewing the available primary (research-based) and conceptual (theory-based) literature
   (c) identifying research ideas, questions, statements or hypotheses
   (d) all of the above.

9. The last part of the research process involves:
   (a) analysing collected research data
   (b) determining research results/findings
   (c) disseminating research findings
   (d) all of the above.

10. The research design (plan) is dependent upon the following starting points:
    (a) the purpose and the question/s being asked
    (b) the nature of the issue or problem being investigated
    (c) what is likely to offer the 'best fit' and potential outcomes
    (d) all of the above.

Additional resources

Beckstead J W, Beckstead L G 2006 A multidimensional analysis of the epistemic origins of nursing theories, models, and frameworks. *International Journal of Nursing Studies* 43:113–22

Clark A M 1998 The qualitative-quantitative debate: moving from positivism and confrontation to post-positivism and reconciliation. *Journal of Advanced Nursing* 27:1242–9

French B 2005 The process of research use in nursing. *Journal of Advanced Nursing* 49:125–34

Guba E, Lincoln Y 1994 Competing paradigms in qualitative research. In: Denzin N K, Lincoln Y S (eds) *Handbook of Qualitative Research*. Sage, Thousand Oaks, CA, pp 105–18

References

Arslanian-Engoren C 2001 Gender and age differences in nurses' triage decisions using vignette patients. *Nursing Research* 50:61–6

Arslanian-Engoren C 2002 Feminist poststructuralism: a methodological paradigm for examining clinical decision-making. *Journal of Advanced Nursing* 37:512–17

Cody W K 2003 Nursing theory as a guide to practice. *Nursing Science Quarterly* 16:225–31

Dalton J M 2003 Development and testing of the theory of collaborative decision-making in nursing practice for triads. *Journal of Advanced Nursing* 41:22–33

Denzin N K, Lincoln Y S (eds) 2005 *Handbook of Qualitative Research*, 3rd edn. Sage, Thousand Oaks, CA

Edin K E, Högberg U 2002 Violence against pregnant women will remain hidden as long as no direct questions are asked. *Midwifery* 18:268–78

Edwards H, Chapman H, Davis L M 2002 Utilization of research evidence by nurses. *Nursing and Health Sciences* 4:89–95

Evans D 2003 Hierarchy of evidence: a framework for ranking evidence evaluating healthcare interventions. *Journal of Clinical Nursing* 12:77–84

Fawcett J, Watson J, Neuman B et al. 2001 On nursing theories and evidence. *Journal of Nursing Scholarship* 33:115–19

French B 2005 Contextual factors influencing research use in nursing. *Worldviews on Evidence-Based Nursing* 2:172–83

Graham I W 2003 The relationship of nursing theory to practice and research within the British context: identifying a way forward. *Nursing Science Quarterly* 16:346–50

Hudson-Barr D 2004 Scientific inquiry: how to read a research article. *Journal for Specialists in Pediatric Nursing* 9:70–2

Hutchinson A M, Johnston L 2004 Bridging the divide: a survey of nurses' opinions regarding barriers to, and facilitators of, research utilization in the practice setting. *Journal of Clinical Nursing* 13:304–15

Kitson A 2001 Approaches used to implement research findings into nursing practice. Report of a study tour to Australia and New Zealand. *International Journal of Nursing Practice* 7:392–405

Leddy S K 2000 Towards a complementary perspective on worldviews. *Nursing Science Quarterly* 13:225–33

Maggs-Rapport F 2001 'Best research practice': in pursuit of methodological rigour. *Journal of Advanced Nursing* 35:373–83

Marrs J-A, Lowry L W 2006 Nursing theory and practice: connecting the dots. *Nursing Science Quarterly* 19:44–50

National Health and Medical Research Council (NHMRC) *Pilot program guidelines for 2007*. Online. Available: www.nhmrc.gov.au/publications/synopses/cp65syn.htm [accessed 15 January 2007]

Olade R A 2003 Attitudes and factors affecting research utilization. *Nursing Forum* 38:5–15

Parse R R (ed.) 2001 *Qualitative Inquiry*. Jones & Bartlett, Boston

Roxburgh M 2006 An exploration of factors which constrain nurses from research participation. *Journal of Clinical Nursing* 15:535–45

Salmon D 1999 A feminist analysis of women's experiences of perineal trauma in the immediate post-delivery period. *Midwifery* 15:247–56

Turris S A 2005 Unpacking the concept of patient satisfaction: a feminist analysis. *Journal of Advanced Nursing* 50:293–8

Veeramah V 2004 Utilization of research findings by graduate nurses and midwives. *Journal of Advanced Nursing* 47:183–91

Weaver K, Olson J K 2006 Understanding paradigms used for nursing research. *Journal of Advanced Nursing* 53:459–69

Williamson G R, Prosser S 2002 Action research: politics, ethics and participation. *Journal of Advanced Nursing* 40:587–93

Wittmann-Price R A 2004 Emancipation in decision-making in women's health care. *Journal of Advanced Nursing* 47:437–45

Yam M 2000 Seen but not heard: battered women's perceptions of the ED experience. *Journal of Emergency Nursing* 26:464–70

Answers

TT Tutorial trigger 1

Without this underpinning knowledge, the researcher does not have a conceptual baseline from which they can determine the nature and origin of their research. This makes it more difficult to both rationalise and justify their adopted research method and stance. It also potentially limits the scope of the conducted research.

TT Tutorial trigger 2

When reading further on from tutorial trigger 2 in this chapter, it hopefully becomes apparent that no one research paradigm, design or method is better than another. All research approaches have their strengths and limitations, depending on what it is that the researcher wants to investigate. No one paradigm position is 'superior' to another, despite what some literature might suggest. The only appropriate answer to the question 'Which is the best paradigm to use (quantitative or qualitative)?', therefore, is the one that is best suited to the task at hand.

Learning activities

1. c	**2.** a	**3.** b	**4.** c
5. a	**6.** b	**7.** d	**8.** d
9. d	**10.** d		

Searching the literature

DOUG ELLIOTT

KEY TERMS

bibliographic databases

Cumulative Index
  to Nursing and
  Allied Health
  Literature (CINAHL)

Medline

PubMed

primary source

refereed (peer-reviewed)
  journals

search strategy

secondary source

Learning outcomes

After reading this chapter, you should be able to:

- discuss the different types of literature sources
- differentiate between primary and secondary sources of professional and scientific information
- conduct a focused search of the literature using an explicit search strategy
- evaluate the search strategies of published papers.

Introduction

A systematic approach to searching the scholarly and professional literature is the first step in producing a literature review on a particular topic of interest. Information and communications technology (ICT) has revolutionised the contemporary process of searching the research literature. A range of online resources are now available to anyone with internet access, including websites, electronic books (e-books), literature databases of published journal articles, full-text journal repositories, and e-journals.

This chapter examines sources of academic literature and describes search strategies as a prelude to a critical review of the available literature, primarily from the perspective of a research consumer. Steps of the literature search and review process are:

1. formulating a review question
2. conducting a comprehensive search of the literature
3. assessing studies for inclusion in the review
4. critical appraisal of the selected studies
5. synthesis of findings from individual studies
6. reporting results and recommendations for practice.

Chapter 4 describes the processes for conducting a literature review (steps 4–6 in the list above). A literature review can take various forms, and has a number of purposes, including:

• identifying the knowledge base related to a clinical practice issue
• supporting a clinical practice guideline or a proposal for an evidence-based practice change
• describing the background for an ethics committee proposal, grant application, or a primary research article
• as the focus in a secondary research paper (literature review; systematic review).

Knowledge and skills for both searching the literature and critically reviewing the literature are essential and complementary for both research consumers and primary researchers. In practical terms, searching and reviewing the literature is a continuous and seamless process.

Types of literature resources

Nursing and midwifery have an ever-growing body of scholarly literature that focuses on discipline-specific topics, as well as a range of concepts or variables from other disciplines that also relate to the nature and practice of nursing or midwifery. The resources available to assist in developing a literature review are wide and varied. Common sources of professional disciplinary literature are journal articles, abstracts, critical reviews, textbooks, chapters in books, abstracts published as conference proceedings, professional and governmental reports, audiotapes, videotapes, personal communications (letters or telephone or in-person interviews), and unpublished doctoral and master's theses. Many of these are now available in digital media formats, and commonly accessed through the internet.

The 'internet' is a broad term that describes an international collaboration of participating commercial, educational and government computer-based communication networks. These resources share computer power, software and information to form a global resource. Internet service providers (ISPs) include a web browser, such as Internet Explorer or Netscape Navigator, to enable internet access. The hypertext interface available with the world-wide web enables text, video and audio material to be developed, stored and accessed.

University and health service libraries host access through an intranet (an internal organisation-based network) or the internet for a range of activities including literature searches. Students commonly access these facilities from their computer centre, library or classroom, remotely via a modem, or wirelessly using 'hotspots' or mobile phone networks. Clinicians also have internet access from their health service work stations or offices. Increasingly, households have internet access through dial-up, wireless or broadband services, while public libraries and internet cafés also provide access.

From a literature search perspective, a 'portal' (a user-friendly computer interface) enables students and clinicians to access library catalogues, literature databases and repositories. Clinician support sites maintained by health departments and professional organisations provide these functions as well as other electronic content such as e-books and government documents and reports. These resources assist a research consumer in undertaking a review of the existing literature base on a specific clinical practice question.

> ## Point to ponder
>
> ▶ Identify which portals, literature databases and other resources are available through your university, health service or organisation.

A competent research consumer is expected to demonstrate a particular skills set, including information literacy skills, how to conduct a literature search and select relevant articles or other resources for review, critically evaluate the selected literature, and then write about it in a progressively sophisticated style. This process is the same whether the purpose is critiquing or writing a literature review, and reflects the cognitive processes and practical techniques of retrieving and critically reviewing sources from the literature. Synthesis and analysis of a defined body of literature is an experiential skill commonly developed and assessed in both undergraduate and postgraduate coursework degree programs, and is increasingly required by clinicians for quality improvement and practice development activities.

Primary and secondary literature sources

The resources used to conduct a literature search — 'primary' and 'secondary' sources, refereed journals, literature and bibliographic databases, and websites — are discussed below. Both types of sources are accessible through refereed journals, electronic or print databases, and websites. Experience in working with these knowledge sources is a requirement for nursing graduates in clinical, educational, research and professional settings. A credible literature review reflects the use of mainly primary sources of information — original research or development of theory. Most primary sources are found in published literature, usually as refereed journal articles (see under 'Refereed journals' heading later in this section), although some original research can be reported as a book or monograph. Academic theses are also a primary source. Many journal articles are now accessible through internet sources as full-text papers or abstracts.

A secondary source is commonly a summary and critique of a range of primary studies on a specific topic (e.g. a literature review paper), a theorist's or researcher's work, or an in-depth analysis on an issue, problem or concept. Three common reasons for using secondary sources are:

1. the full-text primary source is literally unavailable — this may occur for early classic papers or those written in publications with a limited distribution
2. a secondary source provides a different interpretation of an issue or problem — secondary sources help students develop the ability to see things from another reader's point of view, an essential aspect of critical reading
3. when the body of knowledge is so extensive that a comprehensive review provides the best available knowledge, enabling clinicians to make practice decisions without undertaking their own full review of the literature review.

Secondary sources published in refereed journals are frequently written by experienced nursing scholars. Secondary sources include all types of literature reviews (see Chapter 4 for further discussion). The advantages of secondary sources are that they are a review of the state of the science, and form an important component in the application of knowledge to practice. These articles usually provide a critical evaluation of, or a response to, a theory or research study, and include implications for practice and/or contributions of the work to the development of the science of nursing. Research consumers do however have to consider potential limitations of biases with secondary sources. For example, reviews may not fully cover the existing knowledge, or purposely promote a particular approach, therefore not providing a balanced view of the literature for that topic area.

A number of resources now focus on facilitating secondary research and resulting publications, including systematic reviews and clinical practice guidelines designed to support

BOX 3.1 Examples of resources facilitating dissemination of secondary sources of professional information

---

Journals
Evidence Based Nursing — http://www.evidencebasednursing.com
International Journal of Evidence-Based Healthcare — http://www.blackwellpublishing.com/
Worldviews on Evidence-Based Nursing — http://www.blackwellpublishing.com/

Organisations
Campbell Collaboration — http://www.campbellcollaboration.org/ (US-based)
Cochrane Collaboration — http://www.cochrane.org (UK-based) and http://www.cochrane.org.au
  (Australasian site)
Joanna Briggs Institute — http://www.joannabriggs.edu.au (Australasian-based)
Institute for Healthcare Improvement — http://www.ihi.org
National Institute of Clinical Studies — http://www.nicsl.com.au (Australian site)

Clearinghouses/literature repositories
National Guideline Clearinghouse — http://www.guideline.gov (US-based)
National Quality Measures Clearinghouse — http://www.qualitymeasures.ahrq.gov (US-based)

---

evidence-based practice (EBP) (see Box 3.1). Secondary sources should be used in context (e.g. in clinical practice guideline development), and relate to the purpose of literature reviews.

> **Point to ponder**
> ▶ Secondary sources are an important resource for information for a beginning research consumer or practising clinician.

Refereed journals

Printed journals continue to be the common mode for publishing the latest primary research study, review of literature or theoretical paper, although this is being increasingly supported by internet resources with pre-print publication, and current and archived full-text articles available on publisher or journal websites. Some journals are published only in electronic form on the internet (e.g. *International Journal of Nursing Education Scholarship* — http://www.bepress.com/ijnes), while other journals currently continue to have only paper-based full-text articles.

● **Evidence-based practice tip**
Journal articles available electronically (online) in 'pdf' format (portable document format) maintain the page format and table and figure images of the printed version of the article. Articles formatted in 'html' (hypertext mark-up language) do not have the format or image of the printed article.

For a beginning research consumer, refereed (peer-reviewed) journals are the first source for accessing primary scholarly literature. A refereed journal has an editor or co-editors, an editorial board of experts in the discipline, and uses a panel of reviewers to peer-review submitted manuscripts for possible publication. Two or three peer-reviewers are commonly assigned to critique a submitted manuscript. The aim is to judge that the quality, clarity and rigour of the content and writing are suitable for publication in the selected journal.

An indicative (but not exhaustive) list of scholarly and professional nursing journals is presented in Table 3.1. These and other disciplinary and professional journals publish primary research and review papers on the state of current knowledge, including articles on practice, theory and education. Chapter 21 discusses the manuscript preparation, submission and review processes.

● **Evidence-based practice tip**
Publishers now publish a range of texts as e-books on the internet for organisational subscribers such as universities and health departments (e.g. *Mosby's Nursing Consult* — http://www.nursingconsult.com). This format enables regular web-based updates, rather than waiting for the next edition of the book to be revised on a routine three-to five-year publication cycle.

Increasingly, the impact of published studies and journals on policy and practice are being examined, particularly as a means of informing government funding for the research

TABLE 3.1 Examples of nursing and midwifery journals

Australasian-sourced journals	
Asian Journal of Nursing Studies	International Journal of Mental Health Nursing
Australian Critical Care	International Journal of Nursing Practice
Australian Journal of Advanced Nursing	Kai Tiaki
Australian Journal of Emergency Nursing	Nursing.Aust (College of Nursing)
Australian Journal of Rural Health	Nursing Inquiry
Collegian	Women and Birth
International Journal of Evidence-Based Healthcare	
European-sourced journals	
Birth	Journal of Clinical Nursing
European Journal of Cardiovascular Nursing	Journal of Professional Nursing
Intensive and Critical Care Nursing: The International	Midwifery
Journal of Practice and Research	Nurse Education Today
International Journal of Nursing Studies	Nurse Researcher
Journal of Advanced Nursing	Research in Nursing and Health
North American-sourced journals	
Advances in Nursing Science	Journal of Obstetric, Gynecologic and Neonatal Nursing
American Journal of Critical Care	Journal of Nursing Scholarship
Applied Nursing Research	Journal of Qualitative Research
Clinical Nursing Research	Nursing & Health Care Research
CIN: Computers, Informatics, Nursing	Nursing Science Quarterly
Holistic Nursing Practice	Nursing Research
Issues in Mental Health Nursing	Qualitative Health Research

and scholarly activities of universities. There are a number of ways to 'rate' the quality of a journal or an individual article. One controversial process is the use of bibliometrics to calculate a journal's 'impact factor' (IF) and an article's 'citation rate'. An impact factor is calculated by identifying the number of articles in a journal that were subsequently cited by other articles (in that or different journals); that is:

$$IF = \frac{\text{number of articles in a journal cited by other articles}}{\text{total number of articles in the journal}}$$

A citation rate reflects the number of times an individual article is cited by other authors in subsequent articles. Both of these indices are influenced by what databases are used, the range of journals indexed in the database, the time-lag between an article being published and it being subsequently cited by a more recent article, and inflation of citations by self-citation (an author referencing their own previous work).

A number of authors have therefore highlighted the limitations, bias and dangers in using this type of rating (Cheek et al. 2006;

Garfield 2006; Kam 2005). While a number of databases are available for checking citation rates (e.g. CINAHL, Google Scholar, Journals@ OVID, Scopus), the impact factor measurement is currently dominated by one US-based corporation (Thomson Scientific's Institute of Scientific Information [ISI] and their Web of Knowledge database) in this rating process. This issue is discussed from an author's perspective in Chapter 21.

Literature databases

Two types of 'bibliographic' databases are used as tools for the primary research or research consumer processes. Literature databases are a repository of published literature — primarily journal articles. This section discusses the common 'literature repository' bibliographic databases used by nurses, midwives and other health professionals to examine the research literature. A 'portal' such as PubMed or OVID provides user friendly access and search functions for a range of user-selected databases. Portal/database access is commonly via a university or health service server, with the search facilities password-protected (restricted to enrolled students or employees with internet access). 'PubMed', a service of the US National Library of Medicine, provides free public access through the internet for Medline searches, supplying bibliographic information including the abstract with access to free full-text journal articles when available.

Databases are developed by various companies or government agencies, and there is market competition in gaining organisational (university, health department) subscriptions.

BOX 3.2 Common literature databases

Cochrane Collaboration: prepares, maintains and promotes the accessibility of systematic reviews of the effects of healthcare through a variety of documents and facilities; e.g. systematic reviews, clinical guidelines, databases — http://www.cochrane.edu.au.

Cumulative Index to Nursing and Allied Health Literature (CINAHL): first published in 1956 as print-based Cumulative Index to Nursing Literature; CD-ROM database from 1982; online from 1995; indexes over 1600 journals; contains the most comprehensive nursing information for reviewing the literature for research and research consumer purposes.

Medline (Index Medicus): the oldest health-related literature index, first published in 1879; spans medicine, allied health, biophysical sciences, humanities, veterinary and nursing literature; indexes over 4600 journals, primarily English-language or with English-translation abstracts; managed by the US National Library of Medicine (http://www.nlm.gov); also provides free public access to PubMed for Medline searches — http://www.ncbi.nlm.nih.gov.au/entrez/.

MIDIRS (http://www.midirs.org): the Midwives Information and Resource Service is a subscriber information resource for maternity healthcare professionals. Resources include an online database and *Midwifery Digest*, a quarterly publication of best midwifery information collated from a range of sources.

OVID (http://gateway1.ovid.com/): a portal to scientific literature databases (e.g. CINAHL, Cochrane, Medline; 'journals@ovid'); provides abstracts or full-text articles for a selection of nursing and midwifery journals sourced mainly from publishers and professional societies.

Psyclit: (online PsycINFO) database of psychology journals; managed by the

American Psychological Association (APA); the APA has a widely used reference format which is a variant of the Harvard (author/date) style.

Educational Resources Information Center (ERIC): first published in 1969 in co-operation with Current Index to Journals in Education (CIJE).

Other databases: include AIDSLINE (AIDS literature online), CancerLit (Cancer literature), HealthSTAR (Merged: AHA, Health Planning and Administration [HEALTH] and Health Services/Technology Assessment Research [HSTAR]); EMBASE (international biomedical and drug literature); Australasian Medical Index (indexes over 100 Australasian health and medical journals not abstracted on Medline); OSH-ROM (occupational health and safety databases).

Publisher-based databases: most multinational publishers maintain a website providing a database and repository of full-text articles for the journals they publish; commonly accessed as a subscription service by university libraries for access to the full-text articles (as pdf documents); examples include:
- Blackwell 'Synergy' — http://www.blackwell-synergy.com/
- Elsevier 'Science Direct' — http://www.sciencedirect.com/
- Informit / Meditext — http://www.informit.com.au/
- Lippincott — http://www.nursingcenter.com
- Sage 'CSA Illumina' — http://www.csa.com/
- Springer Verlag — http://www.springerlink.com
- Swetswise — http://www.swetswise.com

Note: Website addresses in this box and throughout the book were functional and accurate at the time of writing. As addresses do change, if the site address does not work and there is no automatic redirection, use a generic search engine to locate the new site.

Each database sources a range of journals particularly relevant to the related discipline/s of the database. Box 3.2 lists the common databases relevant for nursing, midwifery and health students and clinicians. There is overlap when a journal article is indexed to a number of different databases, while other journals will be indexed in one database but not another. Increasingly, international publishers are developing online literature databases for their own suite of journals. Availability of full-text article access to a journal relates to whether your organisation has a current subscription or you have a personal subscription.

Databases that were established prior to digital storage (e.g. CINAHL, ERIC, Index Medicus, PsycINFO) all provided their information on journal articles as print-based books to university and hospital libraries. These databases have been progressively adding early articles to their online versions, although there are some limitations. The online CINAHL database does not provide any information on articles published before 1982, while Medline goes back to 1966.

Publisher alerts are available for selected journals after registering free online. The contents of forthcoming issues for nominated journals are then emailed to the registrant. Full-text download is also available with individual or organisational subscription to that journal.

Bibliographic databases

The other type of bibliographic database is PC-based software designed to create your own reference library. Bibliographic databases are a useful tool in managing the literature search and review processes, as they store bibliographic details of journal articles, reports and other print materials. Examples of these databases include Endnote, Reference Manager, Pro-Cite and Papyrus (Conn et al. 2003; Nicoll et al. 1996). Some universities provide research students with access to this type of bibliographic database as part of a site-licence agreement with the software vendors, or it can be purchased individually.

Most literature databases provide an export function to common bibliographic databases, or the search results can be saved in a format that allows importing by a bibliographic database. This function eliminates re-keying of bibliographic information into the database fields, although details should be checked to correct any errors during the import process. These databases also interface with word-processing software. Linkage of the two programs allows insertion of references into the body of a word-processed document (such as a literature review). The in-text citation and list of references can then be formatted automatically to a selected reference style.

Websites

Table 3.2 lists selected Australasian examples of the hundreds of nursing and midwifery sites, internet home pages and chat rooms available. Most university schools or faculties, professional organisations and journals have websites. These sites do not provide literature search and retrieval capabilities similar to the literature databases previously described, but may provide certain information or documents useful for inclusion in a literature search and review.

Remember that the quality and accuracy of information available from the internet also needs to be assessed in a systematic manner. Compared to journal articles and textbooks, there may have been no peer-review process undertaken prior to the publication of internet material. Therefore consider the source of the website when judging the merits of any information.

- Is the source a well-known, reputable organisation?
- What is the purpose of the information dissemination?
- Is the information substantiated by references?
- How does this information relate to other published material?
- Is there any inherent bias in the statements?

Clinical trials registers are now available for researchers to register their current primary or secondary studies. Prospective study registration is a common requirement from journal publishers for publication of the research (see Chapter 20 for further discussion, including details of common registers). These registers are accessible online, enabling research consumers to examine the

TABLE 3.2 Selected examples of Australasian nursing and midwifery websites

Australian College of Midwives, Incorporated	www.acmi.org.au
Information provided on issues such as competency standards, code of practice, independent practice accreditation, educational preparation, professional development, conferences, and membership.	
Australian Nursing and Midwifery Council, Incorporated	www.anmc.org.au
Information provided on professional issues, such as codes of conduct and ethics, competency standards, assessment of overseas qualifications, as well as projects, position statements and publications.	
College of Nursing	www.nursing.aust.edu.au
Provides professional information for members on current news, education, library facilities, research and membership.	
Council of Deans of Nursing & Midwifery, Australia & New Zealand	www.cdnm.edu.au
Represents deans and heads of nursing in universities; provides position statements and information on education, research and health policy.	
Joanna Briggs Institute	www.joannabriggs.edu.au
Provides public access to 'Best Practice Information Sheets', executive summaries of systematic reviews, research protocols, a regularly updated noticeboard, a research area to post current research information and a links page to other useful nursing and evidence-based practice websites. Subscription (individual or institutional) provides access to all publications, including full-text systematic reviews.	
New Zealand Nurses Organisation	www.nzno.org.nz
Professional information provided on the organisation's network of sections and colleges, including the research section with statements on research and ethics, and an index of research. Also included on the site are current issues, services, publications, and education pages.	
Royal College of Nursing, Australia	www.rcna.org.au
Professional information and access to college resources — chapters, networks, online forums, publications, policies, scholarships, conferences, and membership information.	

methods of current studies, although of course no results are available (Conn et al. 2003).

TT Tutorial trigger 1

Many healthcare professionals and consumers now use the internet to search for healthcare information. Before going on the web, develop a set of questions that would be useful to critique the scientific merit of the healthcare information obtained.

Conducting a literature search

As noted earlier, formulation of a question or topic is the important first step (Fineout-Overholt & Johnston 2005). Chapter 4 describes the construction of a focused clinical question relevant for a review of the literature, while Chapter 5 discusses the development of a research question or hypothesis for the purpose of a primary study. Once the question is constructed and refined, a number of subsequent steps guide the search process:

selecting a database; refining the search strategy using keywords and filters; and examining and managing the search results. These steps are discussed below as a prelude to the literature review process.

In preparing to conduct a literature search, research consumers frequently ask 'How many articles do I need?', or 'How far back in the literature do I need to go?' The number of articles required depends on the purpose of the search and the topic being investigated. The aim is to address the assigned or selected topic in a comprehensive manner. If the review is a student assessment task, you need to demonstrate to the marker that you have canvassed a broad and relevant body of literature.

With the rate of knowledge expansion increasing exponentially (Conn et al. 2003), searching beyond five years is probably not required for an undergraduate essay, unless a particular period was known for seminal articles. These papers are identified in the reference lists of later papers. It can also be handy if you come across an extensive literature review on a particular topic, as this usually means you can begin your search a year or two before the last reviewed citation in the reference list. Check whether the publication years searched are stated in the paper.

Selecting a database

A range of literature (bibliographic) databases exist that list nursing, midwifery and related health and medical literature. Selection of an appropriate database/s relates to the purpose and topic of the search. Some portals enable searching of multiple databases simultaneously. Alternatively, a search strategy can be saved and/or re-executed with another database, if the initial results of your database search were not satisfactory.

Keywords

The abstraction and indexing process for each literature database relies on the use of keywords provided by the article authors, or abstractors assigning keywords to the paper. This process has some limitations and the issue of keywords needs to be considered. Each database usually has a specific online search guide that provides information on the organisation of the entries and the keyword terms. For example:
- 'Medical Subject Headings' (MeSH) were developed by the US National Library of Medicine and are used in Medline and PubMed
- CINAHL uses nursing-specific terms that may differ from those used in Medline or other databases.

Finding the right keywords (or variables/concepts/terms) to include in a search is therefore an important element. The keyword function of a database have 'explode' or 'focus' features for terms, and user-entered terms are mapped to the nearest keyword (e.g. 'mental health nursing' maps to 'psychiatric nursing' in CINAHL).

Search filters

In addition to keywords, other important steps can narrow the focus of a search strategy. Numerous filters (database limits) are available as 'check boxes' to include only publications most relevant to your keyword search. Commonly used filters include:
- selecting a range of publication years (e.g. 2001–2006)
- English-language publications only
- human-research studies only
- available as full-text papers (the entire paper is available for reading, rather than just the abstract).

Searches can be conducted for author, keyword, title, and journal, using a range of search filters to refine a search. Individual databases have different search filter features. The use of filters will of course exclude papers, some of which may be useful to your search. It is therefore prudent to undertake a step-wise search, where the focus becomes progressively narrower as more filters are added. Box 3.3 provides an example of a search.

The resulting search results list the bibliographic details, abstracts (and possibly reference lists) of published articles from a specified list of journals, and may link to full-text versions of the journal article. Bibliographic details of a journal article include author/s, publication year, article title, journal name, journal volume number, journal issue number and page numbers.

Reading the abstract is an important step, as this provides more information about the study than what is included in the article title. The abstract enables you to decide whether to include the paper in your list of references and seek to retrieve the full-text article, or discard it as being outside the scope of your search topic (see Chapter 4). There are many aspects related to learning an effective search strategy (Conn et al. 2003). The search in Box 3.3 was a simple illustration of a complex task that requires good training and experiential learning (Shorten et al. 2001; Walters et al. 2006).

Point to ponder

▶ You have noticed an increased incidence of bedsores on your ward and decide to search the literature for the latest information on prevention and treatment. Identify at least three keywords/phrases that you could use to begin the search.

BOX 3.3 Conducting a literature search

- Access the preferred database (e.g. 'CINAHL') on the computer search menu (library systems enable searching of multiple databases simultaneously).
- Type in the search words (e.g. 'nursing research').
- 'nursing research' mapped to a subject heading 'Research, Nursing'; click 'continue', mark 'include all subheadings' (unless you want to search a specific aspect of the subject) and continue; results were 11,263 citations.
- Repeat the search strategy for 'mental health nursing'; this maps to the subject heading 'Psychiatric Nursing'; include all subheadings and continue.
- Type '1 and 2' to combine the search to capture all articles with both subject headings as keywords.
- Limit the search from 2001 to 2006; this results in an output similar to:

#	Search History	Results
1	Research, Nursing/	11263
2	Psychiatric Nursing/	10790
3	1 and 2	295
4	limit to yr=2001–2006	92

- The search resulted in 92 articles abstracted to CINAHL with 'nursing research' and mental health ('psychiatric nursing') for the years 2001–2006.
- Examine the 'display' of the results, reading the title and abstract to decide whether to keep the article and access a full-text copy for further review; mark the entry you want to keep by checking the box.
- There are numerous facilities available — bibliographic details and abstracts can be emailed, imported into a bibliographic database or printed; and full-text articles can be printed in a variety of formats; use a bibliographic database to manage your references and reference format.

(Search conducted using OVID-based CINAHL, 1982 to August 2006.)

Note: Boolean operators are words (such as 'and', 'or', 'not') used to combine and refine the results of searches. The term 'and' was used as a Boolean in the above example to find articles related to both 'Research, Nursing' and 'Psychiatric Nursing'. If 'or' was used, then the sum of the two individual searches would be combined (i.e. resulting in 22,053 articles!).

Reporting the search strategy

All the relevant elements of a search strategy should be reported in a secondary research paper (literature review) — databases accessed; keywords used; publication years; inclusion and/or exclusion criteria for papers; and search filters incorporated. This enables you to critique the rigour and comprehensiveness of the process.

Research in brief

A review paper searched for English language papers between 1992 and 2003, using three databases — CINAHL, Medline and Proquest (Wang & Moyle 2005). The initial search identified 42 papers, which were then assessed against the inclusion criteria — a focus on physical restraint, explicit research methods described, within the long-term aged care setting. This resulted in identification of 22 papers for review.

Literature searches using computerised databases are limited by the range of journals indexed and potential lack of precision in abstracting of keywords. Researchers may therefore also conduct 'hand' or 'manual' searches of the table of contents of relevant journals, to identify other relevant publications that may have been missed during journal indexing in the databases (Conn et al. 2003).

For example, another review paper conducted an electronic search of the Medline, EMBASE, CINAHL and Psych-Review databases for articles published between January 1998 and December 2003. The keywords used were: quality of life; health-related quality of life; outcomes; quality of life outcomes; post traumatic stress; health status; intensive care; and critical illness (Adamson & Elliott 2005). However, other strategies were also reported to identify additional articles: a review of reference lists of articles, conference proceedings and a manual search of relevant journals including *Australian Critical Care, Intensive and Critical*

Care Nursing, Critical Care Medicine and *Intensive Care Medicine*. Publications were included in this review if they were in English-language, studied adult patients and were available in Australia. In total, 74 papers were identified of which 34 related to the general ICU population (Adamson & Elliott 2005).

Tᴛ Tutorial trigger 2

Clinical researchers are usually interested in solving clinical problems regardless of whether the solution is for immediate or future use. When faced with a problem in clinical practice it is important to find out what others have learned about it. To do this it is necessary to firstly go to the literature. List *five* journals that publish reports or research studies that a clinician might use to find out more about a problem.

Summary

This chapter identified the processes involved in conducting a literature search. A range of resources are available for examining a specific clinical practice question. The search strategy is an explicit process for identifying all literature applicable to addressing the research question. The components of a search strategy include databases accessed, keywords used, and search filters activated (e.g. publication years, English-language, human studies). The following chapter discusses the critical review process once an effective literature search has been completed. In practice, the search and review processes are seamless and continuous in their execution.

ⓚEY POINTS

- Primary sources are published articles reporting an original piece of research. Secondary sources (secondary research) are reviews of a series of primary studies on a specific topic.

- Primary sources are essential for literature reviews.

- Secondary sources from peer-reviewed journals provide important synthesised information on a topic of interest, and are useful for developing clinical practice guidelines and modelling critical evaluation skills.

- Strategies for efficiently retrieving scholarly literature include experiential learning, seeking advice from a reference librarian and using a literature (bibliographic) database to manage your references.

Learning activities

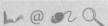

OF THE FOLLOWING, WHICH IS THE MOST EFFICIENT RESOURCE TO USE WHEN PERFORMING A LITERATURE SEARCH ON A CLINICAL RESEARCH TOPIC?
(a) a web browser
(b) online journals
(c) a generic search engine
(d) a university library catalogue.

2. You have conducted an online search of the literature using two databases concurrently, CINAHL and Medline. The keywords used selected 1704 citations. What can you deduce from this?
(a) there has been a lot of research conducted on the topic

(b) using CINAHL and Medline has duplicated all of the publications
(c) the keywords used were not sufficiently focused to narrow the search
(d) a third database is needed to limit the search.

3. Which of the following is an example of a primary source?
(a) a published commentary on the findings of a study
(b) a doctoral thesis that critiques all research on a specific clinical topic
(c) a textbook on critical care nursing

(d) a journal article about a study that used previously unpublished data.

4. The following words or phrases describe either primary or secondary sources. Place a P next to those describing primary sources and an S next to those describing secondary sources.
   (a) summaries of research studies
   (b) first-hand accounts of participant interviews
   (c) biographies
   (d) textbooks
   (e) patient records
   (f) reports written by the researcher
   (g) doctoral or master's theses.

5. A refereed journal:
   (a) publishes both articles and critiques of studies
   (b) is indexed in a bibliographic database
   (c) uses a panel of reviewers to review submitted papers for possible publication
   (d) is retrievable online.

6. Print indexes are useful for finding:
   (a) lists of secondary sources
   (b) the latest unpublished research
   (c) the keywords to use in an electronic search
   (d) sources that have not been entered into an electronic database.

7. When beginning an online literature search:
   (a) use at least two recognised electronic databases
   (b) start with non-research literature
   (c) read only abstracts from primary sources
   (d) use the fewest keywords possible.

8. How many years is it necessary to go back in the literature for an evidence-based project?
   (a) one year is sufficient
   (b) five years is preferred
   (c) ten years is expected
   (d) all literature is to be included.

9. Which one of the following is an example of a secondary source?
   (a) a doctoral thesis
   (b) the Nurse Practitioner Act, describing the scope of practice in the state
   (c) a chapter in a book critiquing a research study

(d) a published report conducted ten years ago, written by the original researcher.

10. The CINAHL Print Index must be used for literature searches of material before which year?
    (a) 1972
    (b) 1982
    (c) 1992
    (d) 2002

Additional resources

Brettle A, Gambling T 2003 Needle in a haystack? Effective literature searching for research. *Radiography* 9:229–36

Doig G S, Simpson F 2003 Efficient literature searching: a core skill for the practice of evidence-based medicine. *Intensive Care Medicine* 29:2119–27

Garg A, Turtle K M 2003 Effectiveness of training health professionals in literature search skills using electronic health databases — a critical appraisal. *Health Information & Libraries Journal* 20:33–41

Hart C 2001 *Doing a literature search: a comprehensive guide for the social sciences*. Sage, London

Walters L A, Wilczynski N, Haynes R B 2006 Developing optimal search strategies for retrieving clinically relevant qualitative studies in EMBASE. *Qualitative Health Research* 16:162–8

References

Adamson H, Elliott D 2005 Quality of life after a critical illness: a review of general ICU studies 1998–2003. *Australian Critical Care* 18:50–60

Cheek J, Garnham B, Quan J 2006 What's in a number? Issues in providing evidence of impact and quality of research(ers). *Qualitative Health Research* 16:423–35

Conn V S, Isaramalai S, Rath S, et al. 2003 Beyond Medline for literature searches. *Journal of Nursing Scholarship* 35:177–82

Fineout-Overholt E, Johnston L 2005 Teaching EBP: asking searchable, answerable clinical questions. *Worldviews on Evidence-Based Nursing* Third Quarter 157–60

Garfield E 2006 The history and meaning of the journal impact factor. *Journal of the American Medical Association* 293:90–3

Kam P C A 2005 Impact factor: over rated and misused? [editorial] *Anaesthesia and Intensive Care* 33:565–6

Nicoll LH, Ouellette TH, et al. 1996 Bibliography database managers. *Computers in Nursing* 14(1):45–6

Shorten A, Wallace M C, Crookes P A 2001 Developing information literacy: a key to evidence-based nursing. *International Nursing Review* 48:86–92

Walters L A, Wilczynski N, Haynes R B 2006 Developing optimal search strategies for retrieving clinically relevant qualitative studies in EMBASE. *Qualitative Health Research* 16:162–8

Wang W-W, Moyle W 2005 Physical restraint use on people with dementia: a review of the literature. *Australian Journal of Advanced Nursing* 22(4):46–52

Answers

TT Tutorial trigger 1

Answers will vary — a list of sample questions include:

1. What is the source of the material? (Note: Look at the last term in the URL address for American sources and the second last when the source is outside the USA, to find the organisational 'type' name (it is three letters long); possibilities include: 'com' for commercial organisation, 'edu' for educational institution, 'gov' for government body, 'int' for international organisation, 'net' for networking organisation, and 'org' for anything else.

   You can feel comfortable with information gathered from an 'edu' or 'gov' source such as www.joannabriggs. edu.au that takes you to the Joanna Briggs Institute in Adelaide, or from www.acnm.org.au which will take you to The Australian Council of Nursing and Midwifery, or http://cinahl.com for CINAHL information systems based in the USA.)

2. Is the source a well-respected medical or nursing institution or government agency, or is the source an individual putting out his/her own opinion? Critique the source.
3. Is the name of the researcher, or researchers and their qualifications given?
4. Is there a mechanism given to obtain further information about the study or the information presented?
5. Is enough data given in the web publication to make a critical analysis about the material such as the analysis that can be made about a research article using the critiquing criteria in the textbook? (Note: In a refereed, professional journal there are usually two or three independent nursing experts in the field who have reviewed the article in a blind-review process to determine that the material merits publication.)

TT Tutorial trigger 2

Answers will vary. A list of five journals publishing clinical research articles could include those listed in Table 3.1.

Learning activities

1. b   2. c   3. d
4. (a) S
   (b) P
   (c) S
   (d) S
   (e) P
   (f) P
   (g) P
5. c   6. d   7. d   8. b
9. c   10. b

4

Reviewing the literature

DOUG ELLIOTT

KEY TERMS

integrative review
meta-analysis
meta-narrative
meta-synthesis
methodological quality
narrative review
systematic review

Learning outcomes

After reading this chapter, you should be able to:

- discuss the review of literature in relation to nursing theory, research, education and practice
- discuss the use of the literature in relation to specific research designs and methodological approaches
- identify the characteristics of a relevant literature review
- differentiate between the different types of literature review
- apply criteria to evaluate (summarise and critique) a research article at a beginning research consumer level
- develop a structured critical review of the literature on a specific topic at a beginning research consumer level.

Introduction

A review of the literature is a systematic and critical review of published papers on a particular topic of interest in a discipline. Two contemporary issues have highlighted the importance for high quality reviews of original research: first, the recent proliferation of nursing and midwifery knowledge through print and online publications and other sources and repositories of information; and second, the emphasis of clinical practice based on the best available evidence. Knowledge, generated by researchers and theorists, builds a coherent and distinct 'body of knowledge' through scholarly publications and presentations.

This chapter introduces the review of literature as a concept essential to the development of our disciplines; a thread that relates practice, research, education and theory (see Figure 4.1). In relation to these four concepts, a critical review of the literature presents:
• new knowledge that can lead to the development, testing or refinement of theories
• gaps or limitations in the literature that can lead to new directions in original research
• the existing knowledge about a particular topic, concept or problem of clinical interest
• research findings that inform evidence-based practice activities (development of clinical practice guidelines; practice development projects).

FIGURE 4.1 Relationship of the review of literature to theory, research, education and practice

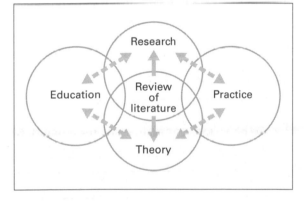

Concepts introduced in this chapter are further developed in the remaining chapters of this book. The preceding chapter described the processes for examining the sources of academic literature and a defined search strategy. The focus of this chapter is primarily from the perspective of a research consumer in conducting a literature review and preparing a written report. The essential components for the production of a structured and critical literature review are discussed, and various types of review are described (e.g. integrative review, systematic review, meta-analysis). Some types of review are complex, and require significant expertise and experience to complete. Issues related to study quality and grades of recommendations for a body of literature are also introduced, although it

is acknowledged that the necessary skills-set for these latter activities are advanced, and beyond the requirements of a beginning or intermediate level research consumer.

Purposes of a literature review

The overall purpose of a review of the literature is to examine the knowledge base to inform a defined area of clinical practice or theoretical perspective, or guide original research. The common forms of a review include use as:
• a systematic summary of a series of original research papers; for example, a systematic review — 'secondary research'
• a supporting background section for a clinical practice guideline or evidence-based recommendation — 'secondary research'
• the background section of an original research proposal, grant application or published paper — 'primary research'.

Point to ponder

▶ Secondary research is the process of reviewing previous original research to produce a more comprehensive or unique understanding of a topic of interest. Primary research is the process of undertaking an original study and collecting new data.

A literature review therefore serves a purpose for both research consumers and primary researchers. The following two subsections consider the literature review from these differing perspectives — from a research consumer's viewpoint as secondary research; and as the basis for supporting proposed original primary research.

Conducting a literature review as secondary research

In clinical practice, the knowledge from a critical review of the literature contributes to the implementation of research-based practice interventions, protocols and evaluation programs that improve the quality of patient care. Undertaking a literature review is therefore a common learning and assessment task in preparing undergraduate students for clinical practice. Literature reviews are also undertaken by graduate coursework and research students for various learning purposes. The process for completing this challenging task needs to be explicitly modelled and learned within the educational setting. Increasingly, clinicians also conduct literature reviews to inform the development and refinement of clinical practice guidelines.

The major research consumer focus of the literature review is therefore to uncover knowledge for use in clinical practice and educational settings. Table 4.1 illustrates a few examples of scholarly activities related to reviews of the literature in educational, practice and professional settings. Each outcome reflects the need for critical thinking and scholarly writing, and the academic and professional expectations for a beginning and developing research consumer in the discipline.

> ### Point to ponder
> ▶ A literature review is central to developing and implementing research consumer activities, and is an essential element in implementing a research-based practice. A practice protocol or nursing intervention implemented in a healthcare setting should be based on a 'critical' review of the contemporary research literature.

The styles of a literature review for secondary research are discussed in more detail later in this chapter.

Conducting a literature review for primary research

A review of the literature is essential in all aspects of the primary research process. Researchers and research students commonly undertake a literature review as a beginning step in the primary research process, including for research proposals submitted to human research

TABLE 4.1 Examples of the uses of the literature for research consumer purposes: educational and practice settings

Educational setting	Clinical practice/professional setting
Undergraduate and graduate coursework students: • develop academic scholarly papers on a specific topic, problem or issue • prepare oral presentations or debates on a topic, problem or issue; clinical projects.	Clinicians: • implement research-based nursing interventions • develop or adapt clinical practice guidelines for use in a local clinical setting • develop, implement and evaluate hospital-specific quality improvement or practice development projects related to patient outcome data.
Research higher degree students: • develop research proposals • develop systematic reviews, research-based practice protocols and other scholarly projects.	Professional nursing organisations/governmental agencies: • position statements • discussion papers.
Faculty: • develop research proposals and grant applications • develop review or theoretical papers • develop and revise curricula.	

ethics committees (HRECs) and funding bodies (see Chapter 19). The review develops a strong knowledge base to inform primary research or other disciplinary scholarly clinical practice and educational activities (see Box 4.1). Each section of Box 4.1 relates to the content in other chapters of this text, highlighting the various connections and amount of background knowledge needed to effectively review the literature. Note that for some qualitative approaches (e.g. grounded theory), the literature review may be performed after the primary data are collected (see Chapter 9).

TT Tutorial trigger 1

The review of literature is usually easy to find in a primary research paper. Most frequently, one of the early sections of the paper is labelled 'Review of Literature' or 'Background' or some other comparable term, or there may be no label to the section. Review the paper by Middleton and colleagues (2005) in Chapter 16. In small groups, briefly discuss the way in which the review of the literature is presented.

Summarise the main points that reflect the purposes of a literature review from the research consumer's perspective.

Research in brief

A short literature review was provided to justify a study of the effectiveness of a brief midwife-led counselling intervention after childbirth perceived by mothers as being emotionally traumatic (Gamble et al. 2005). The authors described the causes, symptoms and adverse psychological outcomes, including depression and post-traumatic stress, related to traumatic childbirth. The paucity of studies on the topic of interest was then discussed, including noting the inconsistent findings and methodological criticisms and potential harmful outcomes described by other authors. These study authors therefore provided justification for this present study.

BOX 4.1 Use of a literature review in relation to the primary research process

Source of knowledge and paradigmatic position:
* reviews conceptual frameworks, theories or models from nursing, midwifery and related fields used to examine a topic, concept or clinical problem
* highlights the context for studying the problem
* can be viewed as a concept map for understanding the relationships between variables
* provides a rationale for the variables and develops propositions about individual variables within the theoretical framework of the study.

Question, problem or hypothesis:
* determines what is known and not known about a topic, concept or problem
* uncovers gaps, consistencies or inconsistencies
* reveals unanswered questions in the literature about a subject, concept, theory or problem
* generates useful questions and hypotheses of clinical importance to the discipline.

Design and method:
* identifies the strengths and weaknesses of designs and methods of previous research studies
* informs selection of a feasible and ethical design, data collection method, sample size, valid and reliable instruments
* reveals the appropriateness of a study's design and assists a researcher in determining whether a previous study should be replicated and/or refined
* identifies the need for instrument refinement or development through continued psychometric testing.

Outcome of the analysis (findings, discussion, implications and recommendations):
* interprets and discusses the results/findings of a study in relation to other previous studies, using examples from the literature
* develops implications of the findings for practice, education and further research
* promotes development of a new practice intervention or provides evidence for current practice.

Characteristics of a critical review

A review includes a critical evaluation of both primary and secondary literature related to the clinical practice question or proposed study, as well as a summary of the overall strengths or weaknesses of the reviewed studies' conflicts and gaps in the literature. It concludes with a statement relating the proposed clinical practice guideline or study to the reviewed research.

From a student perspective, a critical review of the literature is essential to acquiring knowledge for the development of academic papers, presentations and debates. Academic staff expect students to include cited literature in support of their rationale for each clinical practice activity. For example, a student assignment might involve retrieving and critically reviewing the primary sources listed for a particular clinical practice guideline, to determine the degree of support found for the interventions outlined in the guidelines. An effective literature review will reflect the characteristics listed in Table 4.2. All levels and types of review should explicitly describe the search strategy and inclusion criteria for including primary studies in the review (Whittemore 2005a).

While peer-reviewed journals are the major source of studies for inclusion in a review, one issue to consider relates to the access of 'grey literature'. This term refers to studies that are published in sources with limited distribution that may not be included in bibliographic databases (e.g. obscure journals, some online journals, unpublished reports, theses, conference abstracts, policy documents) (Conn et al. 2003). The 'search strategy' for a comprehensive review should therefore include attempts to identify relevant studies from grey literature sources. A review of studies examining the quality of life for survivors of a critical illness used a search of electronic databases as the initial approach in identifying studies. The search strategy however also included a manual search of the proceedings for the annual disciplinary conference to identify abstracts of relevant studies that may have not been subsequently published (Adamson & Elliott 2005).

The development of skills in writing a literature review is experiential — more exposure to literature and more practice in writing will improve the quality and depth of a review. As your experience grows, the style of review will transform from a descriptive summary of individual studies to a more integrated synthesis and analysis of the collective of studies.

Evidence-based practice tip

Comprehensive understanding of a study requires multiple readings — read and re-read selected studies, clarify unfamiliar terms or processes, and discuss or seek advice from clinical and academic colleagues.

TABLE 4.2 Characteristics of a written review of literature

Levels of review	Criteria
Description	• Sufficient number of sources are identified, based on the clinical question, related keywords and appropriate range of publication years. • Review mainly consists of primary sources. • Summary of studies is presented in a logical flow using themes or categories. • Summary is succinct and adequately represents the reviewed literature/knowledge base of a specific topic. • Summaries/paraphrasing of material (direct quotes of content used only for specific purposes and referenced appropriately).
Analysis	• Critical review of study methods, outcomes and applicability to clinical practice. • Assessment of study quality, using accepted review 'criteria' to analyse strengths, weaknesses or limitations and conflicts or gaps in information.
Synthesis	• Linking studies together to form a new whole. • Use of summary tables to facilitate critique of articles in sections or themes and uncover questions or gaps in the literature.

Steps in the review process

As noted in the previous chapter, the six steps involved in the literature search and review process are: formulating a review question, conducting a comprehensive search of the literature, assessing studies for inclusion in the review, critical appraisal of the selected studies, synthesis of findings from individual studies, and reporting results and recommendations for practice. Critical appraisal, synthesis of findings from the studies reviewed, and analysis of the body of literature to inform practice is the focus of this chapter. Many of the remaining chapters examine methodological issues related to various research designs, and Chapter 16 explicitly discusses the critical evaluation of research studies.

Once the relevant studies have been selected from the literature search (described in Chapter 3), a step-wise process for reviewing the literature includes:

- preliminary reading of available abstracts, which allows articles to be selected or discarded from the original search results
- obtaining a full-text print or electronic copy of all included articles to enable organisation for priority critical reading and eventual sorting into themes or categories
- an initial read/scan of all papers that will identify a set of core papers, others that are useful and peripheral to your questions, and perhaps some that are not as useful as first thought, and which may be discarded from the review
- describing the justification for discarding studies
- organising papers into themes, allowing comparison and links between coherent studies during the review (perhaps using summary tables as a guiding and organisational tool)
- critical reading, which requires several readings, a certain level of knowledge

across a broad range of methodological approaches, and is aided by the use of a set of criteria to evaluate the studies.

Other steps or components of the review process relate to the type of review being conducted, and are discussed in the next section, after a discussion of summary tables.

Summary tables

For most styles of literature review, after an initial review of papers it may be useful to construct some working summary tables to provide key characteristics of individual studies — design, sample, variables, outcomes (Whittemore 2005a). A table facilitates effective critique of studies in sections or themes, and identifies questions and gaps in the literature. Initially, column headers are selected to allow analysis of the various papers under specific themes (see Table 4.3).

> **Evidence-based practice tip**
>
> A summary table allows summary information to be noted for each study (description), and enables identification of similarities and differences between the studies (synthesis), and limitations (analysis).

The development and sophistication of the table then progresses as the review of papers continues. Summary tables may be used only as a tool in the preparation of a literature review, or may evolve into an integral component of the final review report or manuscript. Table 4.4 illustrates an example summary table.

Styles for literature reviews

A variety of approaches for conducting a literature review have recently emerged in response to the proliferation of primary research in nursing, midwifery and related health disciplines. This variation has however

TABLE 4.3 Example of summary table column headers

Author/date	Participants	Method/procedure	Outcome variables	Findings
Paper A				
Paper B				
Paper C				

TABLE 4.4 Example of a beginning summary table: recent Australian patient outcome studies for cardiac surgery

Study	Design/Sample	Method	Major findings
Gardner et al. 2003[1]	Prospective observational/93	No pre-surgery measurement; pain, self-efficacy, depression, HR-QOL[3] @ 1 and 6 months; valid and reliable instruments	Significant improvement in QOL @ 6 months compared to 1 month; 22% reported chronic pain @ 6 months, and had lower scores for physical function, general health, social functioning and mental health
Gardner et al. 2005[2]	Exploratory qualitative/8	Memories and experiences during recovery; content analysis of transcripts of interviews @ 6 months	Varying degrees of pain and physical dysfunction continued @ 6 months; emerging themes included comfort/discomfort, hope/hopelessness, acceptance/apprehension, life changes
Elliott et al. 2006	Prospective observational/101	HR-QOL[3] measured prior to surgery, hospital discharge and 6 months; valid and reliable instruments	HR-QOL improved significantly @ 6 months compared to prior measurements except mental health and social functioning; scores continued to be lower than population norms
LeGrande et al. 2006	Prospective observational/182	HR-QOL[3], mood, functioning 1 month before and 2 and 6 months post-surgery; valid and reliable instruments	Physical recovery is earlier than psychological recovery; improvement is not linear or applicable to all patients

Notes:
1. Conference paper — example of 'grey literature'.
2. Qualitative paper — different purpose, method and analyses to other studies presented here.
3. Health related-quality of life (HR-QOL) measurement — common across some studies; may enable meta-analysis of pooled findings.

contributed to inconsistency and confusion in methods and terminology. The types of reviews currently evident in the literature are listed in Table 4.5 (Dixon-Woods & Fitzpatrick 2005; Fingeld 2003; Mays et al. 2005; Whittemore 2005a; Whittemore & Knafl 2005).

Conducting a review of contemporary research without bias or error is a challenging activity, requiring an explicit and transparent process. It is also sometimes difficult to distinguish between the styles of review, as there may be overlap in the terms and processes described. The four common types of review used in nursing and midwifery — narrative, systematic, meta-synthesis and integrative; are described below. Most of these approaches are complex, requiring a certain level of expertise and experience in the content area and methods used in the primary studies (Whittemore 2005a). Readers are also directed to the cited references and 'additional resources' for further in-depth discussion of the processes involved in conducting these reviews, particularly for the latter two types.

Narrative review

A traditional narrative review was the original type of literature review which is still common in contemporary literature. The topic is usually broad, and does not include a focused clinical question or defined search strategy. Analysis of the primary studies is classified as 'narrative' or 'thematic' — a narrative is purely descriptive, while a thematic analysis produces a rudimentary synthesis of findings

Research in brief

A narrative review discussed parasuicide, self-harm and suicide in rural Aboriginal peoples in relation to implications for mental health nursing practice, and recommended a whole-of-community approach for the continuity and integration of mental health services. (Proctor 2005). However, no search strategy or assessment of study quality was presented to substantiate the selection of literature.

TABLE 4.5 Types of literature reviews

Label	Description
Narrative review	A description of studies using narrative analysis; commonly lacks transparency and standards in selection of studies and review processes; findings and conclusions may be open to bias and subjectivity.
Systematic review (SR)	A summary combining findings from quantitative studies with similar hypotheses and methods, to inform research and practice using narrative or statistical analysis.
Meta-analysis	Commonly a component of a SR; combines data from quantitative studies that employ statistical methods; data from individual studies are pooled for quantitative summary analysis.
Meta-synthesis, meta-summary	A summary combining findings from multiple qualitative studies to inform research and practice using narrative analysis.
Integrative review	A broad review that combines findings from quantitative and qualitative studies, theoretical and methodological literature using narrative analysis.

by identifying important and recurring themes (Mays et al. 2005). The result is a broad review of a topic, which probably does not provide enough information on the literature search and review strategies for a reader to judge the potential for bias or subjectivity in the findings and conclusion (Dixon-Woods & Fitzpatrick 2005; Whittemore 2005a).

Another narrative review examined the use of physical restraints for people with dementia (Wang & Moyle 2005), but described the explicit search strategy and inclusion criteria and the results of the search (previously noted in Chapter 3). Using a thematic analysis, four dominant themes were identified: the relationship between restraint use and cognitive decline; falls/related injuries and mortality; alternative to physical restraint use; and nurses' attitudes to restraint use. There was, however, no evidence of judging the methodological quality of the reviewed studies.

Systematic review

A systematic review (SR) is now a common strategy for examining an explicit issue in clinical practice, particularly for 'cause-and-effect' studies where the effect of an intervention or treatment is tested. This style of review minimises the potential for bias, and is now the most common type of review published, particularly for studies of clinical effectiveness. A systematic review explicitly reports all aspects of the literature search and review process — commonly using a:

- focused clinical question (see below)
- defined search strategy (as described in the previous chapter)
- critical appraisal form (checklist) to assess study quality for inclusion in the review
- data extraction form to abstract relevant characteristics of the study (e.g. design, sample, intervention, outcome measures, results)
- data pooling and analysis process to enable a meta-analysis
- classification system to determine the level of evidence.

The SR process can encompass other quantitative designs, but does not include qualitative approaches because of the diverse methodological approaches and the lack of an appropriate framework for assessing the quality of studies and grading the evidence (see 'Body of evidence and grades of recommendations' section later in this chapter).

Point to ponder

▶ The Cochrane Collaboration conducts SRs of randomised controlled trials (RCTs) for cause-and-effect questions. See the website for examples of study protocols and reports of systematic reviews — http://www.cochrane.org.

Focused clinical question

A clinical question for an SR includes specific components, reflected in the acronym PICO:

P Patient population of interest (and clinical setting)
I exposure to an Intervention
C Comparison or Control group used to assess the intervention
O measurable Outcome of interest (end-point)

Evidence-based practice tip

A template for a question is: 'What is the effectiveness of … [*a specific intervention*] … for … [*a defined patient type*] …, as measured by … [*a measurable outcome*]?'.

Meta-analysis

When the data from studies in an SR are sufficiently equivalent, a meta-analysis of the pooled data can be examined, using common quantitative analysis procedures (discussed in Chapter 14). A standardised measure of the effect of the intervention (effect size) is calculated for the outcome measures as:

- mean values (differences) between groups — d
- correlation (association) between two variables — r
- odds ratio between groups exposed and not exposed to an intervention — OR.

Effect sizes of small, medium and large are interpreted for d as 0.20, 0.50 and 0.80, and r as 0.10, 0.30 and 0.50, respectively (Whittemore 2005a).

Other types of reviews have since been developed to enable inclusion of different study methods and to overcome the narrow focus of SRs.

Meta-synthesis

A meta-synthesis is an umbrella term of a process aimed at producing a new and integrative interpretation of individual qualitative studies to form a unitary model or over-arching framework (Fingeld 2003). The term actually encompasses a number of similar approaches — meta-summary (Sandelowski & Barroso

Research in brief

One review of stabilisation techniques for oral endotracheal tubes (ETT) identified seven primary studies, although only three provided enough information to allow a meta-analysis to be conducted. No single method of ETT stabilisation was identified as superior in minimising tube displacement and unplanned or accidental extubations. Randomised controlled trials were therefore recommended to establish best practice and evaluate the cost-effectiveness of stabilisation techniques (Gardner et al. 2005). An example of the meta-analysis is illustrated in Figure 4.2. The pooled data (of two studies only) indicated that fewer patients had lip excoriation from an oral endotracheal tube when a commercial device was used compared to adhesive tape (OR 0.2, 95% confidence interval = 0.1 — 0.5, p = <0.001) (Gardner et al. 2005).

2003), meta-ethnography (McCormick et al. 2003) and grounded formal theory, to provide a more substantive and informative position than findings from separate qualitative studies (Fingeld 2003; McCormick et al. 2003; Thorne et al. 2004). There continues to be disagreement about whether a meta-synthesis is actually a form of systematic review (Sandelowski & Barroso 2003) or not (Fingeld 2003).

All data are converted to text for qualitative analysis, and matrices or tables are used to compare studies and create a new interpretation of the collective data (Jensen &

FIGURE 4.2 Example of a meta-analysis

| Comparison: | commercially manufactured device (CMD) versus adhesive tape | | | | | |
| Outcome: | incidence of lip excoriation | | | | | |
Study	CMD n/N	adhesive n/N	OR (95% CI Fixed)	Weight %	OR (95%CI Fixed)
Kaplow & Bookbinder 1994	4 / 30	11 / 30		36.1	0.27 (0.07, 0.96)
Tasota et al. 1987	5 / 59	18 / 56		63.9	0.20 (0.07, 0.57)
Total (95%CI)	9 / 89	29 / 86		100.0	0.22 (0.10, 0.50)

Test for heterogeneity chi-square=0.13 df=1 p=0.72
Test for overall effect z=−3.60 p=0.0003

.01   .1   1   10   100
Favours CMD   Favours adhesive

(Source: Gardner A, Hughes D, Cook R, et al. 2005 Best practice in stabilisation of oral endotracheal tubes: a systematic review. *Australian Critical Care* 18, p 164, used with permission.)

Allen 1996; Mays et al. 2005). The complex process includes a systematic and transparent approach to review included studies (see for example Greenhalgh et al. 2005).

Integrative review

This approach enables inclusion of studies with diverse methods, as well as theoretical and methodological papers. One study examining the concept of 'integration' in nursing identified 56 published papers — 36 were empirical and 20 were theoretical (e.g. Whittemore 2005b). Stages of the review process — problem identification, literature search, data evaluation, data analysis and reduction, and data comparison — are explicit and transparent (Whittemore & Knafl 2005). Data analysis, reduction and comparison reflect qualitative analysis of primary data as described later in Chapter 9. A recent and evolving approach uses a 'narrative synthesis' (Mays et al. 2005) approach to link complex evidence from multiple paradigms.

> ### Research in brief
>
> A review that examined patient recovery following severe trauma identified over 80 studies from the search strategy. A number of themes were noted including inadequate support for injured individuals along the recovery trajectory, with long-term loss of productivity, a high incidence of psychological sequelae, and a link between poor recovery and increased drug and alcohol consumption. The heterogeneous nature of the studies' methods and outcomes precluded any meta-analysis of the findings (Halcomb et al. 2005). No quality assessment of the primary studies was conducted.

Assessing study quality

Assessment of the study quality of individual studies for a review is a complex task, particularly when a range of methods are used in the primary studies. While criteria for the methodological quality for intervention studies are well developed, the ability to assess descriptive and qualitative studies is less clear (Dixon-Woods & Fitzpatrick 2005; Thomas,

Harden et al. 2004). This section describes the current position for assessing a body of literature, using levels of evidence, a body of evidence assessment matrix and grades of recommendations.

A number of multidisciplinary organisations with members acknowledged as experts experienced in methodological critique are currently examining the complex issue of assessing study quality. These groups include the Cochrane Collaboration, GRADE Working Group, Joanna Briggs Institute, UK National Health Service, US Agency for Healthcare Research and Quality, New Zealand Guidelines Group, Oxford Centre for Evidence-Based Medicine, and the Australian National Health and Medical Research Council (NHMRC). A range of tools for evaluation of the literature have been developed through these groups (see 'Additional resources' at the end of this chapter).

The focus in the following subsection is on developing documents from the NHMRC. With the strong connection between reviewing the literature, clinical practice guideline development and evidence-based practice, readers are also directed to Chapter 17.

Body of evidence and grades of recommendations

At the time of writing, the NHMRC was refining guidelines for reviewing research to assist developers of clinical practice guidelines (NHMRC 2005). A hierarchy for the levels of evidence has been produced for various types of research question — intervention, diagnosis, prognosis, aetiology and screening. Clearly this focus remains on medicine, and does not address other types of questions that are also of interest to nurses, midwives or other health professionals. Table 4.6 outlines the hierarchy of evidence for cause-and-effect studies of clinical interventions, with the primacy of SRs and RCTs clear.

Note that this classification does not acknowledge or value findings from research methods common to nursing and midwifery, such as qualitative or descriptive observational designs. Opinions of respected authorities based on clinical experience, descriptive studies, or reports of expert committees were designated as Level IV evidence in previous

TABLE 4.6 Hierarchy of evidence for cause-and-effect studies of therapeutic interventions

Level	Description
I	A systematic review of level II studies (randomised controlled trials).
II	A randomised controlled trial.
III-1	A pseudo-randomised controlled trial (alternate participant allocation to study groups).
III-2	A comparative study with concurrent controls (e.g. non-randomised experiment, cohort study, case-control study, interrupted time series with a control group).
III-3	Evidence obtained from comparative studies with historical control, two or more single-arm studies, or interrupted time series without a parallel control group.
IV	Evidence obtained from case series (post-test or pre-test/post-test).

(Source: adapted from NHMRC 1999, 2005. Copyright Commonwealth of Australia, used with permission.)

classifications, but these forms of knowledge have now been removed, as the findings do not arise directly from scientific investigation. When evidence from scientific investigation is lacking, any recommendation based on expert opinion must be acknowledged, and should be reviewed as new evidence becomes available (NHMRC 2000).

When assessing study quality, values can be assigned to certain characteristics of study design and methods (Atkins et al. 2004; Brown et al. 2003; Conn & Rantz 2003), commonly in relation to sample size justification, use of reliable and valid measuring instruments, comparison of study groups at baseline for equivalence, withdrawals, drop-outs and other study losses accounted for, and any bias or influencing factors minimised (Thomas, Ciliska et al. 2004; Whittemore 2005b).

Table 4.7 outlines a draft classification system which rates the body of literature in terms of the volume of evidence, the consistency of findings, the clinical impact, generalisability and applicability of the studies' methods and outcomes (NHMRC 2005). This classification

TABLE 4.7 Body of evidence assessment matrix

Component	A Excellent	B Good	C Satisfactory	D Poor
Volume of evidence	Several level I or II studies with low risk of bias	1 or 2 level II studies with low risk of impact, or an SR/multiple level III studies with low risk of bias	Level III studies with low risk of bias, or level I or II studies with moderate risk of bias	Level IV studies, level I to II studies with high risk of bias
Consistency	All studies consistent	Most studies consistent, and inconsistency can be explained	Some inconsistency reflecting genuine uncertainty around clinical question	Evidence is inconsistent
Clinical impact	Very large	Substantial	Moderate	Slight or restricted
Generalisability Study samples are:	Same as the target population for the guideline	Same as the target population for the guideline	Different to target population, but clinically sensible to apply the evidence	Different to target population, and hard to judge whether to generalise to target population
Applicability	Directly applicable to Australian healthcare context	Applicable to Australian healthcare context with few caveats	Probably applicable to Australian healthcare context with some caveats	Not applicable to Australian healthcare context

(Source: adapted from NHMRC 2005. Copyright Commonwealth of Australia, used with permission.)

enables a broader inclusion of study design for intervention studies beyond the randomised controlled trial. This categorisation is similar to one proposed by the GRADE Working Group (Atkins et al. 2004, 2005). A recent Australian paper called for additional categories of study quality assessment, including biological plausibility and reproducibility of findings in subsequent studies, during the necessary continued refinement of these assessment tools (Bellomo & Bagshaw 2006).

The overall body of evidence can then be graded in relation to guiding clinical practice (see Table 4.8). These draft NHMRC guidelines were developed to support clinical guidelines development, and will be refined in the future following feedback from users. These grades reflect the strength of evidence supporting that specific area of clinical practice (NHMRC 2005).

TABLE 4.8 Grade of recommendation

Grade	Description
A	Body of evidence can be trusted to guide practice
B	Body of evidence can be trusted to guide practice in most clinical situations
C	Body of evidence provides some support for recommendation but care should be taken in its application
D	Body of evidence is weak and recommendation must be applied with caution

(Source: NHMRC 2005. Copyright Commonwealth of Australia, used with permission.)

Evaluating a literature review

Critical appraisal of a literature review is a challenging task for a research consumer. Box 4.2 provides questions to consider when reviewing secondary research (a literature review).

T_T Tutorial trigger 2

In small groups, discuss then summarise the main points that reflect the purposes of a literature review from a research consumer's perspective.

BOX 4.2 Critical review of a literature review

1. Are all the relevant concepts and variables included in the review?
2. Are primary sources mainly used?
3. Does the literature review uncover gaps or inconsistencies in knowledge?
4. Does the summary of each reviewed study reflect the essential components of the study design, research process and analysis techniques?
5. Does the critique of each reviewed study include: strengths, weaknesses or limitations of the design; conflicts; and gaps or inconsistencies in information in relation to the area of interest?
6. What overall conclusions can be drawn from the synthesis of the literature?
7. Does the organisation and synthesis of the reviewed studies follow a logical sequence that justifies why there is a need for a particular study?
8. How does the review reflect critical thinking?

Summary

Being able to critique a review of the literature is an acquired skill. The main objectives for a research consumer in relation to a review of the literature are to acquire the ability to: conduct a computer data-based search, efficiently retrieve a sufficient amount of scholarly materials for a literature review, and critically evaluate the selected literature using accepted reviewing criteria. This chapter has described the steps, styles, and limitations of a literature review. The remaining chapters of this book all contribute to further depth and breadth of understanding when reviewing the range of primary studies undertaken by nurses and midwives. This information provides the knowledge to enable the beginning critical evaluation and synthesis of published studies on a specific topic of interest.

(K)EY POINTS

- A review of the literature is a comprehensive, in-depth, systematic and critical review of scholarly publications, unpublished scholarly print materials, internet materials, audiovisual materials and personal communications.
- A literature review provides information for both research consumers and researchers.

- Systematic reviews (SRs) provide an explicit protocol for the search strategy, inclusion criteria for article selection and critical appraisal in the examination of explicit aspects of methodological rigour.
- The ability to critically review data-based literature is necessary for implementing a research-based practice in nursing or midwifery.

Learning activities

1. Reviews of the literature are conducted for both primary research purposes and for secondary research (research consumer) purposes. In what way are these reviews similar?
   i.   the amount and scope of literature reviewed
   ii. the search strategy used
   iii. the degree of critical reading required
   iv. the purpose of the review.
   (a) i and ii
   (b) iii and iv
   (c) ii and iii
   (d) i, ii, iii and iv.

2. You find that most of the articles retrieved during an electronic search of the literature are not useful. Which of the following is the next best step to follow?
   (a) use the articles obtained, knowing that there has been little research in this area
   (b) change the keywords and do another search
   (c) change the study and focus of the literature review
   (d) use a print index to retrieve older papers.

3. Which of the following is an example of 'grey literature'?
   (a) abstracts from an online bibliographic database
   (b) abstracts in a printed proceedings from a conference

   (c) full-text papers in a published journal
   (d) an abstract of a primary study in a textbook.

4. In what circumstances would a literature review be conducted after data were collected?
   (a) when the researcher was unable to formulate the study question
   (b) a qualitative design was used
   (c) there were no significant findings
   (d) too many participants dropped out of the study.

5. A summary table assists in:
   (a) collecting a broad range of literature
   (b) summarising the weaknesses of studies
   (c) tracking the generalisability of studies
   (d) synthesising information from studies.

6. A non-experimental descriptive study provides what level of evidence, according to a cause and effect classification system?
   (a) level II
   (b) level III
   (c) level IV
   (d) lower than level IV.

7. A systematic review (SR) is the most appropriate type of review to examine:
   (a) descriptive and exploratory studies
   (b) cause and effect studies
   (c) studies in a meta-synthesis
   (d) level III studies.

8. In the hierarchy of evidence for cause and effect studies, the opinions of respected authorities or expert committees are:
   (a) graded level II
   (b) graded level III
   (c) graded level IV
   (d) not graded.

9. The 'C' in the acronym PICO stands for:
   (a) Contamination
   (b) Control
   (c) Comparison
   (d) Confounding.

10. The characteristics of a literature review include:
    i. evidence of a comprehensive search of the literature
    ii. a review of mainly secondary sources of literature
    iii. summaries are succinct, with minimal direct quotes
    iv. a logical flow using themes or categories.
    (a) i, ii and iii
    (b) i, iii and iv
    (c) ii, iii and iv
    (d) all of the above.

Additional resources

Agency for Healthcare Research and Quality, US Department of Health and Human Services 2002 Systems to Rate the Strength of Scientific Evidence Summary, Evidence Report/Technology Assessment, number 47. Online. Available: http://www.ahrq.gov

Cochrane Collaboration. Online. Available: http://www.cochrane.org; http://www.cochrane.org.au

Critical Appraisal Skills Program (CASP), UK National Health Service Critical Appraisal Tools — systematic reviews. Online. Available: http://www.phru.nhs.uk/casp

Grading of Recommendations Assessment, Development and Evaluation GRADE Working Group. Online. Available: http://www.gradeworkinggroup.org

Guidelines International Network. Online. Available: http://ww.g-i-n.net

Joanna Briggs Institute. Online. Available: http://www.joannabriggs.edu.au

Magarey J 2001 Elements of a systematic review. *International Journal of Nursing Practice* 7:376–82

National Health and Medical Research Council (NHMRC) 1999 *A guide to the development,* *implementation and evaluation of clinical practice guidelines.* Canberra, NHMRC

—— 2000 *How to use the evidence: assessment and application of scientific evidence.* Canberra, NHMRC

National Institute of Clinical Studies (NICS). *NICS Guide to the Cochrane Library.* Online. Available: http://www.nicsl.com.au/cochrane/index.asp

—— *A guide to finding online evidence to inform clinical decisions.* Online. Available: http://www.whereistheevidence.nicsl.com.au/

New Zealand Guidelines Group (NZGG). Online. Available: http://www.nzgg.org.nz

Oxford Centre for Evidence-Based Medicine (CEBM). Online. Available: http://www.cebm.net

Whittemore R 2005 Combining evidence in nursing research: methods and implications. *Nursing Research* 54:56–62

References

Adamson H, Elliott D 2005 Quality of life after a critical illness: a review of general ICU studies 1998–2005. *Australian Critical Care* 18:50–60

Atkins D, Best D, Briss P A, et al. for the GRADE Working Group 2004 Grading quality of evidence and strength of recommendations. *British Medical Journal* 328:1490 (8 pages)

Atkins D, Briss P A, Eccles M, et al. for the GRADE Working Group 2005 Systems for grading the quality of evidence and the strength of recommendations II: pilot study of a new system. *BMC Health Services Research* 5:25 (12 pages)

Bellomo R, Bagshaw S M 2006 Evidence-based medicine: classifying the evidence from clinical trials. *Critical Care* 10:232 (8 pages)

Brown S A, Upchurch S L, Acton G J 2003 A framework for developing a coding scheme for meta-analysis. *Western Journal of Nursing Research* 25:205–22

Conn V S, Rantz M J 2003 Managing primary study quality in meta-analyses. *Research in Nursing & Health* 26:322–33

Conn V S, Valentine J C, Cooper H M et al. 2003 Grey literature in meta-analyses. *Nursing Research* 52:256–61

Dixon-Woods M, Fitzpatrick R 2005 Qualitative research in systematic reviews (editorial). *British Medical Journal* 323:765–6

Elliott D, Lazarus R, Leeder S R 2006 Health outcomes of patients undergoing cardiac surgery: repeated measures using Short Form-36 and 15 Dimensions of Quality of Life questionnaire. *Heart & Lung* 35:245–51

Fingeld D L 2003 Metasynthesis: the state of the art — so far. *Qualitative Health Research* 13:893–904

Gamble J, Creedy D, Moyle W, et al. 2005 Effectiveness of a counselling intervention after a traumatic childbirth: a randomized controlled trial. *Birth* 32:11–19

Gardner A, Hughes D, Cook R, et al. 2005 Best practice in stabilisation of oral endotracheal tubes: a systematic review. *Australian Critical Care* 18:158–65

Gardner G, Blaszczyk M, Boyle M, et al. 2003 Pain and health status of cardiac surgery patients six months post-discharge. Proceedings of the 28th Annual Scientific Meeting on Intensive Care, Cairns, 17 October

Gardner G, Elliott D, Gill J, et al. 2005 Patient experiences following cardiac surgery: an interview study. *European Journal of Cardiovascular Nursing* 4:242–50

Greenhalgh T, Robert G, MacFarlane F, et al. 2004 Diffusion of innovations in service organizations: systematic review and recommendations. *The Milbank Quarterly* 82:581–629

Greenhalgh T, Robert G, MacFarlane F, et al. 2005 Storylines of research in diffusion of innovation: a meta-narrative approach to systematic review. *Social Science & Medicine* 61:417–30

Halcomb E, Daly J, Davidson P, et al. 2005 Life beyond severe traumatic injury: an integrative review of the literature. *Australian Critical Care* 18:17–24

Jensen L A, Allen M N 1996 Meta-synthesis of qualitative findings. *Qualitative Health Research* 6:553–60

Le Grande M R, Elliott P C, Murphy B M, et al. 2006 Health related quality of life trajectories and predictors following coronary artery bypass surgery. *Health & Quality of Life Outcomes* 4:49

McCormick J, Rodney P, Varcoe C 2003 Reinterpretation across studies: an approach to meta-analysis. *Qualitative Health Research* 13:933–44

Mays N, Pope C, Popay J 2005 Systematically reviewing qualitative and quantitative evidence to inform management and policy-making in the health field. *Journal of Health Services Research & Policy* 10 (supplement):6–20

Middleton S, Donnelly N, Harris J, et al. 2005 Nursing intervention after carotid endarterectomy: a randomized trial of co-ordinated care post-discharge (CCPD). *Journal of Advanced Nursing* 52:250–61

Morse J M 2005 Beyond the clinical trial: expanding criteria for evidence (editorial). *Qualitative Health Research* 15:3–4

National Health and Medical Research Council (NHMRC) 1999 *A guide to the development, implementation and evaluation of clinical practice guidelines*. Canberra, NHMRC

—— 2000 *How to use the evidence: assessment and application of scientific evidence*. Canberra, NHMRC

—— 2005 *NHMRC additional levels of evidence and grades of recommendations for developers of guidelines*. Canberra, NHMRC

Proctor N G 2005 Parasuicide, self-harm and suicide in Aboriginal people in rural Australia: A review of the literature with implications for mental health nursing practice. *International Journal of Nursing Practice* 11:237–41

Sandelowski M, Barroso J 2003 Creating metasummaries of qualitative findings. *Nursing Research* 52:226–33

Saunders L D, Soomro G M, Buckingham J, et al. 2003 Assessing the methodological quality of nonrandomized intervention studies. *Western Journal of Nursing Research* 25:223–37

Soeken K L, Sripusanapan A 2003 Assessing publication bias in meta-analysis. *Nursing Research* 52:57–60

Thomas B H, Ciliska D, Dobbins M, et al. 2004 A process for systematically reviewing the literature: providing the research evidence for public health nursing interventions. *Worldviews on Evidence-Based Nursing* 1:176–84

Thomas J, Harden A, Oakley A, et al. 2004 Integrating qualitative research with trials in systematic reviews. *British Medical Journal* 328:1010–12

Thorne S, Jensen L, Kearney M H, et al. 2004 Qualitative metasynthesis: reflections on methodological orientation and ideological agenda. *Qualitative Health Research* 14:1342–65

Wang W-W, Moyle W 2005 Physical restraint use on people with dementia: a review of the literature. *Australian Journal of Advanced Nursing* 22(4):46–52

Whittemore R 2005a Analysis of integration in nursing science and practice. *Journal of Nursing Scholarship* 37:261–7

—— 2005b Combining evidence in nursing research: methods and implications. *Nursing Research* 54:56–62

Whittemore R, Knafl K 2005 The integrative review: updated methodology. *Journal of Advanced Nursing* 52:546–53

Answers

TT Tutorial trigger 1

The paper by Middleton et al. (2005) provided a section titled 'Background' to describe the relevant literature that supported their primary study. The key points described focused on stroke prevention and management, coordinated care models post-surgery, gaps in evaluation of these models and limitations of previous equivalent studies. The authors provided a justification for the study using the literature.

TT Tutorial trigger 2

A literature review can provide the following information for a research consumer:

- determines what is known and not known about a topic, concept or clinical problem
- identifies gaps, consistencies and inconsistencies in the literature about a topic of interest
- examines unanswered questions about a subject, concept or problem
- identifies conceptual traditions and methods used to examine this type of clinical problem
- uncovers a new practice intervention or provides support for a current intervention
- promotes development of new, or revision of existing, practice protocols, policies or projects/activities related to nursing.

Learning activities

1. c	**2.** b	**3.** b	**4.** b
5. d	**6.** d	**7.** b	**8.** d
9. b and c are both correct		**10.** b	

Identifying research ideas, questions and hypotheses

Zevia Schneider and Dean Whitehead

KEY TERMS

hypothesis
null hypothesis
operational definitions
paradigm
population
research idea
research problem
research question
theory
variables

Learning outcomes

After reading this chapter, you should be able to:

- describe the process of identifying and refining a research idea, question, problem, statement or hypothesis
- identify the issues in matching a research question to an appropriate research approach
- identify the criteria for determining the significance of a research problem.

Introduction

The philosophical basis of a researcher derives from a specific paradigm. A paradigm is a position or view of understanding the world that is shared by a community of scholars or scientists. This world-view shapes one's approach to a variety of activities, including research. The formulation of the research problem (research question, problem statement or hypothesis) is a key preliminary step in the research process, regardless of the method used. The first task of research consumers is to examine the consistency between the research problem and the methods used to address that problem.

An early crucial stage of the research process is where the researcher identifies an appropriate research idea, question or statement in their area of investigation. The process involves finding a research idea, formulating the research problem, and reviewing the literature (to see if the idea has already been investigated), followed by a clear and comprehensive statement of the purpose of the research. Additionally, with certain methods of quantitative research, the key variables (research objectives) and a prediction about the relationship between these variables (hypotheses) will apply.

Deciding on the purpose and direction of a research project is important because there are many issues to be considered during this preliminary stage. For example, is the research for a higher degree, part of coursework requirements, part of an application for a research grant, part of a consortium with nurses or other health professionals, patient-focused or professional-focused, clinical or academic/theoretical? If external funding is being sought, an important consideration is knowing what topics the funding agencies are prepared to fund, or, if in the academic setting, what the implications are for higher education resources and supervision. If in the clinical area, is hospital management prepared and able to create the opportunity for clinical research? These kinds of questions should be discussed with colleagues before making any final decisions about a topic or applying a specific research question/hypothesis (see Chapter 2).

Developing and refining a research idea

Many nurses and midwives already have a reasonable idea of the topics they would like to research, usually centred on a specialty issue or a problem to address. With a research problem the general idea is to try and solve the problem, or at least contribute to further understanding and possible solutions. Mitchell (2004) prompts researchers to ask the 'so what' question prior to conducting their studies — So what difference will the study make to our understanding, to improving health of individuals, and to developing new methods, tools or technologies to solve the clinical problem?

When the researcher is prepared to commit to a certain topic, this is the time for them to talk their ideas through with colleagues, faculty and any other interested parties. It is also important to read around the topic to gauge the feasibility and practicability of undertaking research in that particular area. Research program time, facilities and resources will greatly influence the type of research possible. In many nursing and midwifery educational programs this level of choice may not be available, as often the choice of a research topic will be influenced by the existing research strengths of the faculty, school or department.

Another important factor to consider is what is called 'symmetry of potential outcomes' (Phillips & Pugh 1994 p 86). This is to say that whatever the outcome, your findings will make a contribution to the knowledge base of your discipline, and is as true today as it was when coined by Phillips and Pugh some 13 years or more ago. Following on from this, the next stage is to discuss ideas with faculty or clinical managers to ensure that suitable supervision and facilities can be provided. It is possible that at some time during a Bachelor of Nursing/Midwifery program, an undergraduate nurse may be asked to take part in a clinical research study. In this situation, however, one would need to ensure that the student was surrounded by research mentors. Undergraduate students would not normally initiate a research study, nor are they relied on to make a significant contribution overall. The main point to emphasise here though is that, regardless of status, inexperienced nurse and midwifery researchers should avoid venturing into the research area without adequate expert support and resources.

Further clarification of ideas will occur in initial discussions with research supervisors. Creating a concept map for each research idea is a profitable activity in the early stages of idea development. Concept mapping may be used to show understanding of meaningful relationships and associations among concepts. Gul and Boman (2006) consider concept maps to be powerful meta-cognitive tools that facilitate the acquisition of knowledge through meaningful learning strategies, promoting and evaluating critical thinking. The number of concepts used can be great or small and are limited only by one's imagination. The research question for the map could be 'An exploration of factors that influence self-care in a group of young adults with arthritis'. Figure 5.1 shows an example of a concept map for self-care and the kinds of concepts related to self-care. This kind of detail will clarify your thinking and go a long way to assist you in making a reasoned and realistic choice. Table 5.1 identifies some factors that may influence the development of a research idea.

Developing and refining a research idea into a research question

A researcher spends a great deal of time refining a research idea into an examinable research question, statement or hypothesis. Unfortunately, the reviewer of a research study is not privy to this creative process, because it occurs during the study's conceptualisation. As illustrated in Table 5.1, research problems or topics originate from a variety of sources. Research problems should indicate that practical experience and a critical appraisal of the scientific literature or interest in untested theory have provided the basis for the generation of a research idea. The problem statement should reflect a refinement of the researcher's initial thinking. The reader of a research study should be able to discern that the researcher has:

- defined a specific problem area
- reviewed the relevant literature
- highlighted the potential significance of the problem to nursing or midwifery
- examined the feasibility of studying the research problem.

Often, however, this stage is not adequately examined by researchers. Green and Ruff (2005) are critical of the fact that many clinical researchers experience problems in answering their research questions, because they do not formulate them properly in the first place.

FIGURE 5.1 Self-care concept map

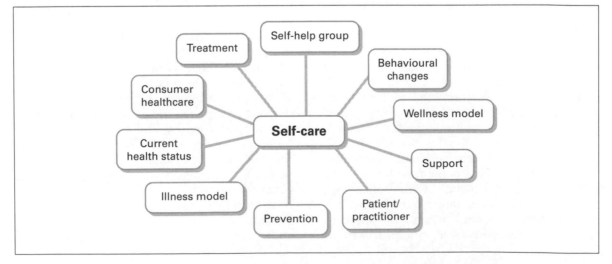

TABLE 5.1 Factors influencing the development of a research idea

Factors	Influence	Example
Practical experience	Clinical practice provides a wealth of experience from which research problems can be derived. The nurse may observe the occurrence of a particular event or pattern and become curious about why it occurs, as well as its relationship to other factors in the patient's environment.	Mothers who received home visits were more likely to be satisfied with postpartum care than women who did not receive this care. Home visits were planned for mothers from two hospitals. Unstructured home visits to women did not provide positive health outcomes (Jirojwong et al. 2005).
Critical appraisal of the scientific literature	A review of studies appearing in journals may indirectly suggest a problem area by stimulating the reader's thinking. A nurse may observe a conflict or inconsistency in the findings of several related research studies and wonder which findings are most valid.	Studies in hospital care of children have identified differing attitudes, perceptions and expectations of nurses and parents regarding their role in the delivery of care (Espezel & Canam 2003; Shields & Nixon 2004; Ygge & Arnetz 2004). Recommendations for further research into staff/parent interactions and education programs for both staff and parents.
Gaps in the literature	A review may identify gaps in the literature and suggest areas for future study. Research ideas can also be generated by research reports that suggest the value of replicating a particular study to extend or refine the existing scientific knowledge base.	Studies published on severe acute respiratory syndrome (SARS) have focused on diagnosis and treatment. This study (Mok et al. 2005) is the first to explore how nurses with SARS perceived and experienced their illness.
Interest in untested theory	Verification of an untested nursing theory provides a relatively uncharted area from which research problems can be derived. Although theories themselves may not be tested, a researcher may investigate a particular concept or concepts related to specific theory. A deductive process would be used to generate the research problem, with questions posed such as, 'If this theory is correct, what kind of behaviour would I expect to observe in particular patients and under which conditions?' or 'If this theory is valid, what kind of supporting evidence would I find?'.	Dalton (2003) extends Kim's theory of collaborative decision-making in nursing practice, in constructing and testing a new theory that moves from Kim's dyadic theory towards a triadic theory — by means of a modified version of Walker and Avant's theory-derivation process.

ττ **Tutorial trigger 1**

A review of the literature has identified limitations of the research studies you have reviewed. The gap you identified relates to pregnant couples' dissatisfaction with antenatal education classes because of limited information about infant care and behaviours. Create a concept map to assist you in formulating a research problem. The map should show your particular interests in antenatal education and may be quite different from the example shown in the answer section at the end of this chapter.

Defining a specific problem area

Researchers generally begin with an interest in some broad topic area, such as pain management, family communication patterns, self-care activities of the aged or management of urinary incontinence. When nurses ask questions such as 'Why are things done this way?', 'I wonder what would happen if ...?' or 'Is this the best way to ...?', they are often well on their way to developing a researchable question. Using qualitative methods, researchers may explore individuals' responses to treatment, or experiences of a clinical condition or health/illness state, and the meanings attached to these experiences (see Chapter 7). With quantitative designs, the research may focus on defined variables of interest and their relationship to each other (see Chapter 10). Regardless of the approach used, the researcher engages in an inquiry process linked to their choice of research approach and experience, as well as the research question under consideration. For example, Annells et al. (2005) aimed to identify district nursing research priorities in Australia using a mixed method approach (see Chapter 15), and Campbell and Torrance (2005) quantitatively explored self-reported changes in coronary risk factors, of Australian patients, three to nine months after coronary artery angioplasty. Figure 5.2 illustrates how the development of a research idea is influenced by practical experience, scientific literature and untested theory.

Research in brief

Following a review of the literature which revealed very few studies relevant to their topic of interest, Rossiter and Yam (2000) aimed to explore, from Vietnamese women's perspectives, factors influencing their choice of infant feeding practices and their views on how health professionals in general could promote and support breastfeeding. A convenience sample of 124 women completed a face-to-face interview in their own homes. Inclusion criteria were that the women, born and reared in Vietnam, had their last infant in Sydney 6 months before data collection. Content analysis was used to analyse the data. Findings showed that factors affecting choice of feeding method were language difficulties in communicating with health professionals about breastfeeding, lack of social support and follow-up care, and attitudes of health professionals.

The research consumer may not see a formal statement of the research question or hypothesis in a research article because of space constraints or stylistic considerations in particular publications. This may also be due to the fact that it is often seen as a 'basic'

step in the research process, although others more appropriately highlight it as one of the most challenging steps (Fineout-Overholt & Johnston 2005). What does appear more often in published articles instead is a statement of the aim, purpose or goal of the research study. Nevertheless, it is equally important for both the consumer and producer of research to understand the importance of the problem statement and hypothesis as foundation elements of the study, as they are components that set the stage for the development of the research study.

Points to ponder

▶ Research ideas, questions or hypotheses should indicate that the researcher has a clear understanding of what they plan to do.

▶ Research ideas, questions or hypotheses determine the design of a study.

▶ Clear research ideas, questions or hypotheses can assist in determining the feasibility, rigour, appropriateness and relevance of research studies.

Reviewing relevant literature

Consistent with the study design, the literature searching and review process is a systematic and rigorous exploration of the extant (existing) literature related to the concept(s) of interest (see Chapters 3 and 4). In the first instance, the review may inform the researcher that their intended course of investigation has occurred previously. This may, early on in the process, steer the researcher away from their intended course of exploration towards a new direction or approach. This may not, however, always be the case as there are valid cases for 'replication' studies — such as different contexts or environments or, simply, to update older studies.

Accomplished reviews provide syntheses of findings from studies and analysis of themes and methods identified from the literature, written in a clear and concise form. There are numerous styles and steps to a literature review, which are discussed more fully in Chapter 4. The literature review should reveal that the literature relevant to the problem area

FIGURE 5.2 Process of formulating a research problem

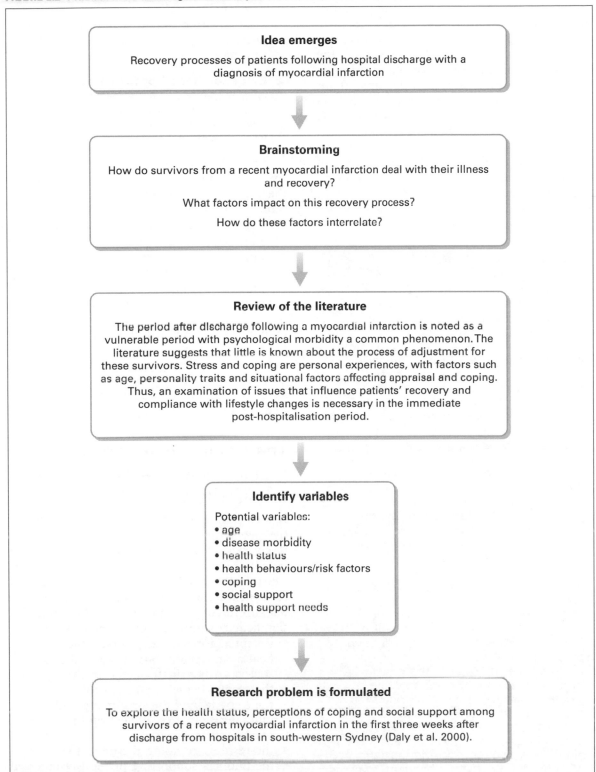

Idea emerges

Recovery processes of patients following hospital discharge with a diagnosis of myocardial infarction

Brainstorming

How do survivors from a recent myocardial infarction deal with their illness and recovery?

What factors impact on this recovery process?

How do these factors interrelate?

Review of the literature

The period after discharge following a myocardial infarction is noted as a vulnerable period with psychological morbidity a common phenomenon. The literature suggests that little is known about the process of adjustment for these survivors. Stress and coping are personal experiences, with factors such as age, personality traits and situational factors affecting appraisal and coping. Thus, an examination of issues that influence patients' recovery and compliance with lifestyle changes is necessary in the immediate post-hospitalisation period.

Identify variables

Potential variables:
• age
• disease morbidity
• health status
• health behaviours/risk factors
• coping
• social support
• health support needs

Research problem is formulated

To explore the health status, perceptions of coping and social support among survivors of a recent myocardial infarction in the first three weeks after discharge from hospitals in south-western Sydney (Daly et al. 2000).

has been critically examined. Often, concluding sections on recommendations and implications for practice in previous articles identify remaining gaps in the literature, the need for replication, or the need for extending the knowledge base about a particular research focus. In the previously cited example about district nursing research priorities in Australia (Annells et al. 2005), the authors report the absence or dearth of publications on the topic. This is good justification for research in the defined area. At this point the researchers in question could have written the following problem statements:

- What is the status of district nursing research in Australia?

Research in brief

Fernandez and Griffiths (2005) reviewed the literature and found that a large number of studies made recommendations for monitoring patients in the recovery room, but little research existed about nursing care of patients following their transfer to the ward. They, therefore, identified a 'research gap'. The authors decided that the most appropriate research design was a randomised controlled trial to compare the incidence of untoward events in the first 24 hours following return to the ward. Patients were randomly assigned to one of two groups: One group was monitored according to standard protocol while the second group was monitored according to experimental protocol. Experimental protocol included monitoring of vital signs on return to the ward, then one hourly for two hours followed by standard protocol. Oxygen saturation and level of arousal were monitored and recorded on return to the ward, then one hourly for two hours followed by standard protocol. The research question asked 'What is the effect of a modified regime compared to existing practices for monitoring vital signs in postoperative patients on their return to the ward from the recovery unit?'. Findings showed no statistically significant difference in the incidence of abnormal vital signs between the groups in the first 24 hours following return to the ward.

- What are the research priorities of district nurses in Australia?
- What research design would provide the most effective way of obtaining this information?

Evidence-based practice tip

When reading a research paper, the research consumer must decide if the stated purpose, aims and objectives are congruent with the research question.

Research readers should be able to identify the interrelatedness of the initial definition of the topic area, the literature review and the refined question or statement. The reader of a research paper examines the end product of this formulation process and might glean an appreciation of how time-consuming it actually is. For example, Arthur et al. (2005) identified the paucity of research on the lived experiences of nurses providing primary healthcare (PHC) in the Philippines. The authors, who examined PHC nursing practised by two rural universities in the Philippines over a five-year period, were moved by the 'impressive work of their colleagues' (p 108) and, subsequently, wanted to publish the findings of the PHC nurses.

The significance of research problem statements to nursing or midwifery

Before proceeding to a final formulation of the problem statement, it is crucial for the researcher to have examined the problem's potential significance to nursing or midwifery. The research problem should have the potential for contributing to and extending the scientific body of nursing or midwifery knowledge. The significance should be in relation to:

- potential for patients, nurses, the healthcare community in general and society to benefit from the study
- the results being applicable for extending the knowledge base of nursing and midwifery practice, education or management
- the results providing theoretical relevance
- the findings supporting previously untested theoretical assumptions, extending or challenging an existing theory or clarifying a conflict in the literature

- the findings informing the formulation or revision of nursing or midwifery practices or policies.

If the research problem has not met any of these criteria, then the significance is questionable. In their exploration of birth expectations of a cohort of Western Australian women, Fenwick et al. (2004) suggested the following recommendations for midwifery practice:
- a need to examine the influence on pregnant women of healthcare providers regarding birth interventions
- further research is needed to develop strategies to assist women to cope with anxiety and fear of the birth experience.

The paucity of published research on preparation for childbirth and parenthood programs in Australia during the past 20 years motivated a qualitative study into first-time pregnant women's experiences and perceptions of pregnancy (Schneider 2002). Findings revealed that while antenatal education classes were a major source of information for pregnant couples they did not provide information on infant care and behaviours and self-care and that conflicting and sometimes unhelpful information was given that resulted in confusion. Recommendations included the establishment of national guidelines for childbirth and parenting programs, the appointment of suitably qualified educators and discussions with pregnant couples regarding need for support, issues of control, and coping mechanisms.

Refining the problem statement

The final problem statement may be written in declarative (a positive, explicit statement) or interrogative (forming or conveying a question) forms as illustrated in Table 5.2. The style chosen is largely a function of the researcher's preference, experience and originating paradigm (see Chapter 2). An effective problem statement exhibits the following three characteristics:
- provides clear identification of the concept of interest (concepts, phenomena or variables under investigation)
- specifies the population being studied

TABLE 5.2 Problem statements in declarative and interrogative forms

Research focus	Problem statement
Declarative	
The childbirth expectations of a self-selected cohort of Western Australian women.	This study reported on tape-recorded telephone interviews with 202 women who were pregnant or had birthed within the past 12 months (Fenwick et al. 2004).
The New Zealand development and trial of mental health nursing clinical indicators — a bicultural study.	Development and validation of bicultural clinical indicators designed to measure achievement of mental health nursing practice standards in New Zealand (O'Brien et al. 2003).
An exploration of how patients and practitioners from linguistically and culturally different backgrounds make decisions in healthcare.	This study reported the experiences of families who have a family member in hospital (Perry et al. 2005).
Interrogative	
Competency Standards for critical care nurses; do they measure up?	How effective and valid is the tool for assessing clinical practice of specialist level critical care nurses? (Fisher et al. 2005).
A comparison of an evidence-based regime with the standard protocol for monitoring postoperative observation: A randomised controlled trial.	How effective is the current standard for monitoring postoperative practice compared with an experimental protocol? (Fernandez & Griffiths 2005).
An investigation of the spiritual care perceptions and practice patterns of Hong Kong nurses.	What are the spiritual care perceptions of Hong Kong nurses and how do these perceptions influence their spiritual care practice? (Chan et al. 2005)

- demonstrates the focus of the study (i.e. examination of experiences, exploration of variables and relationships, or empirical testing).

These components can also be used to develop statements for secondary research approaches such as systematic reviews (see Chapter 4).

> ### Point to ponder
> ▶ When is a researcher likely to use a declarative research question, and when an interrogative research question?

Concept of interest

The concepts of major interest in studies are called phenomena (qualitative) or variables (quantitative). From a quantitative perspective, variables exhibit different values (i.e. the properties of the variable can vary, e.g. pain, anxiety). Properties that differ from each other, such as age, weight, height, religion and ethnicity, are other examples of variables. Quantitative research attempts to understand how and why differences in one variable are related to differences in another variable (i.e. how a change in one variable might affect change in another). A cross-sectional study design by Jirojwong et al. (2005) was used to assess health outcomes of home follow-up visits after postpartum discharge among women who birthed at two Queensland regional hospitals. The concept of interest was to examine the effects of unstructured home visits on the women. Rather than using structured protocol during home visits, nurses and midwives simply responded to the women's circumstances and identified needs. The findings showed that unstructured home visits did not provide positive health outcomes; however, the authors recommend caution in interpreting the result because they were unable to control for some extraneous factors. In addition, sources of information given to the women during pregnancy and health education content by midwives were not explored or assessed.

In qualitative studies, the concept (phenomenon) of interest is explored within a more holistic and humanistic context. Relationships or experiences are explored within the real-world setting. This philosophical-based perspective has an interpretive, emancipatory and transformative intent. Interpretive methodologies include phenomenology, grounded theory, ethnography, historical methods and feminist research (see Chapter 7). A feminist perspective was used by Yarwood et al. (2005) in their New Zealand-based study of the physical activity experiences of women in midlife. Here the concept of interest clearly relates to the participants' ability to maintain physical activities over time at the midlife period. In the study, themes of 'exercise is part of me, part of my life', 'the importance of being fit and healthy', 'exercise interweaves and changes with life situations', and 'constraints and conflicts', emerged. Talking about their experiences, participants unearthed the notion that regular physical exercise was intrinsically connected to family, relationships and work.

It is worth noting that concepts of interest can also be examined through documentary evidence, as in historical research, or sometimes with other approaches which are discussed in Chapter 7.

Population of interest

The terms *population* and *sample* are commonly used in research studies to identify the societal group of interest. The people or elements being studied need to be specified in the problem statement. If the scope of the problem has been narrowed to a specific focus and the variables have been clearly identified, the nature of the population will be evident to the reader of a research report. For example, Jenkins and Elliott (2004) developed a problem statement aimed at investigating levels of stressors and burnout of qualified and unqualified nursing staff in acute mental health settings. The reader can immediately identify that the population of interest is nurses working in acute mental health settings.

With qualitative approaches, participants in the study reflect a particular group or community within societal settings. For example, in the study by Mok et al. (2005), the aim was to explore how ten self-selected nurses, who had contracted Severe Acute Respiratory Syndrome (SARS), experienced their illness. The problem statement was the need to explore how nurses who had contracted SARS

Research in brief

Ygge and Arnetz (2004) aimed to gain a deeper understanding of factors that influence parental involvement with their children in hospital. Semi-structured interviews were conducted with 14 parents of chronically ill children. The research question was 'What is the parental role in the hospital care of their chronically ill children?'. The identified themes relating to support, professionalism, work environment, and responsibility describe the experience and perceptions of parents who regularly spend time with their children in the hospital. The authors concluded that clinical practices which included parental involvement need to be established to optimise hospital care of chronically ill children.

perceived and experienced their illness since previous studies had concentrated on diagnosis, treatment and controlling the infection.

● Evidence-based practice tip

If the concept of interest, the population, and the focus of the study are not clearly defined, the relevance and meaningfulness of the study will be questionable.

Operational definition

An operational definition refers to measurements used to observe or measure a variable and to the delineation of the procedures or operations required to measure, analyse or evaluate a concept. This procedure is necessary to provide clarity.

Hoffman and Elwin (2004 p 9), for instance, state that the definition of critical thinking is diverse so, in their study, critical thinking in nursing is defined as 'the ability to analyse problems through inferential reasoning and reflection on past situations that share similar clinical indicators'.

It is possible that another researcher may provide either a more restricted or broader definition. What is important is that by stating a particular operational definition, the researcher has identified the empirical referents, enabling the research consumer to judge the results of the study accordingly.

● Evidence-based practice tip

An operational definition must clearly delineate the measurements and procedures necessary to measure the concept.

Hypothesis testing

An hypothesis is a quantitative prediction about a relationship between two or more variables or phenomena that suggests an answer to the research question. Hypotheses provide the underpinning source from where quantitative studies originate and great effort is applied to testing them, thus maintaining focus. They are not, however, always stated explicitly in a research article. Hypotheses flow from the problem statement, literature review and theoretical framework. Hypothesis testing is the most commonly used purpose of inferential statistics. Inferential statistics are a set of statistical analytic procedures that permit inferences to be made about a population using results from a representative sample, thus enabling generalisability of findings (see Chapter 11). Hypothesis testing is used to answer such questions as 'Is there a difference between the two groups?' or 'What is the relationship between the two variables?' or 'What are the changes over time?'. Regardless of the specific format used to state the hypothesis, the statement should be worded in clear, simple and concise terms. The three important points to include in the statement are:

1. the variables of the hypothesis
2. the population being studied
3. the predicted outcome of the hypothesis.

Relationship between hypotheses and research design

Regardless of whether the researcher uses a statistical hypothesis (null hypothesis) or a research hypothesis (scientific hypothesis), there is a suggested relationship between the hypothesis and the research design of the study. For example, when an experimental design is utilised, the research consumer would expect to see hypotheses that reflect relationship statements, such as the following:

● X_1 is more effective than X_2 on Y
   (dressing A is more effective than dressing B on decubitis ulcers)

- the effect of X_1 on Y is greater than that of X_2 on Y (the effect of dressing A on decubitis ulcers is greater than the effect of dressing B)
- the incidence of Y will not differ in participants receiving X_1 and X_2 treatments (the incidence/occurrence of decubitis ulcers will be the same for participants receiving dressing A as for those receiving dressing B)
- the incidence of Y will be greater in participants after X_1 than after X_2 (the incidence/occurrence of decubitis ulcers will increase more in participants receiving dressing A than those receiving dressing B).

Such hypotheses indicate that an experimental treatment will be used and that two groups of subjects — experimental and control groups — are being used to test whether the difference predicted by the hypothesis actually exists. In contrast, non-experimental designs reflect associative relationship statements, such as the following:

- X will be negatively related to Y (excessive pain will be negatively related to wound healing)
- X will be positively related to Y (a good nutritional diet will be positively related to wound healing).

Directional versus non-directional hypotheses

Hypotheses can be formulated directionally or non-directionally. A directional hypothesis is one that specifies the expected direction of the relationship between the independent and dependent variables. An independent variable (also termed an explanatory variable) has a presumed effect on the dependent variable (also termed outcome variable). In this case the existence of a relationship is proposed as well as the nature or direction of that relationship. An example of a directional hypothesis is: 'Hospitalised children will feel less anxious if their parent is permitted to remain with them'. A non-directional hypothesis indicates the existence of a relationship between the variables, but does not specify the anticipated direction of the relationship. An example of a non-directional hypothesis is: 'There will be a difference in anxiety levels in children

if their parent is permitted to remain with them'. Other examples of hypotheses can be found in Table 5.3.

In addition to directional and non-directional hypotheses, there is a causal hypothesis. As the name implies, a causal hypothesis postulates a cause for any change and is frequently used in the evaluation of interventions and new drugs. Buist et al. (2004) examined the psychological and social aspects of first-time mothers' transition to motherhood, including care received. Two hundred and thirteen women from two regions in suburban Melbourne participated. It was hypothesised that the two regions' 'differing socioeconomic profiles and support available would impact on the mother's psychological wellbeing' (p 21). Findings showed that being married reduced the risk of distress by half and suggests some support of marital status. Ethnicity appeared to be a strong predictor of postnatal distress; Asian women being less likely to be distressed. Rates of distress decreased over time in the more affluent eastern region but increased in the western developing region. A main limitation of the study was the high attrition rate of participants.

T_T Tutorial trigger 2

You have discovered that you do not concentrate well at lectures the day after night duty and you would like to test your hypothesis. Write (a) a directional hypothesis, and (b) a non-directional hypothesis for the research study.

T_T Tutorial trigger 3

You would like to investigate the reasons why some undergraduate students concentrate less well at lectures the day after night duty.
1. What research question/s might you ask the nurses?
2. What research approaches could you use to answer the research question?

Statistical versus research hypotheses

Readers of research reports may observe that an hypothesis is further categorised as either a research hypothesis or a statistical hypothesis. A research hypothesis, also known as a scientific hypothesis, consists of a statement about the expected relationship between the variables. A research hypothesis indicates what the outcome of the study is expected to

TABLE 5.3 Examples of wording of hypotheses

Hypothesis	Variables*	Type of hypothesis	Type of design suggested
1 There will be a relationship between self-concept and suicidal behaviour.	IV: Self-concept DV: Suicidal behaviour	Non-directional research	Non-experimental
2 Synchrony of maternal and newborn sleep rhythms will be negatively related to postpartum blues.	IV: Synchrony of maternal and newborn sleep rhythms DV: Postpartum blues	Directional research	Non-experimental
3 Structured preoperative education is more effective than structured postoperative education in reducing the patient's perception of pain.	IV: Preoperative education IV: Postoperative education DV: Perception of pain	Directional research	Experimental
4 The incidence and degree of severity of subject discomfort will be less after administration of medications by the Z-track intramuscular injection technique than after administration of medications by the standard intramuscular injection technique.	IV: Z-track intramuscular injection technique IV: Standard intramuscular injection technique DV: Subject discomfort	Directional research	Experimental
5 Progressive relaxation will be more effective in reducing indices of physiological arousal than hypnotic relaxation or self-relaxation in patients undergoing cardiac rehabilitation.	IV: Progressive relaxation IV: Hypnotic relaxation IV: Self-relaxation DV: Physiological arousal indices	Directional research	Experimental
6 There will be a relationship between years of nursing experience and attitude towards patients with human immunodeficiency virus (HIV) disease.	IV: Years of experience DV: Attitude towards HIV patients	Non-directional research	Non-experimental
7 There will be a positive relationship between trust and self-disclosure in marital relationships.	IV: Trust DV: Self-disclosure	Directional research	Non-experimental
8 There will be a greater decrease in post-test state anxiety scores in subjects treated with non-contact therapeutic touch than in subjects treated with contact therapeutic touch.	IV: Non-contact therapeutic touch IV: Contact therapeutic touch DV: State anxiety	Directional research	Experimental

*IV, independent variable; DV, dependent variable.

be. If the researcher obtains statistically significant findings for a research hypothesis, the hypothesis is supported. For example, in a study (Webster et al. in press) designed to assess the safety of changing peripheral venous cannulas when clinically indicated, the research hypotheses were:

- that more unplanned IV cannula re-sites will occur in the 3-day change group (control group) than in the group having their cannula changed only when necessary (intervention group)
- the cost of IV cannulation will be greater in the control group.

Findings showed that the risk of a complication is unaffected when cannulas are re-sited based on clinical parameters and that cost savings may be considerable if cannulas are re-sited only when necessary. The examples in Table 5.4 are examples of statistical hypotheses. When critically analysing research reports, it is important to make sure that the study is adequately powered as the findings may influence clinical practice.

A statistical hypothesis (very commonly known as a null hypothesis) states that there is no relationship between the independent and dependent variables. The examples in Table 5.4 illustrate statistical hypotheses. If, in the data analysis, a statistically significant relationship emerges between the variables, the null hypothesis is rejected. Rejection of the statistical hypothesis is equivalent to acceptance of the research hypothesis. For example, in the quasi-experimental study by Chien et al. (2006), which investigated the effects of a needs-based education program for family carers with a relative in an intensive

Research in brief

An example of a research (statistical) hypothesis is found in the study on the relationship between critical thinking and confidence in decision-making (Hoffman & Elwin 2004). The hypothesis stated that there would be no relationship between critical thinking ability and confidence in decision-making for new graduate nurses. The findings showed that critical thinking ability and confidence in decision-making were negatively related; that is, as scores on critical thinking increased, scores on confidence in decision-making decreased. The findings suggest that nurses who think more critically are more hesitant in clinical decision-making and that those nurses who scored higher on critical-thinking ability would be likely to spend more time looking for answers to clinical problems.

care unit, null or statistical hypotheses were implied. An example of a null hypothesis that could be implied for this study could be that:

> there is no difference in 'reduction of anxiety' or increase in 'needs satisfaction' (the two hypothesised predictors being tested) for family carers receiving a needs-based educational program, when compared to a control (routine care without the needs-based educational program) group.

Chien et al. (2006) reported that there was significant difference in relation to the tested

TABLE 5.4 Examples of statistical hypotheses

Hypothesis	Variables*	Type of hypothesis	Type of design suggested
Oxygen inhalation by nasal cannula of up to 6 L/min does not affect oral temperature measurement taken with an electronic thermometer.	IV: Oxygen inhalation by nasal cannula DV: Oral temperature	Statistical	Experimental
The incidence of pregnancy in adolescent girls attending birth control education classes will not differ from that of girls who do not attend birth control education classes.	IV: Birth control education classes DV: Adolescent pregnancy	Statistical	Experimental
*IV, independent variable; DV, dependent variable.			

variables. The level of statistical significance was less than 5%, meaning that there was little chance of falsely accepting the null hypotheses — thus the null hypotheses were rejected supporting the two stated study hypotheses.

Some researchers refer to the null hypothesis as a statistical contrivance that obscures a straightforward prediction of the outcome. Others state that it is more exact and conservative statistically and that failure to reject the null hypothesis implies that there is insufficient evidence to support the idea of a real difference. Readers of research reports will note that, in general, when hypotheses are stated, research hypotheses are more commonly used than statistical hypotheses. In any study that involves statistical analysis, the underlying null hypothesis is usually assumed without being explicitly stated. Figure 5.3 illustrates the decision path for determining the type of hypothesis presented in a study, as well as the study's readiness for an hypothesis testing design.

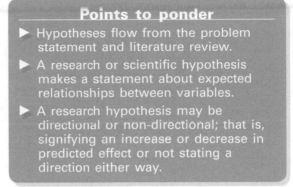

Points to ponder

▶ Hypotheses flow from the problem statement and literature review.

▶ A research or scientific hypothesis makes a statement about expected relationships between variables.

▶ A research hypothesis may be directional or non-directional; that is, signifying an increase or decrease in predicted effect or not stating a direction either way.

Summary

Identifying the most appropriate research idea, problem, question, statement or hypothesis is an integral and key part of successful research. It is fundamental in determining the nature and design of a research project. Researchers undertaking this part of the research process are advised to ask key questions of their research, in order to determine if the right idea,

FIGURE 5.3 Hypothesis testing decision path

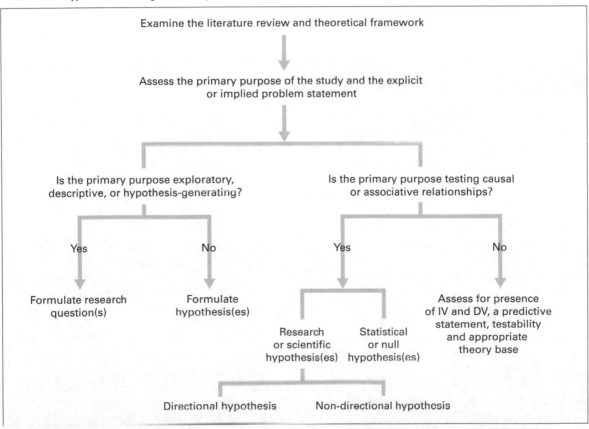

problem, question, statement or hypothesis has been considered. These would include:

- the results being applicable for extending the knowledge base of nursing or mid-wifery practice, education or management
- the results providing theoretical relevance
- the findings supporting previously untested theoretical assumptions

- the findings informing the formulation or revision of nursing or midwifery practices or policies.

If the research idea, problem, question, statement or hypothesis has not met most of the above-stated types of criteria, then the significance of the research is questionable and the rest of the research process will be compromised.

(K)EY POINTS

- Qualitative and quantitative methods have differing philosophical bases, approaches, terminology and evaluation criteria.
- Identification of the research question, statement or problem is an important key preliminary step in the research process. The extent to which this is properly structured often determines the accuracy and appropriateness of the research.

- Refinement of the research problem includes examination of the previous research literature, and discussion of the potential significance of the problem to nursing or midwifery practice, education or theory.
- The research problem should have the potential for contributing to the body of nursing and midwifery knowledge.

Learning activities

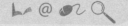

1. The purpose of a literature review is to:
   (a) identify different ways of writing research studies
   (b) identify gaps and limitations in research studies
   (c) identify the best method of reading articles
   (d) identify as many articles as possible.

2. Nursing and midwifery research studies should contribute to:
   (a) a list of the authors' publications
   (b) specific areas of practice they consider important
   (c) the faculty's research profile
   (d) extending the knowledge base of nursing and midwifery practice and education.

3. Why is it that many clinical researchers experience problems in answering their research questions?

   (a) they do not formulate them in the first place
   (b) because the researchers lack experience
   (c) it isn't really necessary to have research questions in the first place
   (d) it is difficult to formulate research questions.

4. An operational definition:
   (a) explains an operation
   (b) specifies the measures, procedures and operations required to measure a concept
   (c) helps clarify the research problem
   (d) answers the research question.

5. Hypothesis testing is used to answer such questions as:
   (a) is there a reason for doing the research study?
   (b) will the findings be valid?

(c) are the predictions reliable?

(d) is there a difference between the two groups?

6. In qualitative studies the phenomena of interest are explored:

(a) within an holistic and humanistic context

(b) only in a community context

(c) only in the clinical area

(d) with a single group of people.

7. A research hypothesis is also known as:

(a) directional hypothesis

(b) a scientific hypothesis

(c) a non-directional hypothesis

(d) null hypothesis.

8. Research questions can be used instead of hypotheses in:

(a) only qualitative studies

(b) qualitative, exploratory and descriptive studies

(c) only quantitative studies

(d) any study where neither research questions nor hypotheses are needed.

9. The wording of the research question should be different from:

(a) the objectives of the study

(b) a description of the design

(c) the purpose or aim of the study

(d) the context of the study.

10. If a study does not show a statistical significance:

(a) it should not be published

(b) it can still contribute to the database of nursing and midwifery knowledge

(c) the study should be replicated immediately

(d) the findings should not be disclosed.

Additional resources

Edwards H, Courtney M, Finlayson K, et al. 2005 Improved healing rates for chronic venous leg ulcers: Pilot study results from a randomized controlled trial of a community nursing intervention. *International Journal of Nursing Practice* 11(4):169–76

Lincoln Y S 1992 Sympathetic connections between qualitative methods and health research. *Qualitative Health Research* 2(4):375–91

Rodger M, Hills J, Kristjanson L 2004 A Delphi Study on Research Priorities for Emergency Nurses in Western Australia. *Journal of Emergency Nursing* 30:117–25

References

Annells M, DeRoche M, Lewin G 2005 A Delphi study of district nursing research priorities in Australia. *Applied Nursing Research* 18:36–43

Arthur D, Drury J, Sy-Sinda M T, et al. 2005 A primary health care curriculum in action: the lived experience of primary health care nurses in a school of nursing in the Philippines: A phenomenological study. *International Journal of Nursing Studies* 43:107–12

Buist A, Milgrom J, Morse C, et al. 2004 Metropolitan Regional Differences in Primary Health Care of Postnatal Depression. *Australian Journal of Advanced Nursing* 21(3):20–7

Campbell M, Torrance C 2005 Coronary Angioplasty: impact on risk factors and patients' understanding of the severity of their condition. *Australian Journal of Advanced Nursing* 22(4):26–31

Chan M F, Chung L Y F, Lee A S C, et al. 2005 Investigating spiritual care perceptions and practice patterns in Hong Kong nurses: results of a cluster analysis. *Nurse Education Today* 26(2):139–50

Chien W-T, Chiu Y L, Lam L-W, et al. 2006 Effects of a needs-based education programme for family carers with a relative in an intensive care unit: a quasi-experimental study. *International Journal of Nursing Studies* 43:39–50

Dalton J M 2003 Development and testing of the theory of collaborative decision-making in nursing practice for triads. *Journal of Advanced Nursing* 41:22–33

Daly J, Elliott D, Cameron-Traub E, et al. 2000 Health status, perceptions of coping and social support immediately after discharge of survivors of acute myocardial infarction. *American Journal of Critical Care* 9(1):62–9

Espezel H J E, Canam C J 2003 Parent–nurse interactions: care of hospitalised children. *Journal of Advanced Nursing* 44(1):34–41

Fenwick J, Hauck Y, Downie J, et al. 2004 The childbirth expectations of a self-selected cohort of Western Australian women. *Midwifery* 21:23–35

Fernandez R, Griffiths R 2005 A comparison of an evidence based regime with the standard protocol for monitoring postoperative observation: a randomised controlled trial. *Australian Journal of Advanced Nursing* 23(1):15–21

Fineout-Overholt E, Johnston L 2005 Teaching EBP: asking searchable, answerable clinical questions. *Worldviews on Evidence-Based Nursing*, third quarter 157–60

Fisher M J, Marshall A P, Kendrick T S 2005 Competency standards for critical care nurses: do they measure up? *Australian Journal of Advanced Nursing* 22(4):32–40

Green M, Ruff T 2005 Why do residents fail to answer their clinical questions? A qualitative study of barriers to practicing evidence-based medicine. *Academic Medicine* 80(2):176–82

Gul R B, Boman J A 2006 Concept mapping: a strategy for teaching and evaluation in nursing education. *Nurse Education in Practice* 6:199–206

Hoffman K, Elwin C 2004 The relationship between critical thinking and confidence in decision-making. *Australian Journal of Advanced Nursing* 22(1):8–12

Jenkins R, Elliott P 2004 Stressors, burnout and social support: nurses in acute mental health settings. *Journal of Advanced Nursing* 48(6):622–31

Jirojwong S, Rossi D, Walker S, et al. 2005 What were the outcomes of home follow-up visits after postpartum hospital discharge? *Australian Journal of Advanced Nursing* 23(1):22–9

Mitchell P H 2004 The 'so what' question: the impact of nursing research. *Journal of Professional Nursing* 20(6):347–8

Mok E, Chung B P M, Chung J W Y, et al. 2005 An exploratory study of nurses suffering from severe acute respiratory syndrome (SARS). *International Journal of Nursing Practice* 11(4):150–60

O'Brien A P, O'Brien A J, Hardy D J, et al. Gaskin C J, Boddy J M, McNulty N, Ryan R, Skews G 2003 The New Zealand development and trial of mental health nursing clinical indicators — a bicultural study. *International Journal of Nursing Studies* 40:853–61

Perry J, Lynam M J, Anderson J M 2005 Resisting vulnerability: the experiences of families who have kin in hospital — a feminist ethnography. *International Journal of Nursing Studies* 43(2):173–84

Phillips E M, Pugh D S 1994 *How to get a PhD: a handbook for students and their supervisors*, 2nd edn. Open University Press, London

Rossiter J C, Yam B M C 2000 Breastfeeding: How could it be enhanced? The perceptions of Vietnamese women in Sydney, Australia. *Journal of Midwifery & Women's Health* 45(3):271–6

Schneider Z 2002 An Australian study of women's experiences of their first pregnancy. *Midwifery* 18:238–49

Shields I, Nixon J 2004 Hospital care of children in four countries. *Journal of Advanced Nursing* 45(5):475–86

Webster J, Lloyd S, Hopkins T, et al. (in press) Developing a Research base for Intravenous Peripheral cannula re-sites (DRIP trial). A randomized controlled trial of hospital in-patients. *International Journal of Nursing Studies*

Yarwood J, Carryer J, Gagan M J 2005 Women maintaining physical activity at midlife: contextual complexities. *Nursing Praxis in New Zealand* 21:24–37

Ygge B M, Arnetz J E 2004 A Study of Parental Involvement in Pediatric Hospital Care: Implications for Clinical Practice. *Journal of Pediatric Nursing* 19(3):217–23

Answers

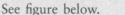 **Tutorial trigger 1**

See figure below.

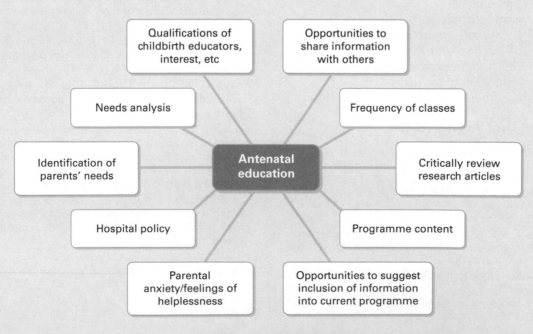

Antenatal education concept map

TT Tutorial trigger 2

(A) Nurses/midwives concentrate less well in lectures on the day following night duty. (directional or causal hypothesis)

(B) Do nurses/midwives concentrate as well at lectures on the day after night duty as they do on day duty? (non-directional hypothesis).

TT Tutorial trigger 3

1. Possible research questions could be:
   (a) Why do you think you concentrate less well at lectures the day after night duty?
   (b) Do you enjoy the lecture material? (use a Likert scale 1 = not at all to 5 = very interesting)
   (c) Do you find yourself nodding off during the lectures?
   (d) Do you have breakfast before attending the lectures?
   (e) Are you distracted during lectures by events that occurred on night duty? (explain)
   (f) Do you sleep well during the day? The usual number of hours or more/less?
   (g) What are your eating patterns on night duty?
   (h) Do noises disturb your sleep during the day?
   (i) Do you manage to get some sleep during your supper break on night duty?
   (j) How would you rate your level of concentration when you go on night duty? (using a Likert scale of 1 = poor to 7 = very good)
   (k) How would you rate your level of concentration when you come off night duty? (using a Likert scale as above)
2. Possible research approaches to answer the research question:
   (a) A 'lived experience' qualitative approach would answer questions requiring reflection and exploration on the part of the nurses. This approach would provide the opportunity to ask in-depth questions and obtain rich personal data.
   (b) A qualitative approach enables exploration of the nurses' responses and the meanings they attach to those feelings and so forth, and provides an opportunity to ask for elaboration. The concepts of interest could be holistically and humanistically explored through the nurses' narratives.
   (c) A quantitative approach would help focus on defined variables of interest and their relationship to each other. Some basic statistical information could be obtained from the Likert scales as well as some important personal information relating to the nurses' self-perceptions. A questionnaire could also be included if participant availability was a concern.
   (d) A mixed-method approach could incorporate both qualitative and quantitative methods.

Learning activities

1. b	**2.** d	**3.** a	**4.** b
5. d	**6.** a	**7.** b	**8.** b
9. c	**10.** b		

Chapter

6

Ethical and legal issues in research

ANNE COUP AND ZEVIA SCHNEIDER

KEY TERMS

animal rights
anonymity
benefits
confidentiality
human research ethics
   committee (HREC)
human rights
informed consent
respect for persons
risk–benefit ratio
vulnerable participants

Learning outcomes

After reading this chapter, you should be able to:

- outline the key historical events that led to the development of ethical codes and regulations for the conduct of research involving human participants
- describe the principles of ethical research involving human participants
- identify the laws, regulations and codes that apply to the conduct of research in Australia and New Zealand
- explain the key elements of an information sheet for prospective research participants
- explain the key elements of a written consent form
- critically comment on the ethical and legal aspects of a published study.

Introduction

Ethical and legal issues in research are concerned with the protection of human participants for whom there are ethical codes and legal regulations to ensure the absence or minimisation of harm, trauma, anxiety or discomfort. Nurses and midwives should be aware of their role in the research process, whether functioning as researcher, research assistant, or health service provider with an advocacy role. This chapter provides an historical background of the development of ethical guidelines and discusses the nature of ethical and legal issues relating to research. The principles that guide ethical decision-making are illustrated with examples, and then follows the role of ethics committees in Australia and New Zealand.

Ethical and legal considerations in research: an historical perspective

Ethical and legal considerations related to research first received worldwide attention after World War II, during the War Crimes Trial in Nuremberg, Germany, conducted by an International Military Tribunal. Among those charged with war crimes were a group of German doctors charged with crimes against humanity that included performing medical experiments upon concentration camp inmates and others without their consent, and with carrying out the so-called 'euthanasia' program that involved murdering hundreds of thousands of humans deemed 'unworthy of life'. The experiments were criminal, a scientific failure (Taylor 1946), and violated international conventions including Article 46 of the Hague Regulations 1907 and criminal law. The doctors also violated the ethical principle in the medical Hippocratic Oath 'to do no harm'. The defendants claimed their medical experiments were lawful; that there was no international law or informal statement that differentiated between legal and illegal human experimentation. In response, an American doctor submitted a memorandum to the United States Counsel for War Crimes which outlined six points defining legitimate research. These six points were expanded and subsequently became known as the 'Nuremberg Code' (see Box 6.1). Unfortunately the legal force of the code was never established during the trial but it did inform numerous international ethics statements developed after the Nuremberg Trials. Links to archives from these trials are available at:

- United States Holocaust Memorial Museum — www.ushmm.org/research/doctors/index.html
- Brig Gen. Telford Taylor — www.law.umkc.edu/faculty/projects/ftrials/nuremberg/NurembergDoctorTrial.html

The first principle in the Nuremberg Code states that 'the voluntary consent of the human subject is absolutely essential'. This requires the person to have the legal capacity to voluntarily give consent, be capable of understanding the information provided, and of making an informed (enlightened) decision about participation. The code's definitions of the terms 'voluntary', 'legal capacity', 'sufficient understanding' and 'enlightened decision' have since been the subject of numerous court cases and commissions involved in setting ethical standards in research (Creighton 1977). In addition, the Nuremberg Code directs that participants must be protected from all unnecessary physical and mental suffering and injury, and have the right to withdraw from the research study at any time. The anticipated benefits of the research should also outweigh the risks. Finally, the code directs that research be conducted by a scientifically qualified person who has a duty to terminate the research if continuation is likely to lead to any form of injury, disability or death of the participant.

After World War II, the World Medical Association (WMA) was established (World Medical Association 1945). The WMA received a report on 'War Crimes and Medicine' and a special committee was set up to prepare an International Code of Medical Ethics which included the Declaration of Geneva (a modernised medical pledge). The code was adopted in 1949 and in 1953 the member

BOX 6.1 Articles of the Nuremberg Code

1. The experimental subject should be of legal age to voluntarily consent to participate in the experiment. The subject must be given all the details of the experiment (nature, purpose, consequences on health) in order that an informed decision to participate can be made in an environment in which there is freedom of choice.
2. The results of the experiment should be of benefit to society and not be achievable by means other than human experimentation.
3. The experiment should be based on the scientific results of animal experimentation and an understanding of the disease process such that the results justify the conduct of the experiment.
4. Every endeavour should be made to avoid undue mental and physical suffering and injury.
5. Experiments that have a known injury to, or result in the death of a subject, should not be conducted. The exception is when investigating physicians are also participating as subjects in the experiment.

6. The importance of the experiment to humanity should be greater than the risk involved.
7. Every precaution should be taken in the experiment to prevent injury, disability or the death of a subject.
8. Only appropriately qualified investigators should conduct experiments.
9. The human subject must be free to withdraw from or discontinue the experiment.
10. The investigators conducting the experiment must be prepared to terminate the experiment at any stage, if there is reason to believe that continuation of the experiment will result in danger, disability or injury to, or the death of, the subject.

Adapted from http://www.raven1.net/nurm Permissible medical experiments. *Trials of war criminals before the Nuremberg Military Tribunals under Control Council Law* No. 10. Nuremberg October 1946–April 1949. (vol. 2, pp 181–82). Washington, US Government Printing Office, (n.d.) Accessed online 30 June 2002.

associations requested a position paper from the WMA Medical Ethics Committee on the ethical and legal requirements regarding human subjects in biomedical research. This declaration was adopted at the 18th General Assembly of the WMA in Helsinki, Finland, in 1964.

The most recent version of the Declaration of Helsinki (2004) (see http://www.wma.net/e/policy/b3.htm) contains principles that add to those in the Nuremberg Code, including:
- the medical researcher has a duty to protect the life, health, privacy and dignity of the human participants
- the research should conform to generally accepted scientific principles, be based on a thorough knowledge of the scientific and other relevant literature and, if appropriate, the results of animal experiments
- the design and performance of any experimental procedure involving human participants should be clearly formulated in a protocol and submitted to an independent ethics committee for review, comment, guidance and approval
- ethics committees exist to ensure that the research conforms to the laws and

regulations of the country in which the research is conducted
- principles for special provisions to protect children or others unable to give consent and state that these groups should only be included if the research is necessary to promote the health of that group
- authors and publishers are reminded of their ethical obligations to report results accurately and to report negative as well as positive results
- publishers are urged not to publish any research reports that do not comply with the declaration principles.

Despite the abovementioned international codes and declarations, post–World War II examples of unethical research continued. One example of unethical research was revealed in New Zealand in the 1980s at the National Women's Hospital in Auckland. The researcher, a gynaecologist, aimed to prove that untreated carcinoma in situ (CIS) would not progress to invasive carcinoma. The prospective trial of conservative treatment (mainly cone biopsy) commenced in 1966. An independent review

Points to ponder

▶ Should we be concerned that some published research articles in international nursing journals make no reference to obtaining ethical approval for their studies?

▶ If prospective participants feel unprotected could this influence their willingness to take part in a study?

Research in brief

The Tuskegee study in Alabama used two groups of poor black males who had been diagnosed with syphilis. The study involved regular medical examinations and blood tests when the men were alive and autopsies when they died. Nurse Rivers played a key role in the continuation of the experiment ensuring that the men in the experimental group were never treated with penicillin (Jones 1981).

of the data for 948 women found that the women who continued to produce abnormal cytology after two years of follow-up had four times the risk of developing invasive cancer; 29 women developed invasive cancer. The authors concluded that the 'study clearly demonstrates that CIS of the cervix had a significant invasive potential' (Cartwright 1988 p 257). In the report of the investigation it was recommended that:

• scientific and ethical assessment for all research meet modern standards
• prospective participants be informed whether the research is therapeutic or non-therapeutic
• written consent be sought when interventionist clinical or non-therapeutic research is planned
• the consent be obtained of the guardian(s) of any child to be included in research (*Report of the Cervical Cancer Inquiry* 1988).

Of concern was that the specialist and the university medical committee that approved the study ignored human participants' rights and the international codes for the ethical conduct of research. The research was allowed to continue despite repeated concerns from other medical researchers at the National Women's Hospital. There have been other examples of unethical medical research (e.g. Tuskegee study) some of which implicate nurses (see 'Research in brief').

In an effort to prevent further unethical biomedical research the United Nations Educational, Scientific and Cultural Organisation (UNESCO) continues to define high standards of integrity, responsibility and accountability in research. The most recent international declaration adopted by UNESCO is the Universal Declaration on Bioethics and Human Rights, 19 October 2005 (available

at http://www.unesco.org/ethics). The aims of this declaration include providing a universal framework of principles and procedures to guide Nation States as they develop legislation, policies and ethics committees. It also guides the actions of individuals, groups, communities, institutions, and public and private corporations, involved in bioethics. The declaration promotes respect for human dignity and protection of human rights and fundamental freedoms. Core principles are:

• respect for autonomy and individual responsibility (informed consent)
• respect for privacy, anonymity and confidentiality
• respect for justice, beneficence
• respect for human vulnerability and personal integrity
• respect for cultural diversity.

Elaboration of these principles follows.

Respect for autonomy and individual responsibility (informed consent)

Respecting a person's autonomy acknowledges their right to hold views and make choices based on personal values and beliefs and acknowledges that they are capable of deciding what happens to them. A person can only exercise their autonomy if they are free from coercion, undue influence and external restraint when making decisions. This means that researchers need to show respectful attitudes and actions to protect the person's autonomy (Beauchamp & Childress 1994). This entails ensuring that research participants have sufficient information about a study, answering their questions until they are satisfied, not influencing their decision, and allowing sufficient time for discussion with their family or significant others. The following elements of informed consent (Box 6.2) ensure respect for autonomy and individual responsibility and are presented to participants in the form of an information sheet (see Appendix 1).

A researcher must determine whether a person is competent to consent before seeking their permission to participate. Competence to consent is determined by the extent to which an individual has the ability to understand sufficiently what the proposed activity involves, their ability to come to a decision about it, and their ability to clearly communicate that decision (Skegg 2003). Learning disabilities or other conditions that affect a person's decision-making ability, such as stroke, dementia or mental illness, do not necessarily mean that the person is not competent to consent; such people should be presumed to have the capacity to consent until professionally assessed and found incompetent (Dye et al. 2004; Griffith 2006). A useful test for assessing capacity to make choices and give consent was developed in England. An individual is not considered competent if they:

- 'are unable to comprehend and retain the necessary information about the procedure or treatment (or in this case the study); and
- unable to weigh the information, balancing risks and needs, and so arrive at a choice' (Johnson 2004 p 93).

If the person is then found incompetent, then either consent must be sought from someone with lawful authority to consent on their behalf or they are excluded from participating. However, Dye et al. (2004) have challenged this 'protection model' of consent that excludes people who lack capacity from participating in research that may provide potential benefits. Instead, they propose a model of supported decision-making that would enable people with learning disabilities to be active partners in participatory research.

An example of an information sheet and a consent form appears in Appendices 1 and 2, respectively.

As noted earlier, special considerations apply when research involves children. In Australia there are no specific legal requirements related

BOX 6.2 Elements of informed consent

- Title of agency (e.g. hospital, university, funding agency)
- Invitation to participate
- Basis for participant selection
- Study purpose or aim
- Explanation of procedures
- Description of potential risks and discomforts
- Access to treatment and compensation if injury occurs
- Potential benefits explained
- Voluntary participation
- Right to withdraw from the study
- Assurance of confidentiality and anonymity
- Conflicts of interest declared
- Offer to answer questions to the satisfaction of the participant
- Names and contact details for researchers, hospital or university involved, and ethics liaison officer/ethics committee administrator
- Concluding consent statement or separate consent form (see Appendix 2)

to a child's participation in research, only for consent to medical procedures. The legal age of minors in most Australian jurisdictions is less than 18 years; for children under this age consent from a parent or guardian is also required (NHMRC 2002). The *Human research ethics handbook* (NHMRC 2002) discusses the ethical importance of consent in relation to a project conducted within a psychology department of an Australian university, where a survey of the experiences of 12-year-old children in relation to puberty was carried out without obtaining parental consent. The outcome was distressed children and angry parents. In New Zealand there are guidelines for health research with children (Ministry of Health 2002), as well as requirements imposed by the New Zealand *Code of health and disability services consumers' rights* (1996).

All research proposals, regardless of approach, should state how consent will be obtained from potential participants. In some cases it may not be appropriate to gain consent in writing, such as when the research involves a sensitive issue (e.g. illegal or stigmatised activities), or if the participant's vulnerability to exposure of significant harm is increased if their identity is inadvertently revealed. In

Research in brief

Powell and Smith (2006) reviewed the current ethics documentation of eight tertiary educational institutions in New Zealand regarding research with children as participants. The focus of the study related to the content of the codes and guidelines. Ethical issues reviewed in the documentation included *consent, protection of child participants, information, confidentiality, anonymity* and *financial inducements*. Findings showed, among other things, that while there was increased consideration of ethical issues, there was variation among the institutions regarding ethics documentation about the child's consent, age or understanding of the child, and parent/guardian's consent. It was noted that little mention was made of confidentiality or anonymity in research involving children.

these cases it may be more appropriate to gain verbal consent only (NHMRC 2002). On the other hand, obtaining consent in 'naturalistic inquiry' methods, such as ethnography, can potentially lead to behavioural changes that might invalidate the study. For example, Taxis and Barber (2003) in their ethnographic study of nurses' drug errors disguised what they were observing. If the nurses had been told what was really being observed this information may have influenced their behaviour and altered the research outcomes. This kind of threat to the validity or accuracy of a study is termed the 'Hawthorne effect' (discussed further in Chapter 12).

An individual's right to autonomy may be violated through coercion, covert data collection and deception. Coercion involves offering a significant reward or threatening some harm if the person does not participate. For example, students may feel pressure to participate in research conducted by academics to ensure good grades. Covert data collection occurs when participants are unaware that research data are being collected. Although covert observation and data collection are usually considered acceptable if undertaken in a public place, the recording of some types of activity could have harmful consequences for the individuals being observed — especially if the activity is illegal (NHMRC 2002).

Humphrey's (1970) controversial observational study of homosexual behaviour that took place in men's public toilets (known as 'tea rooms') is an example of covert data collection. Humphrey, a sociologist, posed as a lookout for the men to warn them if police approached. He noted the men's vehicle registration, traced their address and stored these data in a bank deposit box. A year later he visited them in their homes posing as a researcher for a false survey to gain further information about the men. This systematic deception endangered Humphrey's participants, because if the researcher's data revealing their identities and homosexual practices had been discovered by an unscrupulous person, then blackmail or arrest could have resulted.

TT Tutorial trigger 1

Reports in professional journals often do not provide the reader with detailed information about the ethical procedures used in a study because of word length limitations. However, this does not necessarily mean that the research was in any way unethical. The study reported by Middleton et al. (2005) discusses obtaining informed and written consent from patients. On the basis of information provided in the report about the aims, design and procedures write an information sheet for this study as if you were one of the researchers.

Research in brief

The 'Hawthorne effect' was the term used to explain the unexpected results of a series of industrial psychology experiments at the Hawthorne plant of the US Western Electric Company from 1924 to 1932. Researchers investigated the effects of various physical variables — level of illumination, rest pauses, shorter working hours — on productivity. The workers in both the experimental group (whose work conditions changed) and the control group (whose work conditions did not change) increased their productivity. Productivity levels in the experimental group continued to rise even when lighting was decreased. The workers knew they were being observed. The researchers could not explain these contradictory results. Today this phenomenon would be accounted for as demonstrating social facilitation (Parsons 1974).

Deception involves misinforming participants about the nature and purpose of any intended or actual research. When Taxis and Barber (2003) investigated the incidence and severity of intravenous drug errors in a large hospital, the nurses in the study were told that they were investigating common problems of preparing and administering intravenous drugs. The researchers claimed this deception was valid because it made the study appear less threatening to staff. On the other hand, some research designs necessarily involve some deception, as in randomised control trials where some participants receive a placebo or standard treatment. An important feature of this design is that participants do not know whether they are receiving the experimental treatment or the placebo as this may influence their response and ultimately the results of the experiment. Ethically, what is required is that participants are informed that they may receive a placebo.

Finally, there are some situations where it is ethically acceptable to proceed without obtaining consent from participants. For example, when the research design involves minimal risk and it is not practicable to obtain consent from each participant, such as an observational survey of cycle helmet use. Similarly, consent is not required in the case of de-identified data in epidemiological research, or anonymous surveys (NHMRC 2002).

The NHMRC is responsible for monitoring and providing guidelines for ethical research throughout Australia. Their website (http://www.nhmrc.gov.au) provides a rich source of information on research ethics, whilst in New Zealand, the Health Research Council (HRC; website: http://www.hrc.govt.nz) monitors public research and provides ethical guidelines.

Thus, respect for the autonomy of research participants is a complex issue. The second principle from the UN Declaration on Bioethics and Human Rights concerns the privacy of research participants. A discussion of issues relating to privacy, anonymity and confidentiality follows.

Respect for privacy, anonymity and confidentiality

Respect for privacy

Privacy refers to keeping matters concealed; ensuring they are not widely known or made public. Respect for privacy is both a legal and an ethical requirement in Australia and New Zealand. In Australia, the *Privacy Amendment (Private Sector) Act 2001* (NHMRC 2006) protects personal information held by private sector organisations. In addition, there are two sets of privacy principles to regulate and guide the handling of personal information in Australia. These are the Information Privacy Principles (IPPs), which apply to the Commonwealth public sector, and the National Privacy Principles (NPPs), which apply to the private sector (NHMRC 2006). Most Australian states and territories have also enacted privacy legislation that applies to state public sectors and in some cases the private sector as well (NHMRC 2006). Thus, Australian researchers must access the law relevant to their state or territory as well as the federal guidelines. In New Zealand the *Privacy Act 1993* and its related Health Information Privacy Code 1994 apply to health and disability agencies and organisations in both the public and private sectors (Dawson & Peart 2003).

Ethically, respecting a person's privacy in research involves protecting their *anonymity* and keeping their information *confidential*. For example, the nurses who contracted severe acute respiratory syndrome (SARS) in Hong Kong were assured that their data would remain confidential and anonymous and that no references would be made to them that could result in their identification (Mok et al. 2005).

Anonymity

Complete *anonymity* means that no person, not even the researcher, will be able to identify individuals participating in a study. For example, McLeod et al. (2001) conducted a prospective study of immunisation for a cohort of children registered with a group of medical practices. The children's age, gender and immunisation status were accessed but not their names. The anonymity of the children was therefore protected. In qualitative research, protecting anonymity can be more challenging because the researcher meets the participant face-to-face and needs to develop rapport with the participant in order to elicit information. This is also the case in quantitative research. However, the participant's anonymity can be protected by using invented names (pseudonyms) For example, Fenwick et al. (2005) used a qualitative approach to explore childbirth expectations of a group of women and assured the participants that no identifying features would be present in the interview transcripts or reports of the study.

Tolich (2001) identified another issue relating to privacy in a country like New Zealand, where the small population may have consequences for a research participant. People who live in close proximity share so many stories that the stories themselves may give clues to an individual's identity; even identifying a participant's gender could compromise their privacy. Where maintaining the privacy of organisations and participants becomes particularly challenging, use of pseudonyms will not usually be sufficient. Although Australia's population is much larger, there are also small towns, localised 'neighbourhoods' or communities that may pose similar privacy challenges for a researcher.

Confidentiality

Maintaining *confidentiality* means that the identities of research participants will not be linked to the information they provide. Furthermore, the researcher must ensure secure storage of the data. In qualitative research, maintaining confidentiality can be challenging. For example, a participant's name should not be recorded on an audiotaped interview, and if someone other than the researcher will be transcribing the interview, the participant has

Research in brief

In their study exploring medication knowledge and self-management practices of people with type 2 diabetes, Dunning and Manias (2005) addressed ethical issues in the following way:
- patients were invited to participate when they met the diabetes educator and were given written information about the study
- informed written consent was obtained when they agreed to participate
- an appointment was made to return to the diabetes education centre where the data were collected.

a right to know this and to be assured that the person transcribing will sign a confidentiality declaration. Similarly, if another researcher will be examining the data to confirm the credibility of the study findings, participants should be told this when their consent is being sought. On the other hand, in double blind quantitative studies the researcher would not have access to participants' names.

The basic tenet of respecting participants' identities by keeping the information they provide confidential, applies equally to quantitative research.

Points to ponder
▶ Anonymity is ensured when no one, not even the researcher, can link the participant to the information provided.
▶ Confidentiality is the assurance that a participant's identity will not be linked to the information provided.
▶ Are ethnographic researchers exempt from the usual consent procedures?

Maintaining privacy is an important legal and ethical requirement for researchers who need to familiarise themselves with the specific requirements for their country. Researchers then need to consider the ways that some participants are vulnerable to exploitation and the application of protective ethical principles. The tenet of respect for justice, beneficence, human vulnerability and personal integrity is elaborated below.

Respect for justice, beneficence, human vulnerability and personal integrity

Respect for justice

The ethical principle of justice requires fairness in dealing with others. In research, this means the risks and benefits of the study should be distributed fairly among participants. For example, in a study investigating a nursing intervention after carotid endarterectomy, Middleton et al. (2005) used randomisation to allocate patients to the treatment or control group. The potential positive effects of the intervention were therefore fairly distributed. In the wider sense, the benefits resulting from research and its applications should be shared with society as a whole and within the international community, particularly in developing countries (UNESCO 2005 Article 14).

Participants should be selected for a study because they match specific and clearly stipulated inclusion criteria, not because they are conveniently available or easily exploited. The women in the previously mentioned New Zealand National Women's Hospital study were not treated fairly as they had no choice in their selection.

Research proposals, information sheets and consent forms should clearly explain the participants' involvement, research procedures and the researcher's role and responsibilities. Research procedures should not change without further consent from the participants or participant. If the researcher promises certain benefits for participating in the study, these should be detailed and provided. Such benefits could include being sent a summary of the results or reimbursement of travel costs, but care is needed in this situation because payment of larger amounts could unduly influence the person's decision and potentially be viewed as a possible bribe or inducement to participate.

Beneficence

The ethical principle of beneficence involves doing good, as well as preventing and removing potential harms (Beauchamp & Childress 1994). Harms include any out of the ordinary exposure to the possibility of physical injury or discomfort, psychological injury or distress, social disadvantage, invasion of privacy or infringement of rights (NHMRC 2006). Similarly, the research topic or line of questioning may be psychologically disturbing because it induces fear, anxiety, sadness, or some other distressing emotion in participants. For example, interviewing grandparents about their experience of losing a grandchild is likely to induce painful emotions in the participants. Researchers should identify potential harms or risks in the study proposal and explain what access to debriefing or professional counselling will be provided for participants both during and after the study.

However, given that it is not possible to remove all risks from the research process,

strategies to minimise risks should be used and stated in the research protocol.

> Such strategies may include frequent monitoring of participants; presence of trained personnel who can respond to emergencies; coding of data to protect confidentiality; and 'debriefing' for participants; continuing review and monitoring of data to ensure the study does not continue after the emergence of reliable evidence of reduced efficacy and/ or safety, or actual harm to participants; exclusion of vulnerable individuals or groups from participating in research where necessary and justified; and consideration of whether alternative means for answering the research question are available, and whether participation by humans is really necessary.

(NHMRC 2002 p E4)

Risk–benefit ratio

Some forms of research have the potential to produce a benefit to a patient against the context of risk. For example, a patient with cancer might choose to be part of an experimental treatment that offers some hope of remission. However, a researcher must not understate the potential risks of the experimental treatment nor overstate any potential positive outcomes. Prospective participants should be fully informed about the study, know that it is experimental, and the probability of risks involved. This information should be clear to the participant before their consent is sought. If, on the other hand, the risk–benefit ratio shows that the risks outweigh the benefits, then it will be difficult to justify exposing participants to those risks. However, if the expected harms are minor then the study may still be ethically and legally acceptable because the expected benefits outweigh these lesser harms.

The critical thinking decision path diagram provides an example of the kind of ethical decision-making process that may be used by an ethics committee in evaluating the risk/ benefit of a research study (see Figure 6.1).

Respect for human vulnerability and personal integrity

Some groups of people are more susceptible to physical or psychological hurt or injury and are said to be vulnerable. These are people who have diminished or no capacity to protect

FIGURE 6.1 Critical thinking decision path. Evaluating the risk–benefit ratio of a research study

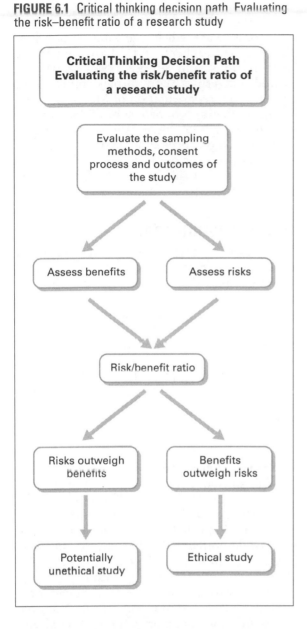

other organisations where strict hierarchy and regulatory procedures exist for 'following orders'). Beecher (1966) published an article describing many examples of unethical or questionably ethical studies that he had identified in the published literature. However, he believed that many of the abuses in the research were due to 'thoughtlessness and carelessness, not a wilful disregard of patients' rights' (Beecher 1966 p 1356). On the other hand, Jessica Mitford's (1973) revelations about experiments behind bars involving drug companies and doctors in the United States showed there was 'wilful disregard' for human rights. The World Medical Association had recommended that prisoners, being captive groups, should not be used as the participants of experiments; the American medical researchers disregarded this. These vulnerable groups have at times been treated badly by researchers; their vulnerability and personal integrity have not always been respected.

Research in brief

Parents who applied to admit their child with severe intellectual disability to Willowbrook State School in the USA in 1964 were sent a letter saying there was no space for new admissions. Soon after they were sent another letter saying there were a few vacancies in the hepatitis research unit if they volunteered their child for that. Children participating in the study were placed in a special isolation unit and were deliberately exposed to hepatitis (Ramsey 1970).

Points to ponder

▶ Research should only be done with children if comparable research with adults could not answer the same question and the purpose of the research is to obtain knowledge relevant to the health needs of children.

▶ Permission from the parent or guardian must be obtained in the case of a child. However, when the child is able to give consent, the consent must be obtained in addition to that of their legal guardian.

themselves from threats to their safety or personal integrity. Respect for personal integrity involves: enhancing the person's self-identity; paying attention to their humanness, acknowledging who they are and treating them well. At times researchers in the past have recruited participants from the most vulnerable groups in society, such as the homeless, prisoners, gay men, children with intellectual disability, dying patients, and ethnic minorities. Other vulnerable groups, where there is a potential power-base inequality, can include pregnant women, children and service-men/women (or

Respect for cultural diversity

There is a further cultural aspect to the 'respect for persons' that was discussed earlier (NHMRC 2002). Individuals are also members of various groups that inform their sense of identity and values. The cultural nature of these groups is not restricted to ethnicity but may also include sexual orientation, religious affiliation, employment status, disability and age.

Indigenous people are a particular cultural group that pose additional ethical concerns because they may have experienced the harmful effects of colonisation. Cram (2001 p 37) argues that research involving indigenous people and conducted by non-indigenous people 'all too often results in judgments being made that are based on the cultural standpoint of the researcher rather than the lived reality of the indigenous population'. Furthermore, this type of research may benefit the researcher more than the indigenous people who are studied. Williams (1998) suggests that conventional ethical procedures may not be appropriate for indigenous peoples because these have the potential to further disable the aspirations and integrity of those who are the focus of the research.

The indigenous peoples of both Australia and New Zealand have lobbied their respective governments and scientific communities to protect them from further exploitation by researchers. In both countries guidelines for research with indigenous people require respect for those cultures, to ensure that the researcher understands how culture may influence the ethical issues and so take steps to protect participants' cultural integrity during the study. In Australia, research involving Aboriginal and Torres Strait Islander peoples is governed by separate guidelines (see NHMRC *Guidelines on Ethical Matters in Aboriginal and Torres Strait Islander Health Research* 1991). The Health Research Council of New Zealand also has separate guidelines for researchers on health research involving Maōri (1998) and Pacific peoples (2004) (website: http://www.hrc.govt.nz). These guidelines are intended to assist researchers undertaking biomedical, public health or clinical research involving Maōri or Pacific participants or research on issues relevant to Maōri or Pacific people's health. Consultation is a key component in the development of research with these groups and is the means of establishing co-operative, collaborative and ethical working relationships between researchers and Maōri or Pacific organisations and groups. New Zealand's accredited ethics committees must have proportional representation of Maōri members to ensure that appropriate consultation occurs. Consultation with these groups also ensures that research practices and outcomes contribute to the health development of Maōri (through the principles of the Treaty of Waitangi) and Pacific peoples.

Ethics committees

While there is international agreement about ethical considerations in research involving human beings, there is evidence that ensuring strict adherence to the guidelines may be problematic. In regard to the cervical cancer project in New Zealand in the 1980s, Judge Cartwright found that an institutional committee failed to adequately review either the scientific merit of the study or protect the participants (*Report of the cervical cancer inquiry* 1988). Consequently, the judge recommended that national ethical standards be developed and independent ethics committees be set up to review all health research proposals and experimental treatments.

The subsequent passing of the *Health Research Council Act 1990* enabled the establishment of New Zealand's first Health Research Council (HRC) and regional health ethics committees. The passage of the *New Zealand Public Health and Disability Act 2000* means there is now a statutory requirement to provide for the establishment of a national ethics committee — the National Ethics Advisory Committee (NEAC) on Health and Disability Support Services (Dawson & Peart 2003).

In Australia, the National Health and Medical Research Council (NHMRC) was first constituted in 1936. The present council was established under the *National Health and Medical Research Council Act 1992*, along with the Australian Health Ethics Committee (AHEC), that has statutory responsibility for developing guidelines for the ethical conduct of health research, the most recent being the *Human Research Ethics Handbook* 2002. The AHEC also produces ethical guidelines covering specific areas of health and research, such as clinical trials, and assisted reproductive technology. The guidelines are available on the website: www.nhmrc.gov.au.

The former Australian council recommended peer-group assessment of experiments involving human participants, by an institutional ethics committee (IEC), as long ago as 1972. Later, the council strengthened this recommendation, by issuing the statement that in order to be eligible to receive funding from the council, a study must be reviewed by an IEC. This proved to be an effective inducement for institutions to establish IECs. These committees are now known as human research ethics committees (HRECs) (NHMRC 2006). Therefore, in both countries, there is a statutory organisation (council) to set national ethical standards and scrutinise research — although only in an advisory capacity. There is no statutory requirement to obtain ethical approval in either country; instead access to government funding is the only inducement to formal ethical review. However, the researcher remains answerable to the respective ethics (human or animal) committee who have the authority to stop a project should concerns emerge. These government-led attempts to protect human research participants have only been partially successful, because some responsibility still rests with the researcher. Issues relating to researcher integrity and honesty will be discussed followed by an examination of laws pertaining to research, and the conduct of clinical trials. The broad role of human research ethics committees appears in Box 6.3 (Crisp & Taylor 2005).

TT Tutorial trigger 2

The Nursing Research and Development Unit (a joint venture between the university and hospital) has been asked to investigate patients' experience of the outreach palliative care service. The title of the study is 'Patients' lived experience of the outreach palliative care service'. What approval process would you need to follow for this study?

Researcher integrity and honesty

The integrity and honesty of a researcher is critical for the conduct, reporting and publication of studies. A number of recent fraudulent studies have been revealed in various

---

BOX 6.3 The broad role of human research ethics committees (HRECs)

- Risks to participants are minimised.
- Risks to participants are reasonable in relation to anticipated benefits, if any, and the importance of the knowledge that may reasonably be expected to result.
- Selection of participants is equitable.
- Informed consent will be sought, as required.
- Informed consent will be appropriately documented.
- Adequate provision is made for monitoring the research to ensure the safety of participants.
- Appropriate provisions are made to protect the privacy of participants and the confidentiality of data.
- When vulnerable subjects are involved, appropriate additional safeguards are included to protect their rights and welfare.

(Reproduced with permission from Crisp & Taylor 2005 *Potter & Perry's Fundamentals of Nursing*, 2nd edn. Elsevier, Sydney. Based on data from National Health and Medical Research Council (NHMRC): *National statement on ethical conduct in research involving humans*, Canberra, 12999, Ausinfo; Code of Federal Regulations: Protection of human subjects, 45CFR46 (1983, revised as of March 1993), Washington, DC, 1993, US Department of Health and Human Services; and Polit & Hungler 1999 *Nursing research: principles and methods*, 6th ed. JB Lippincott, Philadelphia.)

---

countries; in some cases the study was never conducted, in others results were falsified. For example, Michael Briggs, a former Professor of Human Biology at Geelong's Deakin University in Victoria, was found to have faked trials, methods and papers that he published regarding the safety of an oral contraceptive pill (Martin 1989). Another example was the forced resignation of leading international South Korean embryologist, Professor Hwang Woo-suk, who fabricated results of his stem cell research in 2005; research that had the potential to benefit people with diabetes and Parkinson's diseases (Debaets 2006).

The US federal government's concern about the increasing incidence of scientific misconduct resulted in the establishment of the Office of Research Integrity (ORI) in 1989. The ORI continues to update policy, rules and regulations related to scientific misconduct and to manage any investigations of alleged scientific misconduct in the US.

> Research misconduct means *fabrication*, *falsification* or *plagiarism* in proposing, performing or reviewing research, or in reporting research results.
> (a) *Fabrication* is making up data or results and recording or reporting them.
> (b) *Falsification* is manipulating research materials, equipment or processes, or changing or omitting data or results such that the research is not accurately represented in the research record.
> (c) *Plagiarism* is the appropriation of another person's ideas, processes, results or words without giving appropriate credit.
> (d) Research misconduct does not include honest error or differences of opinion.
>
> (US Department of Health and Human Services 2005)

A CINAHL search using the key terms 'scientific', 'fraud' and 'nursing' found no published examples of a nurse acting as a primary investigator who had been accused of scientific misconduct. However, as Hawley and Jeffers (1992) point out, nurses have been implicated in scientific misconduct through their association with medical researchers, whether or not they were actively involved in the research. For example, the nurses at National Women's Hospital were criticised by Judge Cartwright for failing to advocate for their patients (*Report of the cervical cancer inquiry* 1988) and Nurse Rivers was implicated in the unethical Tuskegee syphilis study (Jones 1981). In the UK a research nurse was reported to the UKCC — now the Nursing and Midwifery Council — and admitted falsifying research data in a medical research project and claiming expenses for research work she had not carried out (Castledine 2002).

The continued existence of scientific fraud and failure of peer review (Bevan 2004; Martin 1992; Nylenna & Simonsen 2006) demonstrates that national guidelines and financial inducements to obtain approval from ethical committees are not sufficient. There are no formal penalties if a researcher breaches ethical standards for research. At best, ethical guidelines can be influential in the practice of research but have no legal force. It is noteworthy, however, that in Australia and New Zealand there is a range of acts, regulations and codes with which researchers are obliged to comply; that is, research law.

Points to ponder

► How could you determine whether a published study that provided no evidence of ethical approval had in fact been through an ethics committee?

► If a researcher walked into your hospital ward and said they had come to interview patients what checks could you make to ensure that the study has ethical approval?

Research law

Research law partially comes from traditional areas such as consent, contract, negligence and intellectual property (copyright). There are also specific laws that establish and regulate public research funding agencies. Other laws have a much broader focus that extend well beyond research, for example, privacy and human rights, but they also have important implications for the conduct of research and research relationships (Dawson & Peart 2003). For example, there are specific statutes in Australia and New Zealand that regulate the conduct of clinical trials of new drugs or experimental procedures. There are also statutes requiring consultation with Maōri about research involving their communities or resources, to which Treaty of Waitangi principles apply. Thus, the researcher–human participants' relationship is heavily regulated to protect participants from exploitation and harm (Dawson & Peart 2003).

Clinical trials

Researchers conducting clinical trials in Australia must meet the legal requirements of the *Therapeutic Goods Act 1989*. This act is administered by the Therapeutic Goods Administration (TGA) who produce a number of useful documents for researchers and ethics committees. An Australian research participant can sue the researcher or research institution for compensatory or exemplary damages if they suffer illness or injury as a result of participating in the study (Forrester & Griffiths 2005).

On the other hand, research involving human participants in New Zealand must comply with the *Medicines Act 1981* and *Accident Rehabilitation Compensation Insurance (ARCI) Act 1992*. This compels researchers to complete a declaration to ensure indemnity cover for participants in clinical trials when applying for approval from a regional ethics committee (Ministry of Health and Accident Compensation Corporation 1993). New Zealand has a 'no fault' accident and illness compensation scheme and this legislation severely limits the person's ability to sue a health practitioner or researcher.

TT Tutorial trigger 3

- You represent a hypothetical drug company that recruited healthy volunteers to test an experimental drug. When the researchers administered the experimental drug several of the participants had a severe anaphylactic response and they required intensive care for several weeks.
- You have been asked to respond to media criticism that this drug trial is unethical. What arguments would you give to show that the drug trial was ethical?

O'Brien (2001 p 27) points out that:

> researchers cannot claim to be operating ethically when their research activity is inconsistent with the law and/or when they are exposing research participants to procedures and activities which may either place those participants outside the law or create risks for participants for which there are legal consequences.

Researchers then need to consider which legislation will apply to their study when they are developing the research proposal. Laws that influence the practice of research are the strongest means of ensuring the protection of human participants but even then there are no guarantees. Legal protection is limited by the necessity for both a formal complaint and evidence to be laid with the police, and it may be difficult to prove a causal relationship between the injury sustained and the research.

Professional nursing organisations have a role to play in guiding nurses and midwives in the practice of research. In Australia, the *Standards for Research for the Nursing Profession* were developed by the Australian Nursing Federation (ANF 1997) as guidelines for registered nurses undertaking research.

These standards provide the structure for ensuring accountability for nursing research for the profession and the community and are complementary to the NHMRC guidelines (1991). The role of both guidelines for the ethical conduct of research and the role of institutional research and ethics committees cannot be overstated: both are vitally important as safeguards.

A discussion of ethical and legal issues in research would not be complete without reference to animal experimentation which occurs in many hospitals. Nurses who may encounter animal experimentation should be aware of their rights.

Legal and ethical considerations in animal experimentation

In the 1970s, animal activists and anti-vivisectionist societies drew the public's attention to animal experimentation in research. Following World War II, there was an increase in the use of animals in research and a number of states/territories passed legislation called 'pound seizure laws' that allowed, and even mandated, the release of unclaimed animals from pounds to laboratories. The first pound seizure law was enacted in 1949 and repealed only in 1972. Regulations governing the welfare of animals in research can be found in the *Australian Code of Practice for the Care and Use of Animals for Scientific Purposes* (NHMRC, ARC, CSIRO, AV-CC 2004). The code is legally enforceable in all Australian states and territories. The guidelines are summarised in the NHMRC Statement of Animal Experimentation and outline the principles for the use and care of experimental animals. The code provides guidelines for the humane conduct of scientific and teaching activities that use animals.

This section serves only as an introduction to the concept of legal/ethical issues related to animal experimentation. Principles of protection of animal rights in research have evolved over time, as has a growing body of literature in the area (current literature on animal rights and ethics is available on the Australian website: www.animalethics.org. au). Animals, unlike humans, cannot give informed consent, but conditions safeguarding their welfare must not be ignored. Nurses who encounter the use of animals in, say, medical drug-related research should be alert to the rights of all animals. It is, of course, unlikely that nurses or midwives would be directly involved with research using animals, but they may witness other health professional colleagues doing so, and therefore need to be aware from this perspective.

Sometimes, research studies published in professional journals do not provide the research consumer with detailed information regarding the ways in which ethical procedures were adhered to, however, this does not necessarily mean that the research was unethical. In the absence of documentation regarding ethical issues, the acknowledgment that the research study was approved by an external HREC will assure the reader that the proposal was reviewed and permission given to proceed with the study. The detailed guidelines in Box 6.4 will assist the research consumer in evaluating the legal and ethical aspects of a research study.

BOX 6.4 Criteria for evaluating the legal and ethical aspects of a research study

- Was the study approved by an ethics committee?
- Did participants receive full information about the purpose and nature of the study?
- What evidence is provided to indicate that informed consent was obtained from participants?
- Did the researcher clearly explain any risks and their management?
- Did the researcher discuss the risk–benefit ratio?
- Did the researcher meet legal requirements?
- Is there any evidence of harassment, inducement or coercion during the consent process?
- How was the privacy of the participants maintained?
- What special protection was in place for vulnerable participants?
- Did participants have access to the results or findings of the research study?

Summary

All research projects involving humans and animals are required to be submitted to their respective institutional ethics committees before the commencement of a project. These institutional ethics committees act in the interests of research participants in order to ensure the guidelines developed by the NHMRC are observed. It is incumbent upon nurses and midwives to understand exactly what is meant by ensuring patient 'rights' as they apply to participants and other individuals (including themselves) in the research process. As research consumers, nurses and midwives need to critically evaluate research studies in order to decide whether ethical and legal issues have been appropriately addressed or not.

Adhering closely to ethical principles and procedures is an inherent part of the research process. Researchers should be duty-bound to clearly include details of this process in their disseminated findings — although this is not always the case. It constitutes a vital part of research design. While it is not always explicitly covered in the following qualitative and quantitative methods sections, it is at least implicit that it is an integral part of the overall process.

KEY POINTS

- Internationally agreed ethical principles in research involving human participants are: respect for autonomy; respect for privacy; respect for justice; beneficence; respect for human vulnerability and integrity; and respect for cultural diversity.
- Informed consent procedures ensure the individual's autonomy and right to self-determination are respected.
- Respecting an individual's privacy in research involves protecting their anonymity and treating their information as confidential.
- Some groups of people are more vulnerable to exploitation than others and require special protection; for example, children, prisoners, service people, people with mental health and learning disability issues, pregnant women etc.
- Research misconduct involves fabrication, falsification, plagiarism or other unacceptable practices.

Learning activities

1. When the researcher notifies a person of any proposed participation in research which of the following ethical requirements is being met?
   (a) respect for justice
   (b) respect for privacy
   (c) beneficence
   (d) respect for autonomy.

2. The qualitative researcher used pseudonyms when quoting the participant's narrative in the published study so met the requirement for:
   (a) respect for justice and equity
   (b) respect for privacy
   (c) beneficence
   (d) respect for autonomy.

3. By selecting only unemployed men for the study and promising to pay them a substantial amount of money to be in the experimental group, the researcher did not meet the requirement for:
   (a) respect for justice and equity
   (b) respect for privacy
   (c) beneficence
   (d) respect for autonomy.

4. The researcher acknowledged in the information sheet that talking about experiences of the death of a child might be emotionally painful. By setting up access to counselling services for participants, the researcher met the requirement for:
   (a) respect for autonomy
   (b) respect for justice
   (c) beneficence
   (d) respect for privacy.

5. The role of an institutional or regional ethics committee in Australia or New Zealand is to:
   (a) protect research participants and enforce national ethical standards
   (b) advise on national ethical standards and protect research participants
   (c) enforce national ethical standards and fund research
   (d) fund research in institutions or regions and protect research participants.

6. The statement about vulnerable participants that is not true is:
   (a) vulnerable participants are less able to understand what is involved if they take part in the study
   (b) vulnerable participants find it difficult to understand how risky the study may be
   (c) vulnerable participants cannot communicate their wishes about taking part in the study
   (d) vulnerable participants are those people less likely to be harmed.

7. Research involving indigenous people has special ethical concerns because:
   (a) they are a different culture from the rest of the population
   (b) of their minority group status
   (c) the group's leaders may refuse access to participants
   (d) they tend to live in remote areas.

8. Research misconduct refers to:
   (a) a study that has been poorly conducted
   (b) a study that is unscientific
   (c) errors in data analysis or interpretation
   (d) fabrication or falsification of research results.

9. Informed consent in research involves:
   (a) a person being informed that they are a study participant and about the nature of the study
   (b) a person agreeing to participate in a study after receiving information about the nature of the study and being told the experimental drug may cure them
   (c) a person signing a consent form for a research study after receiving information about the nature of the study and what it will involve for them personally
   (d) a person freely agreeing to participate in a study after receiving information about the nature of the study and what it will involve for them personally.

10. Therapeutic research is:
   (a) research that may benefit future patients but not those acting as research participants
   (b) research investigating different forms of treatment that ranks the most effective (therapeutic) to the least effective treatment
   (c) research that gives the patient an opportunity to receive experimental treatment that may have beneficial effects
   (d) the therapeutic effect experienced by participants sharing distressing experiences in qualitative studies.

Additional resources

Australian Nursing Council *Code of Ethics and Code of Conduct*. Online. Available: www.anc.org.au

Munhall P L 2001 Ethical considerations in qualitative research. In: Munhall P L (ed.) *Nursing research: a qualitative perspective*, 3rd edn. Jones & Bartlett, Sudbury, MA, pp 537–49

National Health and Medical Research Council. Online. Available: www.nhmrc.gov.au

New Zealand Health and Disability Commission. Online. Available: http://www.hdc.org.nz

New Zealand Health Research Council. Online. Available: www.hrc.org.nz

New Zealand Privacy Commission. Online. Available: www.privacy.org.nz

Nursing Council of New Zealand *Code of Conduct for Nurses*. Online. Available: www.nursingcouncil.org.nz

References

Australian Code of Practice for the Care and Use of Animals for Scientific Purposes, 7th edn 2004. NHMRC, ARC, CSIRO, AV-CC. Australian Government, Canberra

Australian Nursing Federation (ANF) 1997 *Standards for Research for the Nursing Profession*. Australian Nursing Federation Publications Unit, Melbourne

Beauchamp T L, Childress J F 1994 *Principles of biomedical ethics*, 4th edn. Oxford University Press, New York

Beecher H K 1966 Ethics and clinical research. *New England Journal of Medicine* 274:1354–60

Bevan D 2004 The changing face of scientific misconduct. *Clinical and Investigative Medicine* 27(3):117–19

Cartright, S 1988 *Report of the cervical cancer enquiry*. Government Printer, Auckland, New Zealand

Castledine G 2002 Research nurse who falsified the results of research. *British Journal of Nursing* 11(17):1119

Cram F 2001 Rangahau Māori: Tona tika, tona pono — The validity and integrity of Māori research. In: Tolich M (ed.) *Research ethics in Aotearoa New Zealand*. Pearson Education, Auckland, New Zealand, pp 35–52

Creighton H 1977 Legal concerns of nursing research. *Nursing Research* 26(4):337–40

Crisp J, Taylor C 2005 *Potter & Perry's fundamentals of nursing*, 2nd edn. Elsevier, Sydney, p 83

Dawson J, Peart N (eds) 2003 *The law of research: a guide*. University of Otago Press, Dunedin, New Zealand

Debaets A M 2006 Korean cloning scandal and scientific fraud. *Ethics and medicine* 22(1):61–2

Dunning T, Manias E 2005 Medication knowledge and self management by people with type 2 diabetes. *Australian Journal of Advanced Nursing* 23(1):7–13

Dye L, Hendy S, Hare D J, et al. 2004 Capacity to consent to participate in research — a recontextualisation. *British Journal of Learning Disabilities* 32:144–50

Fenwick J, Hauck Y, Downie J, et al. 2005 The childbirth expectations of a self-selected cohort of Eastern Australian women. *Midwifery* 21:23–35

Forrester K, Griffiths D 2005 *Essentials of law for health professionals*, 2nd edn. Elsevier, Sydney

Griffith R 2006 Making decisions for incapable adults 4: participation in research. *British Journal of Community Nursing* 11(6):261–5

Hawley D J, Jeffers J M 1992 Scientific misconduct as a dilemma for nursing. *Image: Journal of Nursing Scholarship* 24(1):51–5

Health and Disability Commissioner 1994 *Health and disability consumers' code of rights*. Health and Disability Commissioner, Wellington, New Zealand

Health Research Council of New Zealand 1998 *Guidelines for researchers on health research involving Māori*. Māori Health Committee of the Health Research Council of New Zealand. Online. Available: http://www.hrc.govt.nz [accessed 20 December 2006]

—— 2004 *Guidelines for researchers on health research involving Pacific peoples resident in New Zealand*. Online. Available: http://www.hrc.govt.nz [accessed 20 December 2006]

Humphrey L 1970 *Tearoom trade: impersonal sex in public places*. Aldine, Chicago

Johnson S (general editor) 2004 *Health care and the law*, 3rd New Zealand edn. Brookers, Wellington, New Zealand

Jones J H 1981 *Bad blood: the Tuskegee syphilis experiment — a tragedy of race and medicine*. Free Press, New York

McLeod D, McBain L, Nydham T 2001 A prospective study of immunisation for a cohort of children. *New Zealand Medical Journal* 114:291–4

Martin B 1989 Fraud and Australian academics. *Thought and action* 5(2):95–102

—— 1992 Scientific fraud and the power structure of science. *Prometheus* 10(1):83–98

Middleton S, Donnelly N, Harris J, et al. 2005 Nursing intervention after carotid endarterectomy: a randomised trial of coordinated care post discharge. *Journal of Advanced Nursing* 52(3):250–61

Ministry of Health 2002 *Guidelines for health research with children*. Ministry of Health, Wellington, New Zealand

Ministry of Health and Accident Compensation Corporation 1993 (December) *Compensation for injuries caused as a result of participation in a clinical trial and the role of ethics committees: guidelines*. Ministry of Health, Wellington, New Zealand

Mitford J 1973 *Kind and unusual punishment*. Random House, New York

Mok E, Chung B P M, Chung J W Y, et al. 2005 An exploratory study of nurses suffering from severe acute respiratory syndrome (SARS). *International Journal of Nursing Practice* 11(4):150–60

National Health & Medical Research Council (NHMRC) 1991 *Guidelines on ethical matters in Aboriginal and Torres Strait Islander Health Research*. Commonwealth of Australia, Canberra

—— 2002 *Human research ethics handbook*. Online. Available: www.7.health.gov.au/nhmrc/publications/hrecbook/02-ethics/01.htm [accessed 19 April 2006]

—— 2006 *Privacy Amendment (Private Sector) Act 2001*. Online. Available: http://www.nhmrc.gov.au/publications/index.htm [accessed 23 December 2006]

New Zealand Ministry of Health 1996 *Code of health and disability services consumers' rights*. Online. Available: http://www.everybody.co.nz/page-ccd5ca86-35bd-4ccc-9ffl-dbc8fd8dcbbd.aspx [accessed 23 December 2006]

Nylenna M, Simonsen S 2006 Scientific misconduct: a new approach to prevention. *The Lancet* 367(9526):1882–4

O'Brien M 2001 Doing ethical research legally: research ethics and the law. In: Tolich M (ed.) *Research ethics in Aotearoa New Zealand*. Pearson Education, Auckland, New Zealand, pp 25–34

Parsons H M 1974 What happened at Hawthorne? *Science* 183:922–32

Powell M A, Smith A B 2006 Ethical guidelines for research with children: a review of current research ethics documentation in New Zealand. Kotuitui: *New Zealand Journal of Social Science* 1:125–38

Ramsey P 1970 *The patient as person: explorations in medical ethics*. Yale University Press, New Haven

Report of the cervical cancer inquiry 1988. Judge Cartwright, Government Printer, Auckland, New Zealand

Skegg P D G 2003 Consent and information disclosure. In: Dawson J, Peart N (eds) *The law of research: a guide*. University of Otago Press, Dunedin, New Zealand, pp 233–51

Taxis K, Barber N 2003 Ethnographic study of incidence and severity of intravenous drug errors. *British Medical Journal* 326:684–7

Taylor, Brig. General Telford 1946. Opening Statement at Nuremberg Doctor Trial. Online. Available: www.law.umkc.edu/faculty/projects/ftrials/nuremberg/NurembergDoctorTrial.html [accessed 21 December 2006]

Tolich M (ed.) 2001 *Research ethics in Aotearoa New Zealand*. Pearson Education, Auckland, New Zealand

United Nations Educational, Scientific and Cultural Organisation (UNESCO) 2005 *Universal Declaration on Bioethics and Human Rights*. Online. Available: http://www.unesco.org/ethics [accessed 23 December 2006]

US Department of Health and Human Services (DHHS) Public Health Service 2005 CFR Section 93, 103 p 18

Williams L M 1998 Ethics and nursing research: meeting the needs of indigenous peoples. *Nursing Inquiry* 5:25–31

World Medical Association History. Online. Available: http://www.wma.net/e/history/golden_years.htm [accessed 13 April 2006]

APPENDIX 1 Sample information sheet

(The information sheet is to be printed on the letterhead of the university at which you are enrolled or hospital/health service in which you are employed.)

INFORMATION SHEET

Dear _____

I am currently studying for my (*name of degree*) at (*name of university*). My thesis is by research. The title of my research project is:

'*Women's experiences of pregnancy in an environment of conflicting discourses about health*'

Researcher: (*student's name, department in which enrolled, university, suburb, state and postcode*). Telephone number: _____ Email address_____

The purpose of this exploratory research project is to discover how you experience your pregnancy, and the attitudes and meanings you give to the event. Your **own** interpretation and the meaning and significance you attach to this period are important in this study.

If you agree to participate, you will be asked to attend four interviews conducted at three stages during your pregnancy (8–12 weeks, 20–28 weeks and 36–38 weeks gestation), and once following the birth of your baby. Each interview will take about one hour. The interviews will be conducted at a time and place convenient to both you and me.

Please understand that you are free to withdraw from participation in this research study at any time and ask that all your records be returned to you or destroyed and not used in any way, provided that the request for destruction or return of records be made within four weeks of the completion of the interview.

Any complaint regarding the nature or conduct of this research may be directed to:

Ethics Liaison Officer, Human Research Ethics Committee, (*name of university, suburb, state and postcode*). Telephone: _____

Yours sincerely

(*researcher's name*)

APPENDIX 2 Sample consent form

(*The information sheet is to be printed on the letterhead of the university at which you are enrolled or hospital/health service in which you are employed.*)

Faculty of _____

CONSENT FORM

Title of Project: '*Women's experiences of pregnancy in an environment of conflicting discourses about health*'

Name of researcher, and department address:_____

I *(name of participant)* (please print) have read and understood all of the information on the 'Information Sheet' and any questions that I have asked have been answered to my satisfaction.

I agree to take part in this research study on the understanding that:
- I can withdraw from the study at any stage   Yes/No
- I agree to the four interviews being taped   Yes/No
- I agree to the use of any material which does not identify me
  in any way   Yes/No

Please understand that you are free to withdraw from participation in this research study at any time after *each* interview, and ask that all your records be returned to you or destroyed and not used in any way, provided that the request for destruction or return of records be made within four weeks of the completion of the interview.

Should I wish to discuss my participation with someone not directly involved in the project, particularly in regard to matters concerning policies, information about the conduct of the study, or my rights as a participant, or I wish to make a confidential complaint, I may contact:

Ethics Liaison Officer, Human Research Ethics Committee, (*name of university, suburb, state and postcode*). Telephone: _____

Name of Participant: _____

Date: _____   Signature: _____

Researcher: _____

Date: _____   Signature: _____

Answers

TT Tutorial trigger 1

Your Information Sheet should contain all of the following:

1. An invitation to take part in research.
2. Information about the researcher(s) and how to contact you.
3. Explanation about the aim of the study — 'to evaluate the short-term impact of nursing-led, co-ordinated care for patients after discharge following carotid-endarterectomy'. This could be worded more simply.
4. The study will use an experimental design and a questionnaire written in English.
5. If you decide to participate you will be asked to complete a mailed questionnaire about your health and understanding of factors that influence your health.
6. Then you will be randomly allocated to one of two groups. In both groups you will receive usual care after this procedure. But in only one of the groups you will receive extra input from the nurse.
7. If you are in the group receiving extra care you will receive a phone call from the nurse at 2, 6 and 12 weeks after discharge to ask you about your recovery, lifestyle changes and your understanding of risk factors.
8. We would also like your permission to contact your GP and inform him about the procedure, how it went, and what factors you would like to work on to reduce your risk of stroke.
9. All information you provide will be treated as confidential and your name will not be used in the final report.

TT Tutorial trigger 2

1. The proposal would have to be submitted to the Faculty Research Committee/ Graduate School of Nursing Research Committee and the university Human Research Ethics Committee/Regional Health Ethics Committee.
2. A covering letter (showing support from the Faculty/Graduate School of Nursing and clearance from the university HREC, and Regional Ethics Committee) with the proposal attached must be sent to Hospital X requesting permission to interview a number of patients.
3. The hospital HREC will then review your proposal at their meeting.
4. Once permission has been granted, patients may be invited to participate in the study. Information sheets written in plain language would be distributed by someone other than the researcher and patients would then contact the researcher if they wanted to participate.
5. When the patient contacts you (the researcher), a mutually convenient time to meet should be arranged. This first meeting would be an opportunity to answer any questions and obtain written consent to participate. The consent form would state how patient confidentiality and anonymity would be ensured as well as their right to withdraw from the study at any time without prejudice.
6. Finally, allow each patient sufficient time to ask questions and read the consent form before obtaining written consent.

TT Tutorial trigger 3

1. Firstly, this experimental drug offers enormous hope to a lot of patients afflicted by a dreadful disease.
2. This drug trial was approved by the national ethics committee.
3. In order to establish the safety of experimental drugs for humans we need to test them on humans. Animal experiments are useful but do not show how the drug will behave in a human being.
4. Testing the drug on healthy humans is less risky than testing the drug on the person with the serious medical problem; it might make them worse until we know whether it works and what is an appropriate dosage.
5. The people who took part in this stage of the clinical trial were all healthy volunteers. Although they each received some money for the inconvenience of taking part we do not consider it was so much money that it would influence their decision to take part.
6. The people who took part were all fully informed of the expected risks and assured of free emergency or other healthcare if they had an adverse event. They all signed a consent form.
7. If this serious medical problem could be treated then this will lead to better health

and quality of life for a significant number of seriously ill patients.

8. In addition, if this serious medical problem could be treated this will reduce healthcare costs for individual patients and society, thus, making more money available for other health priorities.

9. Using healthy participants in drug trials benefits the greater good of society or at least the good of patients afflicted with the disease that the drug is designed to treat.

10. Even if a few participants have become ill through taking this experimental drug we have learned something important that will advance our research.

Learning activities

1. d	**2.** b	**3.** a	**4.** c
5. b	**6.** d	**7.** b	**8.** d
9. d	**10.** c		

Research appreciation and application

Common qualitative methods

DEAN WHITEHEAD

KEY TERMS

descriptive exploratory
emancipatory
ethnography
grounded theory
interpretive
phenomenology
qualitative
   research methods

Learning outcomes

After reading this chapter, you should be able to:

- describe the common types of qualitative research approaches in relation to nursing and midwifery issues
- discuss the appropriateness of qualitative frameworks, theories and philosophies
- describe the value of the knowledge gained from qualitative research for practice
- identify the types of health-related issues that are best explored by the use of qualitative research.

Introduction

Qualitative research refers to a series of broadly divergent and related methodologies that cluster under a paradigmatic umbrella (see Chapter 2). No one approach governs qualitative research and so permits multiple ways of exploring different phenomena. Qualitative researchers therefore have a range of research approaches available to them. Which approach they choose to adopt usually depends on the nature of the study and the type of knowledge that the researcher wishes to develop. The three most common qualitative research approaches used in both nursing and midwifery are phenomenology, grounded theory and ethnography. Proportionally, they most probably rank in that order. Each of these approaches holds a set of related but differing ontological (being-related), epistemological (knowledge-related) and methodological beliefs. It is these beliefs that inform and shape qualitative research studies.

One of the main characteristics of qualitative research is that it involves a close relationship between the researcher and participant. This is quite different from research conducted within the quantitative paradigm, where there is frequently no direct contact with participants. Research participants, in qualitative research, are therefore viewed as 'knowers'. That is, they are viewed as possessing the knowledge that the researcher seeks to elicit. This is because the participants will have been selected on the basis that they are part of the phenomena, environment or culture that the researcher is examining — or that they have lived through an experience from which relevant opinions, values or beliefs have emerged (see sampling in Chapter 8). All qualitative research, therefore, links people's subjective experiences, perceptions, thoughts and feelings, and lived phenomena — rather than what is objective; that is, it explores the phenomenon revealed in and through individuals (Crotty 1996).

Qualitative methods are underpinned by specific philosophical or theoretical positions and frameworks. It is necessary to explore these in some detail if we are to understand how, why and when such research is undertaken. This detail also assists in informing us what specific qualitative research processes emerge from philosophical or theoretical positions. This exploration is also necessary because, often, studies will report that they have occurred under the 'umbrella' of qualitative research, but do not specifically define which type (see later in this chapter). An appreciation of the more common methods will allow the reader to make a more informed decision, as to what method/s has/have been used, even if this is not explicitly stated.

This chapter, then, takes the reader through a range of the more common qualitative approaches in health-related research. It is important to note here that this chapter focuses primarily on the theoretical and philosophical underpinnings, frameworks and processes of the most common qualitative methods. It is following chapters which deal with the specifics of further qualitative research process and design — such as data collection, sampling techniques and analysis of data.

Why is qualitative research useful?

Quantitative research, through the collection and analysis of numerical data, generally informs us of how often, when or how effective particular nursing interventions or treatments are. This information relates directly to the research participants or 'elements' (may be non-human i.e. a specific drug or wound dressing) being tested. What quantitative research does not intend to do, however, is seek to understand personal experiences, interpretations and constructs — from the perspective of research participants. Instead, this is the place and intention of qualitative research. Qualitative research, therefore, lends itself far more to symbolic and conceptual utilisation, than to instrumental utilisation often seen in quantitative research (Sandelowski 2004).

Qualitative research, over the years, has proven very useful to the disciplines of nursing and midwifery. They both share basic premises related to beliefs about individuals and their relationship to the care environment. Qualitative research generally adopts an 'interpretive' and 'naturalistic' approach to viewing the world and its contained phenomena. This means that qualitative research is designed to help us understand naturally occurring social phenomena, through exploring the attitudes, beliefs, meanings, values and experiences of research participants. For health-related qualitative research, the research participants will usually be selected on the basis of them being clients, client's caregivers/relatives and/or health professionals. This is where qualitative research possesses the greatest potential to be useful. It has the potential, through such inquiry with its chosen participants, to raise awareness of the need for change. This occurs when health and nursing care situations are critically examined and evaluated from the perspective of the participants' experiences of care situations — either spoken or observed.

Different qualitative methodologies broadly share many similar properties. The scope of all qualitative research is ground within principles that intrinsically value an holistic perspective of experience, and the individual's ability to make sense of, and reflect on, their experiences. Also, qualitative research is essentially 'inductive' in its approach. This means that it is driven by the collected data and the findings and conclusion are drawn directly from this data. Furthermore, in terms of process, all qualitative research demands, of the researcher, the ability to be continuously reflexive and self-scrutinising — while balancing this against the need for both creativity and rigour (Pyett 2003). This said, while sharing properties, different qualitative approaches explore experiences and phenomena in different ways; generally producing different types of research outcomes. For this reason, much of the following text is devoted to the main different research traditions, in turn, used by qualitative researchers in nursing and midwifery-related qualitative research.

TT Tutorial trigger 1

Identify a health-related issue that you think would be best explored using a qualitative approach and devise a suitable research question (see Chapter 5) to investigate that issue.

Point to ponder

▶ Qualitative methods offer researchers the opportunity to gather rich information from their clients and colleagues and, at the same time, develop close and meaningful relationships.

Evidence-based practice tip

Qualitative research is best used where the researcher wishes to gain insights into the way that clients, their caregivers and colleagues engage and interact with each other. In other words, to gain insights into the way that they define, interpret and analyse different situations, events, experiences and phenomena.

Phenomenology
Origins and philosophical underpinnings

Phenomenology, as a framework for research inquiry, has been widely embraced by health professional researchers. It is seen as a way of understanding phenomena that occur within and outside the domain of health professionals. It is still the most common qualitative method adopted by nurse and midwifery researchers and, therefore, the main focus of this chapter. Phenomenology is designed to illuminate phenomena and disclose previously unnoticed or overlooked issues, as it explores the experience and meaning of phenomena. Phenomenology, therefore, reveals meanings embedded in the investigated situation or identifies impact of phenomenon, rather than makes inferences. At the same time, it provides rich descriptions that aid understanding. The result of uncovering such knowledge is that researchers may better understand the possibilities embedded in the experience of phenomena.

Phenomenology has found appeal in nursing and midwifery research because it reflects values and beliefs that are coherent with both these disciplines, and allows questions to be explored that are important to them. Certain questions are most often asked. These tend to focus on understanding experiences of phenomena related to health and illness, treatment and care — from the perspective of both those cared for and those providing care. For instance, Johnson et al. (2006) investigated the experiences of mechanically ventilated patients in a critical care unit setting in Queensland, Australia. They revealed what it meant for the participants to exist, live through, and survive their experience. The main identified theme was 'existing in an uneveryday world'. Similarly, Erlandsson and Fagerberg's (2005) study, of mothers' lived experiences of co-care and post-care after birth, reveals what the experience of childbirth meant to the mothers.

A phenomenon is defined as 'something that is shown, or revealed, or manifest in experience' (Blackburn 1994 p 285). The goal of phenomenology is to develop an understanding of a phenomenon through the specific human experience of the phenomenon, in order to better understand that experience of being in that 'life-world'. It strives to understand a person's experiences, rather than to provide causal explanation of those experiences. The process of phenomenological research, therefore, does not fragment the experience that is being studied. Instead, it provides descriptions that are rich and full and interpretations that illuminate what it means to be a person in their particular world. The phenomenological researcher is committed to understanding the experience of the phenomena holistically. Phenomenology, therefore, is mostly used to develop 'pathic' understanding. This type of understanding is useful for empathetic care and in guiding nursing actions concerned with aspects such as feelings/emotions, interactions, meanings of experiences and responses to phenomena (Annells 1999). Researchers find phenomenology particularly useful for the study of those phenomena that do not lend themselves readily to the processes of quantification, control or comparison. Cheung and Hocking (2004), for instance, in their Melbourne-based 'caring as worrying: the experience of spousal carers' article, use a phenomenological approach. It is difficult to think of another research method that could provide the description required to encapsulate the experience of a spouse's complex emotional relationship with their ill partner and their concerns for the future of both.

> ### Points to ponder
> ▶ Phenomena can be understood through the experiences people have of them.
> ▶ Phenomenology provides an understanding of people and their relationships with their worlds.
> ▶ Language is accepted as a means for understanding others' experience of phenomena.

Research in brief

O'Brien (2001) studied nurse–client relationships, bringing together the perspective of community psychiatric nurses and clients with a mental illness. The nurses identified 'being there', 'being concerned', 'establishing trust' and 'facilitating transition' as central to their experience of the relationship. The clients identified 'having someone looking out for me', 'working in collaboration' and 'being understood and gaining understanding' as central to the relationship. In bringing these themes together, relationships were revealed within an arena in which the clients could 'be' and in which they could explore the 'possibilities of being'. This illuminated distinct similarities in what was important to both clients and nurses about their shared relationships.

Phenomenology was first a philosophy but has subsequently been adapted and used as a structured approach to research inquiry. While phenomenology has provided health professionals with many riches, in terms of understanding human existence and experience, it also provides considerable challenges to the researcher. This is mainly due to the many different philosophical schools of thought and subsequent interpretation that have emerged since the turn of the twentieth century. A phenomenologist, by necessity, requires an overall understanding of several different philosophical schools of thought. Alongside this, they must also possess an in-depth knowledge of their adopted philosophical framework, in order to produce research that is true to the chosen framework. The two most common phenomenological schools of philosophy, adopted by both nurses and midwives, have emerged from the Husserlian and Heideggerian tradition and occasionally from the works of Gadamer (Paley 1998). Other popular, but less used, philosophical interpretations have emerged — such as those of van Manen (1984), Merleau-Ponty (Dowling 2006), and Crotty (Barkway 2001) — but are not included here. Dowling's (2006) article offers a detailed and insightful account of many of the phenomenological schools. This section provides a basic overview of some key concepts that need to be considered when undertaking phenomenological research. These key concepts have implications for how research studies, using certain approaches, are conducted.

Husserlian phenomenology

Phenomenology, as a philosophical movement, has its origins in Ancient Greek philosophy. It is, however, the German philosopher Husserl (1859–1938) who is credited as the founder of the twentieth century phenomenological movement. Husserl's desire was to seek an alternative to positivism (see Chapter 2) that would integrate the world of science alongside the real 'life-world' (*lebenswelt*) of people (Sadala & Adorno 2002). For Husserl, human beings were subjects in a world of objects and it was the study of the consciousness of those objects that he called phenomenology. From this focus, he developed one of the two main schools of phenomenology (descriptive phenomenology) and was primarily interested in the question, 'What do we know …?' (Koivisto et al. 2002). Husserl moved philosophical discussion from the question of whether or not objects in our conscious awareness had a separate existence, to the systematic analysis of consciousness and its objects. He aimed to separate out (bracket) mood, thoughts, memories and emotions to focus on conscious awareness of objects. He believed that understanding about intuition, judgment, and thus logic and truth, emerged as a result of reflecting upon the experiences of life (Dahlberg et al. 2001). Husserl's phenomenology is epistemological in nature. That is, it is concerned with asking questions of knowledge about objects gained through conscious awareness. Husserl concluded that 'essences', as the things that define experience, exist within the conscious experiences of people and this consciousness (and its intention) is presented by people to the world (Koivisto et al. 2002; Sadala & Adorno 2002).

Heideggerian phenomenology

Heidegger (1889–1976), who was a pupil and colleague of Husserl, questioned the relationship between consciousness and objects and thus diverged significantly from Husserl's interpretations. Heidegger's assertions helped to form the other main school of phenomenological philosophy (interpretive phenomenology). For Heidegger, the practical 'situatedness' of human experience is his most important premise. Heidegger focused his efforts on the study of a person's practical situatedness of their human experience and towards the understanding of the necessary conditions for people being or existing in their worlds. Thus Heideggerian phenomenology is 'ontological'. This means that it seeks to understand the conditions whereby human beings can understand their existence and, therefore, the nature and the meaning of 'being'.

The notion of being or 'being-in-this-world' is central to Heidegger's interpretations and is referred to by Heidegger in the commonly used context of 'Da-sein' (Heidegger 1962 p 67). The German verb Da-sein essentially means 'to exist', although there are other variations in interpretation. Therefore, Heidegger asserts that people are aware of their own existence and question what it means to be them in or outside their own world. This state is connected to the concept of 'self' which is, in turn, inextricably woven into the wider context of the person's place in their community, world and the cosmos. Thus people are capable of

---

Research in brief

Erlandsson and Fagerberg's (2005) study adopts a Husserlian phenomenological methodology. It explores the mothers' of premature or sick babies lived experiences of co-care and post-care after birth, revealing what the experience of childbirth meant to the mothers. Several main themes emerged. These being; 'the mothers' strong desire to be close to their baby', 'to be able to be close to your baby', 'not to be able to be close to your baby', 'to be seen', 'not to be seen', 'to be part of a functional team', and 'not to be part of a functional team'. While not common for emerging themes in phenomenological research, it is worth noting here that many of the themes present as 'opposites' to each other. The study identified that, no matter what the circumstances were, mothers wanted to remain close to their babies over a range of maternity services — where, often, they were denied this opportunity.

questioning the meaning of their experiences of being. They can interpret their different worlds, in contextualised ways, in comparison with others around them. People can reflect on the meaning of their experience and can look forward to possibilities of being.

Heidegger also described Da-sein as being in the midst of a world that is familiar and that is understood. This world contains horizons that comprise pre-understandings which enable us to make sense of our situations. This 'hermeneutic circle' (Heidegger 1962 p 119) describes the historical, cultural and personal preconceptions from which understanding is developed. This notion lends itself to the commonly used term 'hermeneutics'. Hermeneutic phenomenology provides a framework that defines a view of persons and their being-in-the-world. It does so through questioning the collected data (text) and moving from parts to the whole of this text, in which each part gives the other parts meaning. It also defines how meaning and language are understood and thus how knowledge, about human beings and their world, is subjective, temporal and historical.

The hermeneutic circle is not a static entity; it is dynamic. Therefore, the preconceptions contained in understanding are challenged by new understandings. It is by making the background preconceptions explicit in language that the testing of assumptions is possible. The process is kaleidoscopic, as different patterns emerge in the process of the illumination of taken-for-granted understandings. People come to a research encounter with a history of culture and experience that is bound in language. This process of understanding brings together perspectives influenced by past and current events and articulated in a shared language. For instance, Whitehead (2002a) refers to the 'phenomenological nod' that he experienced when investigating the academic assignment writing experiences of a group of student nurses. This nod confirmed that the students' experiences were very similar to his past experiences and describes how they relate to the current and future experiences of both parties.

Also important to Heidegger (1962 p 386) was the notion that 'being in the world' is always understood in terms of 'temporality'. Temporality refers to the fact that life, as it is lived now, cannot be divorced from the historical experience of living a life and the potential for that life in the future. Temporality is thus intrinsically involved in the meaning of life experience. So, as we can see, Heideggerian philosophy has at its core the relationships between self, being, meaning, existence and temporality. For those who require a deeper understanding of Heidegger's interpretive phenomenology, an Australian nurse researcher, Mackey (2005), provides a comprehensive description and analysis.

Gadamerian phenomenology

While Heidegger viewed phenomenology and hermeneutics as one and the same, Gadamer challenged this. Gadamer (1976) sought to expand the ideas of Heidegger and his concept of the hermeneutic circle. He did this by suggesting that the realisation of self occurs in the circle of understanding. Wood and Giddings (2005), in interviewing New Zealand-based Research Fellow Brian Phillips, discuss the nature and intention of his PhD study. In this study, he used Gadamerian hermeneutics to interpret men's experiences of suicidality and the relationship of masculinity in shaping their beliefs and understanding of this phenomenon. For this level of self-realisation to occur, the phenomenologist does not simply examine the language of the participant to describe the discovery of Da-sein. Instead, they incorporate their own interpretation and understanding from their own personal world. Therefore, self-understanding does not emerge from transparency of oneself, but by throwing light onto the tendencies and motivations that are exposed in the language spoken. Turner's (2005) study of hope, seen through the eyes of Australian youth, adopts a philosophy of understanding as advocated by Gadamer. They describe this process as including; identification of the researchers' pre-understandings of the explored phenomenon, adopting an attitude of *Bildung* (remaining open to meaning), identification of prejudices and expectations of the whole, using prejudices to develop horizons, and fusion/blending of these horizons to identify explored phenomenon.

> **𝑻𝑻 Tutorial trigger 2**
>
> Referring back to tutorial trigger 1, can you identify a specific phenomenological approach that would be best for you? Would you have to adjust your initial research question?

The purpose and process of phenomenology

Phenomenological studies are 'interpretive' from beginning to end. That is, the researcher first of all identifies the phenomenon and then asks the question. In doing so, they interpret it as an important question to ask. The researcher needs to be able to encourage exploration of the meaning of the experience of the phenomenon, for the interviewed person, and then to ask for concrete examples that can help illuminate the meaning. Undertaking phenomenological research requires a commitment to philosophical understanding. Therefore, researchers need to be able to:

• reflect on what it means to be a person in the world
• reflect on one's own experience and explore one's own understandings of a phenomenon
• think beyond the 'proving of facts', towards a desire to explore the experiences of self and others — of a phenomenon in a particular context
• have sufficient understanding of the phenomenological methodology and framework, in order to explicate how it informs the method of the study and the findings of the study.

To some extent, the reader may find the philosophical concepts of phenomenological research confusing and confounding. They can appear overly complex. In this chapter the presentation of the conventional philosophies can only be superficial. However, to help simplify matters, some phenomenological researchers have devised step-by-step procedures to help interpret and analyse the collected language (data). The two main proponents are Giorgi (1997) (see 'Research in brief') and Colaizzi (1978) (see Chapter 9). Reference to their seminal work and nursing studies that adopt their principles may provide further clarity.

The differences between a Husserlian epistemological tradition and a Heideggerian ontological tradition are important. This is because they impact on the questions that can be asked and the kinds of answers that can be sought. Paley (1998) argues that, while the differences between the two traditions are marked because they both focus on the 'lived experience', there is little to choose between the methodologies adopted by researchers. Questions that can utilise a Husserlian approach to research are epistemological questions of knowing 'How is this phenomenon known?'. Studies using this approach utilise bracketing (distancing oneself from the interpretation of the phenomenon through suspending all biases and preconceived beliefs) of both the researcher's and the participant's prior knowledge of the phenomenon. Questions that can utilise a Heideggerian approach to research are ontological questions of experience: 'How is this phenomenon understood through experience of the phenomenon?' Using different phenomenological methods, therefore, will demand different things of its participants and the researcher. The outcomes will be significantly different. It is vital, therefore, that the phenomenologist researcher understands

---

Research in brief

Kvigne et al. (2005) use a Giorgi-inspired phenomenological method to research the nature of nursing care and rehabilitation of female stroke survivors from the perspective of 14 hospital-based nurses. The analysis of the data used the Giorgi-related steps of (1) gaining a sense of the whole; (2) distinguishing the text into meaning units; (3) generating essential aspects and themes; and (4) synthesising the essential aspect of understandings and reflections into a consistent statement. It is worth noting that Erlandsson and Fagerberg's (2005) study (mentioned in the last 'Research in brief' box) also adopts a Giorgi-inspired Husserlian phenomenological methodology.

Points to ponder

▶ The process of phenomenological interpretation involves both an awareness of the pre-understandings that the researcher brings to the study and close reading of the gathered text.

▶ Phenomenological writing is a creative process that reaches beyond narrative description to reveal meaning and understanding.

this, and understands the most appropriate method to gain the type of insight required.

T_T Tutorial Trigger 3

When critically reviewing a phenomenological study what would you expect to see in place that would denote effective phenomenological process had been applied?

Grounded theory
Origins and theoretical underpinnings

Grounded theory refers to the method initially developed and introduced by Glaser and Strauss (1967), and further discussed and developed by them and other colleagues (Corbin & Strauss 1990; Glaser 1999; Strauss & Corbin 1998). Glaser and Strauss, two non-health professional sociologists, working in a US-based department of nursing doctoral studies in the 1960s, formulated techniques for generating theory about social processes so that the theory became 'grounded'. The theories are grounded by way of where the theory originates and emerges through analysing collected data. The data are collected from where human action and interaction occur over time, through speaking with and listening to those who have been engaged in the action and interaction — and sometimes from documents pertaining to the action and interaction. Essentially, grounded theory is designed to develop theoretical explanation for socially constructed events and ideally generate hypotheses for further research. Theory grounded in this manner is often believed to produce more useful and pragmatic outcomes than what arises from pure theorising alone. Therefore, knowledge may be increased through generating new theories, rather than analysing data within existing theories (Heath & Cowley 2004). Grounded theory has become a widely used qualitative methodology in nursing and

midwifery research, as a means to inductively distil clinical issues of importance by creating meaning about those issues through the analysis and modelling of theory (Mills et al. 2006).

Grounded theory is linked, by some, to the notion of 'symbolic interactionism' — a term coined by Blumer in 1937 (Neill 2006). This form of process aligns an interactionist approach alongside naturalistic inquiry to develop theory. This is where individuals are known to share culturally orientated understandings of their world. These understandings are shaped by similar beliefs, values and attitudes and determine how individuals behave according to how they interpret the world around them. People are seen as being both self-aware and aware of others and therefore can adapt their social interactions and situational behaviour to shape meaning and society (Heath & Cowley 2004). In this context, the focus lies with the symbolic meanings that are unearthed by people's interactions, actions and resulting consequences. This is linked to the fact that many grounded theory research questions start with the premise of asking 'How do people …?'. For instance, Whitehead (2002b p 199) broadly asks the question, in his grounded theory study, 'How do nursing students prepare for their current and on-going health promotion role?'.

It is increasingly accepted that grounded theory does not offer prediction (i.e. if this happens, then that will occur) unlike theory developed in other sciences such as bio-science, where so-called factual laws or 'truths' can be found. According to the Queensland-based researchers Mills et al. (2006 p 12), grounded theory does not seek to provide full individual accounts as evidence. Instead, it aims 'to move a theoretically sensitive analysis of participants' stories onto a higher plane, while still retaining a clear connection to the data from which it was derived'.

The purpose and process of grounded theory

Grounded theory, as a research methodology, is popular among nurse and midwifery researchers. Perhaps this is because it is not necessarily focused only on social processes, but has also evolved to explain human action and interaction in clinically related issues of social, psycho-social or spiritual dimensions of life. Grounded theory research, according to the area of interest, tends to concentrate on either the patient primarily, the nurse involved in nurse–patient action and interaction, or both. A good example is the Western Australia-based study by Henderson (2003), who investigated power imbalances between nurses and patients. A further example is Furber and Thomson's (2006), grounded theory study into the 'deviance and good practice' of mother's baby-feeding practices. The direct patient link is not always the case though. Hylton's (2005) New Zealand-based study sought to theorise the experiences of a sample of predominantly Māori enrolled nurses (ENs) — as they made the transition from this role towards full registration within a degree program.

Research in brief

Roach (2004) reports on a grounded theory study of nursing home staff, working in both Australia and Sweden, and their attitudes towards the sexual behaviour of residents. The findings demonstrated that nursing staff's perceptions and behaviours were directly influenced by both the organisational ethos on sexuality and their own level of comfort related to the issue of client sexuality. The conceptual paradigm was termed 'guarding discomfort' and related to the ways that staff guarded themselves against feelings of discomfort.

Strauss and Corbin (1998 p 25) define theorising as 'the act of constructing, from data, an explanatory scheme that systematically integrates various concepts through statements of relationship'. A grounded theory is most likely to be a middle-range theory. That is, more than some working hypotheses used in everyday life — but not an all-inclusive 'grand' theory, beyond the context of human action and interaction (Glaser & Strauss 1967). Grounded theory is also usually context dependent and substantive, where the resultant theory may be about a substantive area (i.e. seeking solutions to a problem). Alternatively, formal theory may be developed from data across various substantive areas about an abstract over-arching issue. Some formal theory development is occurring in health profession research, such as theorising about the process of 'negotiating' in regard to women carers interacting with professionals in helping systems (Wuest 2000).

Research in brief

Wilkins (2006) reports on a grounded theory study of eight primiparous women, aged between 20 and 39 years, who had given birth normally at term to healthy babies. They were exploring the support needs of first-time mothers as part of a journey towards intuitive parenting. The findings revealed the type of journey that these mothers experienced, as they left behind their 'comfortable and controlled' environments where they were 'experts', facing the unknown world of motherhood. 'Doing it right' emerged as the main theme — as the mothers strived to offer optimal care to their babies.

In grounded theory development, according to Strauss and Corbin (1998), there are three levels:
1. description — using language to convey ideas that purport to describe aspects of the action and interaction.
2. conceptual ordering — organising ideas into abstract concepts and grouping (classifying) these into like-groups (categories) and possibly sub-groups (sub-categories) — in order to make sense of action and interaction.
3. an explanatory scheme — offers plausible but contextualised explanatory relationships between the categories (and includes also the levels of description and conceptual ordering).

Some reports of grounded theory research offer conceptual ordering, rather than explanatory scheme grounded theories. Glaser (1999) says this type of research results in 'theory bits' that lead to 'story-talk' or an 'incident trip', rather than an integrated or multivariate theory. Conceptual ordering can, however, usefully inform nurses and midwives about human action and interaction. For instance, to gain basic understanding that builds empathy or that assists in communicating meaningfully with a patient.

It is generally agreed that the framework for a grounded theory is that which is developed from data analysed to form and support the grounded theory. That is, the theoretical framework 'evolves during the research itself' (Strauss & Corbin 1990 p 49). Grounded theory research can be conducted according to a variety of perspectives, but with the primary ones being 'objectivism' and 'constructivism'. Objectivism considers that, as in the natural sciences, there are realities/truths/facts (an object) to be revealed, albeit that in human social science, reality can only be incompletely revealed. Objectivist grounded theory aims to find and uncover what is believed to be 'there' (to be real) about human action and interaction. It seeks to do so rigorously, thus seeking to limit 'bias' using specified technique. The theory is then thought to purely emerge. In contrast, constructivism considers that, in human social science, there are multiple constructed realities that are subject and relative to the opinion of the person experiencing the situation and the person theorising. Constructivist grounded theorists view their research product (theory) as representing one of multiple, intangible realities about what may be happening regarding human action and interaction. The researchers theorising 'lens' is shaped by factors such as culture, political ideology, moral stance, or discourse as conscious or subconscious.

The classic grounded theory method, as formulated and published originally by Glaser and Strauss (1967), has been modified so that there are now multiple versions (e.g. Strauss & Corbin 1998; Charmaz 2000). Different versions primarily reflect different ideas about how data are analysed to the point that a theory results. This said, some other ideas pertaining to the method differ. Most commonly in nursing and midwifery research either classic grounded theory, or the more recent Strauss and Corbin (1990, 1998) version, is used. Reference to Heath and Cowley's (2004) seminal paper, on comparing Glaser and Strauss's versions of grounded theory, will give the reader additional insight and understanding.

While the variety of versions can be frustrating for someone planning a grounded theory research project, this situation provides choice.

It also enhances the possibility of being able to justify analysis and theorisation steps that suit the researcher's own philosophical, cognitive and meaning–making processes. To adopt and adapt the method is common (Glaser 1999). Lastly, it is also important to understand that, although grounded theory research analyses mostly qualitative data, quantitative data can also be collected and analysed. Therefore grounded theory can be viewed as not only a qualitative research method. It is possible to view grounded theory as the methodology that most closely bridges the 'paradigm gap', or continuum, between quantitative and qualitative research (see Chapter 2).

TT Tutorial trigger 4

Referring back to tutorial trigger 1, could you use a grounded theory method to investigate your chosen clinical issue? Would you have to adjust your initial research question?

Point to ponder

▶ Some grounded theory research may not fully construct a theory (as an explanatory theme) but may offer conceptual ordering about human action and interaction process.

Evidence-based practice tip

Grounded theory research may be conducted according to a variety of philosophical perspectives about what can be known, concerning human action and interaction, and how it can be known. Different approaches will provide different outcomes for practice.

Ethnography
Origins and theoretical underpinnings

The term 'ethnography' originates from the Greek 'ethnos' (custom, culture, group) and the Latin 'graphia' (drawing, writing or description). Therefore it is concerned with describing a custom, group or culture. Ethnography, as the descriptive study of cultures, has emerged as a sub-set of anthropological research (the study of humankind) over the years. Brewer (2000) explains that ethnography is not a particular data collection method, but a style of research with the objective to understand the activities and meanings of a social group.

Research in brief

Duke and Street's (2005) Victoria-based study applies a critical ethnographic approach to uncover the tensions and constraints that nurses face, when delivering care in hospital-in-the-home programs that are often under the auspices of acute-care institutions and double up for them. Nurses had their daily practices observed within patients' homes and were then interviewed afterwards. They conclude that there is significant pressure on nurses who practise in these home programs, imposed by acute hospitals who wish to reduce bed-stay occupancy. In turn, this agenda was seen to clash with the professional commitment to provide holistic care.

Inherent in ethnography is the concept of culture. As meaning systems involve relationships that are not universal, different cultural groups (human societies) perceive these relationships and meanings differently. Culture then is knowledge learned, shared and understood by each member of their societal group, so that their interactions and behaviours can be interpreted and understood by its members. Ethnography is considered holistic, in this sense, as it aims to understand the behaviour of a group of people within the context of its own culture. This is achieved by long periods of observation, the gathering of many kinds of data, and employing multiple methods and hypotheses to cover all aspects of forming a picture of the social whole (Fetterman 2000). This is to say that behaviours and events are studied in relation to other factors that may influence or generate the events and behaviours.

Research in brief

Walsh's (2006) study uses ethnography to study the intuitive 'nesting' and 'matresence' behaviours of pregnant mothers, as they assess the suitability of birth centres. They found that the environment invoked a nesting response and a nurturing orientation of 'becoming mother' (matresence). They suggest that the findings challenge maternity services to review traditional conceptualisations of safety in clinical intrapartum care.

> **Points to ponder**
> ► Ethnography allows in-depth inquiry of a phenomenon within its cultural context.
> ► The strength of ethnographic research is in the emic (insider reality/perspective) and etic (outsider reality/perspective) interpretations of phenomena. An ethnographic researcher may have access to both perspectives — depending on their involvement within the culture.

Evidence-based practice tip
Nurses and midwives can employ ethnography to promote relationships, understanding and collaboration with other healthcare professions to enhance teamwork for the benefit of the patient.

The purpose and process of ethnography

Perry et al. (2006), in applying a feminist (see Chapter 2) ethnography with families who have relatives in hospital, state that a central tenet of ethnographic process is that individuals' experiences are socially organised. As such, the researcher examines these experiences and then proceeds to explore how broader social relationships have shaped them. In order to do this all ethnographers have to enter a research site, be it in a community setting or a hospital unit, to conduct their study. The research setting is the 'conceptual field' and the conduct of research in the field is known as 'fieldwork'. The selection of the field depends on the research topic. In many nursing and midwifery examples, the site is chosen on the basis of convenience and/or familiarity. Manias and Street's (2001) study provides a typical Australasian example. Their research on nurse–doctor interactions during ward rounds occurred in a critical care unit because one of the researchers was a staff member of the unit. While some studies require one site for research, there are studies that may require multiple sites. Hanna's (2001) study on teenage motherhood required observations at different sites, because the five teenage mothers she studied were each living on their own.

Points to ponder

▶ Substantial field work is crucial for adequate sampling of people and events over time.

▶ The different types of data gathered in ethnographic research help to provide the richness in description and interpretation.

Evidence-based practice tip

When conducting ethnographic research, the researcher must be theoretically informed. This is needed to either guide the study or to recognise emerging theories for testing, as well as to be able to build on existing theories as they relate to the practice setting.

T_T Tutorial trigger 5

Referring back again to tutorial trigger 1, could you use an ethnographic method to investigate your chosen clinical issue? Would you have to adjust your initial research question?

Other common qualitative methods

The three most common methodologies described above are all categorised in the interpretive tradition of qualitative research (see Chapter 2). There are other less common research methods of note that are relevant to nursing and midwifery research. Two of these are categorised under the heading of critical (social theory)/emancipatory research. The first, feminist research, is already covered in Chapter 2. The second, action research, is covered extensively in Chapter 15 — as a 'mixed-method' design. One other, also comes under the umbrella of mixed-methods research, that of Delphi — which, again, is covered in detail in Chapter 15. This leaves one particular methodology of note (although others will argue that there are several more — beyond the scope of this chapter); that of historical research.

Historical research

Historical research has been used for many years by nursing and midwifery researchers. It has many uses and a number of different forms. Ultimately, however, historical research is most useful when comparing social systems to see what is common across societies, what makes them unique — and in the study of long-term societal change and connections between divergent social factors (Yuginovich 2000). Of course, for many, historical research simply provides the lens by which the past can be viewed, both positive and negative, in relation to current and future events and cycles. It is known that nursing and midwifery practice has been influenced by ongoing, and sometimes repetitive, trends throughout their formation — and that these trends either change or repeat with each new generation (Kirby 2004).

Most health professionals can probably appreciate why, at times, it is a useful exercise to look back at past events in our healthcare history. To do so provides a form of reference whereby we can identify if we have learnt and moved on from past mistakes, are in a position to re-learn, or if it is appropriate to repeat events of the past. In Madsen's (2005) historical analysis of twentieth century untrained nursing staff in a district of Queensland, she states that findings could influence current relationships between professional nurses and others who undertake nursing work. In investigating more recent history, Biedermann et al. (2001) used oral history interviews to explore the wartime experiences of living Australian Army nurses serving in the Vietnam War (1967–1971). While not directly impacting on practice, the findings increase current knowledge on what it is like for nurses working in war environments.

With historical research, data are collected and analysed from a variety of sources. With more recent history, as noted above, this may be from interviews with the living. This could be those directly involved in investigated events or from descendants/relatives of those passed on. More likely, is that the historical reference is from archived written sources; that is, personal/official letters, diaries, journals, reports, documents, meeting minutes, and so forth. For instance, Meehan's (2003) study of the Irish system of 'careful nurses' of the nineteenth century included the study of letters, biographies, diaries and British Crimean War army correspondence. Other forms of historical representations are from the visual arts and might include paintings, drawings, cartoons and photographs. Mander and Marshall (2003) use historical analysis to study seven paintings (from 1550–1676) depicting dead babies, and compare them to recent photographs — noting similarities in depiction. They report that, back at this time and perhaps through such open representations, mothers and families reacted better to such events.

What if the qualitative methodology or method is not identified?

Where researchers do not specify the exact qualitative methodology (theoretical/philosophical framework) that they have adopted in their research, this is not necessarily a problem. Sandelowski (2000 p 334) suggests that, where qualitative researchers do not claim a specific method (research process) this may be because they wish to stay close to their data and to the 'surface of words and events'. This occurs when straight description of phenomena are more important (qualitative description). She argues that qualitative description studies are atypically eclectic but employ reasonable combinations of sampling, data collection, analysis and 're-presentation' techniques (see Chapters 8 and 9). For instance, Gilmour and Huntington's (2005) New Zealand-based study, into patients coping with dementia and memory loss, is reported as adopting a 'qualitative research design'. The absence of methodological detail means that a specific approach cannot be placed. Sheehan et al.'s (2003) study, investigating Australian women's stories of their baby-feeding decisions in pregnancy, does similar. Annells (2007) argues that this form of 'descriptive exploratory' methodology is fast emerging in nursing and midwifery research and could even take over as the most common qualitative approach in the future. Fenwick et al. (2005), in their study on the childbirth expectations of a self-selected cohort of Western Australian women, are 'up-front' in explicitly stating that they use an explorative descriptive design. This descriptive exploratory methodology of qualitative research, and its associated methods, can also be referred to as 'free-form' — as discussed in Chapter 9.

Keeping abreast of qualitative developments

Different interpretations of using and combining common and less common qualitative approaches are emerging, as we look to investigate different clinical issues in different ways. For instance, Maggs-Rapport (2000) argues the case for combining both ethnography and phenomenology in single studies. Similarly, Henderson (2005) sets the scene for combining the methodologies of dramaturgy, ethnomethodology and ethnography. Cutcliffe et al. (2006) recently presented a 'modified' grounded theory study, while Perry et al. (2006) apply a novel approach to feminist ethnography. It is important for the researcher and research consumer to keep abreast of these developments. For the researcher, they too can aim to design and implement new and novel interpretations, where conventional methods appear not to suit.

Summary

In turn, the common qualitative methodologies of phenomenology, grounded theory and ethnography have been explored in this chapter. Other less common, but important, qualitative traditions are also singled out. Each is an important approach in its own right. Appreciation of them all will assist the beginning researcher in deciding which method fits which research task best. Qualitative research represents an historically important mainstay for nursing research. Its place in nursing research is assured and, if anything, is stronger today than at any time previously. This is especially so with the emergence of mixed-methods research (see Chapter 15). Nursing and midwifery have a vested interest in maintaining this qualitative tradition, as they seek to gain the methodological advantage that accompanies the building on and further development of qualitative method, rigour, scope and outcome. The following two chapters explore and describe method-specific design processes as they apply to qualitative research.

KEY POINTS

- The three most common qualitative methods for nursing and midwifery research are phenomenology, grounded theory and ethnography.
- Qualitative research is by nature usually interpretive, emic, naturalistic and holistic.
- Qualitative methods aim to help us understand naturally occurring social phenomena through exploring the attitudes, beliefs, meanings, values and experiences of the research participants.
- Nurse and midwifery researchers and theorists are continually adapting and recontextualising qualitative methods and techniques, as a means to explore new phenomena in new ways.

Learning activities

1. Qualitative research's main aim is to:
   (a) investigate issues that quantitative research is unable to
   (b) understand naturally occurring social phenomena
   (c) include participants in the research
   (d) determine what patients think about nurses.

2. Qualitative research, by its nature, is usually:
   (a) deductive, emic, naturalistic and holistic
   (b) interpretive, etic, naturalistic and holistic
   (c) interpretive, emic, naturalistic and holistic
   (d) deductive, etic, naturalistic and holistic.

3. What is accepted as the main means for understanding others' experience of phenomena?
   (a) numerical data
   (b) language
   (c) observation
   (d) surveys.

4. Husserlian phenomenology is associated with?
   (a) Lebenswelt, epistemology, bracketing, descriptive phenomenology
   (b) Lebenswelt, ontology, bracketing, interpretive phenomenology
   (c) Da-sein, epistemology, bracketing, descriptive phenomenology
   (d) Da-sein, ontology, bracketing, interpretive phenomenology.

5. Heideggerian phenomenology is associated with?
   (a) Lebenswelt, epistemology, descriptive phenomenology
   (b) Lebenswelt, ontology, interpretive phenomenology
   (c) Da-sein, epistemology, descriptive phenomenology
   (d) Da-sein, ontology, interpretive phenomenology.

6. The hermeneutic circle describes:
   (a) the fact that life experiences go around and around
   (b) the fact that life cycles go around and around
   (c) the historical, cultural and personal preconceptions from which understanding is developed
   (d) the process by which all life is understood.

7. Grounded theory aims to:
   (a) develop a well-rounded theory for use in later research
   (b) develop theoretical explanation for socially constructed events and ideally generate hypothesis for further research
   (c) develop a rationale for linking qualitative findings to quantitative findings
   (d) develop theoretical explanation for experimentally constructed events and ideally generate hypothesis for further research.

8. Grounded theory originates from and has been further developed by:
   (a) Strauss and Corbin
   (b) Strauss and Chopin
   (c) Glaser and Corbin
   (d) Glaser and Strauss.

9. Ethnography has its origins in:
   (a) quantitative research
   (b) feminist research
   (c) historical research
   (d) anthropology.

10. Ethnography typically includes:
    (a) the study of cultures, fieldwork, surveys, insider/outsider reality
    (b) the study of cultures, fieldwork, observation, insider/outsider reality
    (c) the study of individuals, fieldwork, observation, insider/outsider reality
    (d) the study of individuals, laboratory work, observation, insider/outsider reality.

Additional resources

Denzin N K, Lincoln Y S 2005 (eds) *The Sage Handbook of Qualitative Research*, 3rd edn. Sage Publications, Thousand Oaks California

Glaser, B (ed.) 1994 *Examples of grounded theory: a reader*. Sociology Press, Mill Valley, California

Grounded Theory Institute (with a focus on facilitating classic grounded theory method). Online. Available: http://www.groundedtheory.com

Koch T 1996 Implementation of a hermeneutic enquiry in nursing: philosophy, rigour and representation. *Journal of Advanced Nursing* 24:174–84

Strauss A 1995 Notes on the nature and development of general theories. *Qualitative Inquiry* 1:7–18

Wood P J, Giddings L S 2005 Understanding experience through Gadamerian hermeneutics: an interview with Brian Phillips. *Nursing Praxis in New Zealand* 21:3–13

Yegdich T 2000 Clinical supervision, death, Heidegger and Freud come 'out of the sighs'. *Journal of Advanced Nursing* 31:953–61

References

Annells M 1999 Evaluating phenomenology: usefulness, quality and philosophical foundations. *Nurse Researcher* 6:5–19

—— 2007 What's common with qualitative nursing research these days? (guest editorial). *Journal of Clinical Nursing* 16(2):223–4

Barkway P 2001 Michael Crotty and nursing phenomenology: criticism or critique? *Nursing Inquiry* 8:191–5

Biedermann N, Usher K, William A, Hayes B 2001 The wartime experiences of Australian Army nurses in Vietnam, 1967–1971. *Journal of Advanced Nursing* 35:543–9

Blackburn S 1994 *The Oxford Dictionary of Philosophy*. Oxford University Press, Oxford

Brewer J D 2000 *Ethnography*. Open University Press, Buckingham

Charmaz K 2000 Grounded theory: objectivist and constructivist methods. In: Denzin N, Lincoln Y (eds) *Handbook of qualitative research*, 2nd edn. Sage Publications, Thousand Oaks, California

Cheung J, Hocking P 2004 Caring as worrying: the experience of spousal carers. *Journal of Advanced Nursing* 47:475–82

Colaizzi P 1978 Psychological research as a phenomenologist views it. In: Valle R S, King M (eds) *Existential phenomenological alternatives for psychology*. Oxford University Press, New York

Corbin J, Strauss A 1996 Analytic ordering for theoretical purposes. *Qualitative Inquiry* 2(2):139–50

—— 1990 Grounded theory research: procedures, canons, and evaluative criteria. *Qualitative Sociology* 13(1):3–21

Crotty M 1996 *Phenomenology and Nursing Research*. Churchill Livingstone, Melbourne

Cutcliffe J R, Stevenson C, Jackson S, et al. 2006 A modified grounded theory study of how psychiatric nurses work with suicidal people. *International Journal of Nursing Studies* (in press)

Dahlberg K, Drew N, Nyström M 2001 *Reflective Life World Research*. Lund, Sweden

Dowling M 2006 From Husserl to van Manen: a review of different phenomenological approaches. *International Journal of Nursing Studies* (in press)

Duke M, Street A 2005 Tensions and constraints for nurses in hospital-in-the-home programmes. *International Journal of Nursing Practice* 11:221–7

Erlandsson K, Fagerberg I 2005 Mothers' lived experiences of co-care and post-care after birth, and their strong desire to be close to their baby. *Midwifery* 21:131–8

Fenwick J, Hauck Y, Downie J, et al. 2005 The childbirth expectations of a self-selected cohort of Western Australian women. *Midwifery* 21:23–35

Fetterman D M 2000 *Ethnography: step by step*, 2nd edn. Sage Publications, Newbury Park

Furber C M, Thomson A M 2006 'Breaking the rules' in baby-feeding practice in the UK: deviance and good practice? *Midwifery* 22:365–76

Gadamer H G 1976 *Truth and Method*, 2nd edn. Sheed & Ware, London

Gilmour J A, Huntington A D 2005 Finding the balance: living with memory loss. *International Journal of Nursing Practice* 11:118–24

Giorgi A 1997 The theoretical practice and evaluation of the phenomenological method as a qualitative research procedure. *Journal of Phenomenological Psychology* 28:235–60

Glaser B 1999 The future of grounded theory. *Qualitative Health Research* 9(6):836–45

Glaser B, Strauss A 1967 *The discovery of grounded theory: strategies for qualitative research*. Aldine, New York

Hanna B 2001 Negotiating motherhood: the struggles of teenage mothers. *Journal of Advanced Nursing* 34(4):456–64

Heath H, Cowley S 2004 Developing a grounded theory approach: a comparison of Glaser and Strauss. *International Journal of Nursing Studies* 41:141–50

Heidegger M 1962 *Being and Time*. (Macquarie J & Robinson E, trans), Blackwell, Oxford (original work published 1927)

Henderson A 2005 The value of integrating interpretive research approaches in the exposition of healthcare context. *Journal of Advanced Nursing* 52:554–60

Henderson S 2003 Power imbalance between nurses and patients: a potential inhibitor of partnership in care. *Journal of Clinical Nursing* 12:501–8

Hylton J A 2005 Relearning how to learn: Enrolled nurse transition to degree at a New Zealand rural satellite campus. *Nurse Education Today* 25:519–26

Johnson P, St John W, Moyle W 2006 Long-term mechanical ventilation in a critical care unit: existing in an uneveryday world. *Journal of Advanced Nursing* 53:551–8

Kirby S 2004 A historical perspective on the contrasting experiences of nurses as research subjects and research activists. *International Journal of Nursing Practice* 10:272–9

Koivisto K, Janhonen S, Väisänen L 2002 Applying a phenomenological method of analysis derived from Giorgi to a psychiatric nursing study. *Journal of Advanced Nursing* 39:258–65

Kvigne K, Kirkevold M, Gjengedal E 2005 The nature of nursing care and rehabilitation of female stroke survivors: the perspective of hospital nurses. *Journal of Clinical Nursing* 14:897–905

Mackey S 2005 Phenomenological nursing research: methodological insights derived from Heidegger's interpretive phenomenology. *International Journal of Nursing Studies* 42:179–86

Madsen W 2005 Early 20th century untrained nursing staff in the Rockhampton district: a necessary evil? *Journal of Advanced Nursing* 51:307–13

Maggs-Rapport F 2000 Combining methodological approaches in research: ethnography and interpretive phenomenology. *Journal of Advanced Nursing* 31:219–25

Mander R, Marshall R K 2003 An historical analysis of the role of paintings and photographs in comforting bereaved parents. *Midwifery* 19:230–42

Manias E, Street A 2001 Rethinking ethnography: reconstructing nursing relationships. *Journal of Advanced Nursing* 33:234–42

Meehan T C 2003 Careful nursing: a model for contemporary nursing practice. *Journal of Advanced Nursing* 44:99–107

Mills J, Bonner A, Francis K 2006 Adopting a constructivist approach to grounded theory: implications for research design. *International Journal of Nursing Practice* 12:8–13

Neill S J 2006 Grounded theory sampling: the contribution of reflexivity. *Journal of Research in Nursing* 11:253–60

O'Brien L 2001 The relationship between community psychiatric nurses and clients with severe and persistent mental illness: the client's experience. *Australian and New Zealand Journal of Mental Health Nursing* 10:176–86

Paley J 1998 Misinterpretive phenomenology: Heidegger, ontology and nursing research. *Journal of Advanced Nursing* 27:817–24

Perry J, Lynham M J, Anderson J M 2006 Resisting vulnerability: the experiences of families who have kin in hospital — a feminist ethnography. *International Journal of Nursing Studies* 43:173–84

Pyett P M 2003 Validation of qualitative research in the 'real world'. *Qualitative Health Research* 13:1170–9

Roach S M 2004 Sexual behaviour of nursing home residents: staff perceptions and responses. *Journal of Advanced Nursing* 48:371–9

Sadala M L A, Adorno R-C F 2002 Phenomenology as a method to investigate the experience lived: a perspective from Husserl and Merleau Ponty's thought. *Journal of Advanced Nursing* 37:282–93

Sandelowski M 2000 Whatever happened to qualitative description? *Research in Nursing & Health* 23:334–40

—— 2004 Using qualitative research. *Qualitative Health Research* 14:1366–86

Sheehan A, Schmeid V, Cooke M 2003 Australian women's stories of their baby-feeding decisions in pregnancy. *Midwifery* 19:259–66

Strauss A, Corbin J 1990 Basics of qualitative research: grounded theory procedures and techniques. Sage Publications, Newbury Park

—— 1998 *Basics of qualitative research: techniques and procedures for developing grounded theory*, 2nd edn. Sage Publications, Thousand Oaks, California

Todres L, Wheeler S 2001 The complementarity of phenomenology, hermeneutics and existentialism as a philosophical perspective for nursing research. *International Journal of Nursing Studies* 38:1–8

Turner S 2005 Hope seen through the eyes of 10 Australian young people. *Journal of Advanced Nursing* 52:508–17

van Manen M 1984 Practicing phenomenological writing. *Phenomenology & Pedagogy* 2(1):36–69

Walsh D J 2006 'Nesting' and Matresence' as distinctive features of a free-standing birth centre in the UK *Midwifery* 22:228–39

Whitehead D 2002a The academic writing experiences of a group of student nurses: a phenomenological study. *Journal of Advanced Nursing* 38:498–506

—— 2002b The 'health promotional' role of a pre-registration student cohort in the UK: a grounded theory study. *Nurse Education in Practice* 2:197–207

Wilkins K 2006 A qualitative study exploring the support needs of first-time mothers on their journey towards intuitive parenting. *Midwifery* 22:169–80

Wood P J, Giddings L S 2005 Understanding experience through Gadamerian hermeneutics: an interview with Brian Phillips. *Nursing Praxis in New Zealand* 21:3–13

Wuest J 2000 Negotiating with helping systems: an example of grounded theory evolving through emergent fit. *Qualitative Health Research* 10(1):51–70

Yuginovich T 2000 More than time and place: using historical comparative research as a tool for nursing. *International Journal of Nursing Practice* 6:70–5

Answers

TT Tutorial triggers 1 and 2

Personal observation/experience exercise, not requiring suggested answers.

TT Tutorial trigger 3

- Does this study reflect a phenomenological view of persons and their worlds? Are the

participants seen as able to reflect on their experience of the phenomenon and to develop shared meaning with another?
- Does the researcher describe their own experience and perspective of the phenomenon?
- Is the context of the phenomenon and of the participants described in sufficient detail so that the reader can identify similarities and uniqueness in how the phenomenon might be experienced?
- Are the process and the content of the interview described in narrative?
- Does the analysis of the data (language) focus on the meaning of the experience of the phenomena?
- Does the researcher bring together the background understanding of the phenomenon from multiple sources; their own understandings and that of the participants?
- Do the identified themes provide a way of understanding the meaning of the experience for the participants?
- Are the findings discussed in light of their implications?
- Are the findings discussed in light of phenomenological understandings of what it means to be a person in the world?

TT Tutorial triggers 4 and 5

Personal observation/experience exercise, not requiring suggested answers.

Learning activities

1. b	**2.** c	**3.** b	**4.** a
5. d	**6.** c	**7.** b	**8.** d
9. d	**10.** b		

Sampling data and data collection in qualitative research

DEAN WHITEHEAD AND MERILYN ANNELLS

Learning outcomes

After reading this chapter, you should be able to:

- describe the rationale and processes for conducting qualitative sampling techniques
- identify the main methods and modes by which data are collected in qualitative research
- examine the process of qualitative interviewing
- identify the nature of focus groups
- examine the process of qualitative observation
- explain the benefits and limitations of qualitative data collection methods
- describe the notion of mixed method applied to qualitative data collection
- denote qualitative data collection methods other than interview and observation.

Introduction

An integral part of the qualitative research process lies in determining and choosing appropriate examples of populations to study (sample/s). Directly leading on from this process, called 'sampling', the next step in the research process is to collect information (data) from the chosen sample or population — ready for data analysis. These research stages are very closely interrelated. Therefore, any error in one will subsequently impact on the other. There are many different ways of conducting these stages and so this chapter examines, in turn, the rationale and processes for the first two steps (sampling and data collection). The following chapter details the data analysis stage.

Sampling techniques and procedures in qualitative research

Usually, the primary purpose of sampling is the selection of suitable events that require recruitment of participants or items. Sampling then, in qualitative research, is the process of choosing suitable 'units' of interest, so that the focus of the study can be adequately researched. Most qualitative research uses participants (humans) as its sample material. In some studies, sampling will involve a combination of sample types — such as with those involving both participants and items (documents, records, reports, letters, diaries, photographs etc). Other times only items may be selected. This is often the case in historical research (see Chapter 7). Potential participants, in historical research, may no longer be alive, so the researcher tries to gather accounts, recollections and experiences from existing formal and/or personal records or documents. For instance, the case of a study of the historical background of untrained nursing services in the Rockhampton (Queensland) district in the early twentieth century. In this study, Madsen (2005) extracted qualitative data from samples of local government and council records, nurse registration records, hospital committee records and minutes of professional nursing organisation bodies. A sample chosen for a qualitative research study, then, usually contains:

- examples of a specific population of people (e.g. for phenomenological research)
- examples of items, such as minutes of meetings, reports, letters etc (e.g. for historical research)

- a combination of both, where specific events such as population incidents, situations and interactions are complemented with the types of items described above (e.g. for grounded theory research).

TT Tutorial trigger 1

You want to explore the experiences of carers who care for relatives with cancer. What initial considerations might you need to identify in relation to choosing an appropriate participant sample?

In qualitative research, effective sample selection process is very important because inappropriate procedures may jeopardise the integrity, findings and outcomes of a project. However, unlike quantitative research sampling, there are no rigid or established rules for deciding on the 'best' sample size or method. Sample sizes also differ from quantitative samples in that they are usually much smaller in comparison. Despite this, rigour in qualitative sampling is still very important. It still requires the researcher to know how to appropriately and proportionally select participants, or items, that could have been chosen overall. There are a number of ways that sampling can be approached and the choice of qualitative research design will often guide the process. Higginbottom (2004) and Tuckett (2004) both provide useful critical commentary on the processes of qualitative sampling, as they relate to different study designs and procedures.

Types of sampling

Sampling in qualitative research is *non-probability* sampling, in that the participants or items are chosen in a non-random manner.

Therefore, the probability of a participant being chosen for the sample is not known by the potential participant. There are four main types of qualitative sampling: convenience sampling, purposive sampling, snowball sampling and theoretical sampling. *Convenience* sampling occurs when people are selected because they are conveniently (opportunistically) available with regard to access, location, time and willingness. They also all meet predetermined criteria for inclusion in a study (see later in this chapter under 'inclusion and exclusion criteria').

Research in brief

French (2005) uses a convenience sample of specialist nurses to help construct evidence-based policy recommendations for evaluating research use in practice. The specialist nurses were divided into different groups and drawn together for a series of 'clinical workshops' at a local university. Three frames of reference/ evaluative criteria, for decisions related to evaluating research in practice, were identified: the research task and fit of the task (including relevance, effectiveness, quality, practicality, effort and impact); feasibility and fit with the *status quo*; and availability of nursing control and feedback from practice.

Purposive (purposeful) sampling provides information-rich cases for in-depth study. Sometimes referred to as judgment sampling, purposive sampling occurs when the researcher selects people who have the required status or experience or are endowed with special knowledge, to provide the researcher with the vital information they seek. For example, Leung et al. (2005) use a purposive sample of 11 postpartum-depressed Hong Kong Chinese mothers to investigate the lived experience of postpartum stress from the perspective of the depressed mother. Even with this brief synopsis, it is not difficult to ascertain that this purposive sample would need to include participants who were exclusively of Chinese origin, living in Hong Kong, who had recently given birth, and were suffering the effects of postpartum depression.

Snowball sampling occurs when the researcher starts gathering information from a few people and then relies on these people to put the researcher in touch with others who may be friends, relatives, colleagues or other significant contacts. This method of sampling is also referred to as networking. This type of sampling is especially useful where the sample is representative of marginalised or stigmatised individuals. As such, they may normally be reluctant to come forward without the reassurance of knowing someone who has already participated in the study. Sometimes though, research ethics committees may not grant permission for snowball sampling because of either privacy concerns, issues of consent, or the potential for coercion — depending on the type of snowball sampling proposed for a study. Streeton et al. (2004) provide useful discussion on the issues and dilemmas of specific snowball recruitment technique.

Research in brief

Jackson and Mannix (2004) set out to investigate the emotive topic of 'mother-blaming' from the feminist perspective (see Chapter 2) of those who had experienced this phenomenon. Three participants were recruited initially via a women's email network. Following this initial recruitment, a snowball sampling method recruited a further 17 volunteers. Problems of recruiting participants to this study, using other than a snowball technique, are highlighted in the fact that the findings showed that the investigated mother-blaming issue was perpetuated by inappropriate scrutiny from health professionals.

Theoretical sampling is mostly used in grounded theory studies, but is increasingly being used in some modes of qualitative descriptive exploratory studies. It is sampling that occurs sequentially and in tandem with data analysis, when previously analysed data guide what data need to be collected next and where to seek the additional data (see Chapter 9). The first selected events, participants or items, from which initial data are collected, are usually purposively chosen or conveniently available.

TT Tutorial trigger 2

In your tutorial group, if you wanted to explore the phenomenon of client-centred care, which sampling technique would/could you choose? What overall considerations are necessary before making your final choice? What differences emerge between group members and are there any differences based on wanting to explore different aspects of client-centred care?

Inclusion and exclusion criteria

To be suitable for inclusion in a study, sample populations or items usually need to possess specific characteristics and meet certain requirements. These preselected criteria are commonly referred to as *inclusion criteria*. Sometimes *exclusion* (delimitations) *criteria* will also be stipulated, where participant attributes or characteristics are not appropriate for inclusion. Both sets of criteria commonly centre on issues such as age, gender, culture, type of disease, nature of event, or health status. Some criteria may be reasonably assumed and need not be stated, as for the example of not mentioning men in the sample of most midwifery-related studies. This is unless, of course, the researcher wants to study the experiences of fathers-to-be or male midwives. If this were the case, a different and specific set of inclusion/exclusion criteria would need to be identified.

TT Tutorial trigger 3

You intend to research the perceptions of patients with in-dwelling catheters. What might you decide in terms of inclusion/exclusion criteria?

The selection of research participants

In qualitative research, participants are viewed as self-interpreting beings able to reflect upon and articulate their experiences, values, beliefs and opinions. Different qualitative approaches have varying sampling intentions regarding participants. Participants in phenomenological studies, for instance, are chosen because of their experience of the phenomenon being studied and because of their ability to articulate that experience. In grounded theory, because samples of events and incidents involving action or interaction relevant to the research focus are sought, participants must have been or are currently involved in those events. With

ethnographic research the researcher is in the 'field', observing and recording the events and behaviours of participants, where situations and people are either selected or rejected for observation. Therefore, ethnographers engage in a variety of sampling procedures because they are sampling time, people and the context of an observed and recorded situation.

What size sample is required?

Unlike quantitative approaches, which aim to establish statistical significance by sampling a predetermined number of units of interest, qualitative researchers do not usually begin a project with a predetermined sample size. There are no overall formal criteria for determining sample sizes and, therefore, no rules to suggest when a sample size is small or large enough for the task at hand. Essentially, in a qualitative study, the 'richness' of data collected is far more important than the number of participants. This said, the researcher still requires insight to the size most likely to accommodate this required richness. As Patton (2002) states, the sample size in qualitative research should be judged in context and decided on the basis of study rationale and purpose.

Some qualitative research methods have suggested ways of establishing sample size suitability at some point in the research process; that is, such as when data become theoretically saturated or when no new information is being gained (see Chapter 9). Regarding the number of participants in qualitative studies, a common range is usually somewhere from 8 to 15 participants, but can widely vary both inside and outside this range. It is possible to have only one participant, if this can be justified, as for some case study designs (see Chapter 15). On the other hand, quite a large number of participants may be involved. For instance, Crowe et al.'s (2001) New Zealand-based qualitative study accessed 131 community-based client participants, in order to evaluate consumer mental health service provision. With *focus groups* (group interviews), discussed later in this chapter, the overall number will be higher — especially where more than one group is needed for comparison between groups. Check et al.'s (2005) South Australian study, for instance, used 14 different stakeholder focus groups to investigate factors that influenced the decisions of older people living in independent units. Small samples, however, are far more manageable because of the sheer amount of potentially rich and detailed data that can be generated from each single participant.

> ### Point to ponder
> ▶ Without accurate and appropriate sampling procedures, qualitative studies are significantly affected in terms of representativeness, quality and accuracy.

● **Evidence-based practice tip**
When sampling, ensure that steps within a sampling plan include identifying the target population, delineating the population, key characteristics of the population, identifying eligibility criteria, recruitment structures, highlighting possible weaknesses, and sample size justification.

Data collection in qualitative research

As suggested, in the introduction of this chapter, the process of data collection is directly related to the previous stage of sampling. The linked activities are best viewed as complementary. Data (information), therefore, are collected directly from the identified and selected sample population. Data collected from the sample can be either direct data or indirect data. *Direct data* include recordable spoken or written words and also observable body language, actions and interactions. Here, the interactions may be human-to-human, or human responses to inanimate objects such as a haemodialysis machine. Whatever can be observed or communicated are considered to be potential or actual data. This will occur when considering the thoughts, feelings, experiences, meaning of experience, responses, actions, interactions, language and processes of individuals and groups within their social and/or cultural setting. It is this type of data that sets the 'context' of qualitative studies. *Indirect data* are generated initially by some other person or people, such as with documents or photographs reporting an event or an artistic rendition of an event or experience (e.g. novels, songs, paintings, poems). Turner (2005) used photographs, taken by the Australian youth study participants to depict their interpretations and experiences of hope, as a means of collecting indirect data. Direct data though are the most common form in qualitative research.

Depending on the types of data required for a qualitative study, various methods of collecting data can be used singularly or in combination to generate direct data. These methods may include interview, observation, open-ended questionnaire, journaling, or 'think aloud' sessions. Manias et al. (2005) use both interview and observational techniques to gather qualitative data, related to Australian nurses' communication with health professionals when managing patients' medications. Where indirect data need to be collected, these are sought through a variety of methods. These may include systematically searching archives or trawling through the internet — with data collected being either in hard copy form or electronic (see Chapter 3). Direct data can be collected by the participant involved in a study at the request of the researcher (e.g. through writing a personal journal or diary) and then provided to the researcher. Most commonly, however, qualitative approaches acquire data primarily through interpersonal contact with participants (usually an interview) or, secondly, through the presence of the researcher in proximity to pertinent events (usually observation). This is unlike quantitative research where, frequently, there is no interpersonal contact with participants or events. Casey (2006) offers a useful rendition of her experiences in deciding on the most appropriate method of data collection, for her nursing-related health promotion study.

Interviews

Interviews are regarded as the prime method for qualitative data collection; also representing the most common method for gathering qualitative data in nursing-related research (Borbasi et al. 2005). 'Oral narrative', therefore, is the basis of most qualitative research text. There is even a form of research that is devoted to just this form, *narrative research* (Overcash 2004). Narrative is most often gained through a direct encounter between researcher and participant (or occasionally several participants) in in-depth interviews or in group interviews called 'focus groups' (Lane et al. 2001). Scheduled telephone interviews, interviews via email, or non-scheduled informal 'on-the-spot' interviews (chats) may also be used.

Interviews may be unstructured, semi-structured or occasionally structured. With *unstructured* interviews, questions are not preselected and, therefore, this represents the most conversational interview style. The fact that the outcome of the interview is unknown and could follow any possible direction also makes it the most 'free-form' style of interviewing. Turner (2005 p 510) describes the unstructured interviews of Australian youths as 'a free-flowing conversation with a definite focal point'. Most researchers though will conduct unstructured interviews with some idea of the sort of questions that are most appropriate for the study. *Semi-structured* interviews have an interview guide providing some possible questions or topics for discussion. This said, there is freedom to ask any questions in any order, following tangents or seeking clarification of previous answers. Allen and Fabri's (2005) qualitative evaluation of a community aged-care nurse practitioner service, in Victoria, uses semi-structured interviews to elicit data. In both unstructured and semi-structured interviews, questions are non-directive, mainly open-ended, and are designed to trigger and stimulate the participant to talk about the focus of the research. *Structured* interviews follow a list of set questions, usually asked in a certain order, but these questions are still open-ended in qualitative research. This distinguishes them from structured quantitative interviews, which usually only ask closed-ended questions. With *focus group interviews*, the researcher gathers the informants together to engage in dialogue with each other. This means that a unique discussion format is operative.

TT Tutorial trigger 4

Devise an interview schedule for investigating the experiences of clients who have an in-dwelling catheter. What sort of things might you want to ask and know of your participants?

Conducting interviews

The structure and conduct of the interview are important, as a poor interview will yield poor quality narrative data and poor outcomes overall. Conducting interviews is a complex, demanding and exact skill that requires due attention to process and, preferably, prior training. It is unwise to conduct research interviews in terms of 'learn as you go' although the extent to which such training is offered or available to most nurses is often patchy, debatable or unknown. In the absence of structured training, the less desirable options of piloting or performing 'dry or dummy runs' with peers and/or colleagues may compensate to a certain degree.

Where novice or experienced researchers are appropriately equipped to conduct interviews in the clinical setting, certain prerequisites will nearly always need to be in place. A warm and non-judgmental demeanour towards the participant/s should be established and maintained throughout. Questions asked should be balanced, unbiased, non-threatening, sensitive and clear. The majority of interviews conducted in qualitative research are audio-recorded or, less commonly, video-recorded. In Fenwick et al.'s (2005) study, they completely tape-recorded telephone interviews of a self-selected cohort of Western Australian women, experiencing childbirth. Annells (2006), however, chose to video-record interviews for her Australian hermeneutic phenomenology study on the experience of flatus incontinence by people with bowel ostomies. Both of these formats have an advantage over handwritten notes, because it is often impossible to record everything one hears or to observe everything that occurs in an interview situation.

In the interview process, the participant needs to be made to feel as comfortable as possible. It is necessary to ensure adequate privacy and comfort and ensure that all items required for the encounter are available; for example, recording equipment, tapes, consent forms, participant information sheets, tissues and beverages. Researchers should take proactive steps, such as posting 'do not disturb' signs, and disabling telephone or pager devices. This will help to ensure that interruptions are avoided. Appropriate time should be allowed for each interview. Interviews should not be hurried or stopped before they have naturally completed. If, however, the participant wishes to terminate the interview, or the researcher senses that the participant is becoming too tired or distressed, then the interview can be stopped or paused at any time. This may mean setting up a new appointment for another occasion. It is, however, preferable to resume as soon as possible so that flow and recall of previous discussion is not lost. It is recommended that no single interview last more than 1–2 hours as interview fatigue is otherwise likely to occur.

TT Tutorial trigger 5

What are the features of a 'conducive' environment for the conduct of interviews in qualitative research?

During an interview, appropriate responsiveness is required. It should be remembered that the purpose is to gain information from the participant — and not an opportunity for the researcher to express their own thoughts and feelings. In a structured or semi-structured interview, an appropriate range of questions is asked, as perhaps listed on interview guidelines. The purpose of these lists of questions is to provide clarity and assist the participant if stuck or confused. Questions may also be used to prompt expansion and elaboration if further detail is required. An active listening stance is adopted, concentrating on what is being said as well as being alert to other cues; particularly non-verbal cues. The participant is encouraged to be reflective. Soon after, or during the interview, some researchers find it useful to record (memoing) non-verbal aspects of the encounters with participants. Alongside this, they may well note and review their own thoughts and feelings about the interview and any 'extraordinary' situations or events that arise. The memos may then assist later data analysis (see Chapter 9).

Qualitative interviews should allow the interviewee to speak freely and elicit in-depth, lengthy responses through employment of facilitative techniques used singularly or in combination. Possible techniques include:

- Funnelling — beginning the interview with general and broad opening questions and then narrowing down to topic specifics as the interview progresses.
- Story-telling — asking questions in a manner which encourages story-telling and more elaborate answers, for example, 'Tell me about …'
- Probing — eliciting further details or seeking clarification. Price (2002) details an innovative probing technique called 'laddered questions'. This is where appropriate questions are asked in a series leading from the least intrusive questions to the most intrusive. This technique identifies classifications of questions; questions about 'actions' are deemed to be the least invasive, through to questions about 'philosophy' (feelings/values/beliefs) as the most invasive.
- Paraphrasing — where repeating what the participant has said, without changing the meaning of what has been said, facilitates understanding and clarity and acts as a further prompt.

Research in brief

Wynaden et al. (2005) use semi-structured interviews to ask open-ended questions of prominent Western Australian-based Asian community members and Asian healthcare professionals. They were seeking to gain insight into the factors that influenced Asian communities' access to mental healthcare services. The interviews used a form of funnelling; starting with a broad question and then becoming increasingly focused as interviews progressed. Their findings showed that members of the localised Asian population were unwilling to access such services, due to cultural beliefs and associated notions of shame and stigma.

Benefits of interviews

Interviews provide the researcher with a valuable opportunity to enter the world of the participant and reflect on a particular event. Rapport and trust can be developed and are desirable to facilitate the yield of 'rich', extensive, detailed and pertinent data. Interviews should evolve as conversational encounters that offer useful opportunities to clarify issues, as well as probe for ever-deeper insight. Interviews also offer unique data, where interview outcomes will never be exactly the same between participants. Also, particularly with emotional and emotive issues, the interviewer is able to offer appropriate support and referral to counselling if the need exists or arises. Overall then, qualitative interviews potentially offer a productive, meaningful and supportive facility for both researcher and participants.

Limitations of interviews

Price (2002) identifies a range of challenges when it comes to interviewing, such as securing access, making sensitive records, managing power relationships, managing 'space', managing communication, and managing sequelae of interviews. Interviews are not so much limited by techniques and methods used, but mostly by how these are applied by the researcher. Ethically, interview schedules should be challenged if there are questions which are seemingly biased, leading, unbalanced, emotive, imposing, coercive, manipulating or threatening. Therefore, the potential for an increased imbalance in the power relationship between interviewer and interviewee should be avoided although, even in collaborative research designs that are well executed, some degree of power differential will always exist in an interview situation.

Interviews can be time-consuming and resource-intensive to establish; in particular, focus group sessions. Although in qualitative research estimation can be made about how many interviews may be necessary to gather a 'complete' set of data, this is not always correct. Also, limiting data collection to 'one-off' interviews with participants may lead to insufficient in-depth information. The interviewer (despite any effort to 'bracket' out their own experiences, ideas, prejudices and opinions prior to the interview) is always partly generating data as well as the interviewee, so the resultant data will inevitably be partly influenced by the interviewer, whether this is through subtle body language or the nature of questions asked. This can be a problem if an objective approach is being used for the study, although this may not be the case for subjective approaches.

Focus group interviews

Focus groups are useful as they help to explore, develop and refine initial research questions and interview schedules. They can also be useful as part of an illuminative evaluative framework to assess client needs and the outcomes of such investigation (Banning 2005). Focus groups use interview schedules but these differ in scope, nature and intention from other research interviews. This is because of the unique nature of group dynamics and insights gained from interaction between participants. Focus groups offer a collective set of values, experiences and observations of participants that are later interpreted in context. Sometimes group synergy or consensus on issues occurs, but this is not always the case. If a series of focus groups are scheduled, initial interviews usually identify broad factors and perspectives related to the focus of the study, while subsequent interviews seek to prioritise and narrow down generated issues. In Newton and McKenna's (in press) study of the transitional journey of Australian new graduate nurses, they used four different location focus groups and conducted three interviews for each group at regular intervals over an 18-month transition period, in order to narrow down their generated issues.

Focus group interviews are usually more economical to conduct than individual interviews. They may not, however, explore issues as deeply as one-on-one interviews, nor do they tend to expose sensitive or potentially embarrassing information. Researchers generally need quite high levels of interviewing expertise to conduct focus group interviews. For instance, they require 'gate-keeping' skills to help avoid 'group think' outcomes, prevent any individuals from monopolising conversations, as well as teasing contributions from quieter members.

● **Evidence-based practice tip**
Focus groups can be used as a preliminary means of identifying an appropriate research question/issue and/or an appropriate interview schedule for conducting later one-on-one interviews. The focus groups, in this case, act as a means of identification, verification and consensus between a whole range of participants.

Research in brief

Hylton (2005) reports on the New Zealand study that uses focus groups to explore the factors that enhanced or hindered the transition of predominantly Māori enrolled nurses as they progressed through an enrolled nurse to degree program. There were two focus groups (ten students in one and six teachers in another) with each group interviewed separately on two occasions. The focus of this article is centred on the major category to emerge; this being 'relearning how to learn'.

Observation

Observational methods are commonly used in qualitative research designs and may vary between modes. Observation is the process of watching the daily life and behaviours of participants, in their natural setting, in order to record aspects such as social position and function, or actions and interactions. Qualitative observation is conventionally the domain of ethnographers (Borbasi et al. 2005), but is also used in other qualitative approaches. This is especially so with those conducted within an interpretive/constructivist paradigm (see Chapter 2) — where exploring context is often used to interpret and understand behaviour (Mulhall 2003).

In qualitative research, observation methods are mostly unstructured. Here, the researcher enters the 'field' with no predetermined notion or schedule, as to what they may or may not see or hear. Sometimes, however, qualitative observation may have some structure. For instance, observers in a ward or clinic may focus observation on a certain phenomenon of interest, such as episodes of violence or acute hospital admissions. In an example, Zeitz (2005) observed (as a 'non-participant' observer) a total of 81 South Australian post-operative patients, for 282 patient hours, to identify what constituted postoperative nursing monitoring.

Process of observation

Methods of observation range across a continuum from participation to observation where four distinct roles of participation and observation can be distinguished. These being: complete participant, participant-as-observer; observer-as-participant; and complete observer. These roles can also be adopted in quantitative research and are further discussed in Chapter 12. Differences in observer roles revolve around the degree of researcher involvement (intervention) or detachment (concealment) with participants (see Figure 8.1).

In the situation of *complete participation*, the researcher is a functioning member of the community (or group) under observation. Complete participation gives the researcher the best opportunity to observe behaviours as the researcher is integrated into the community. Most anthropological studies use this technique as the researcher is already a member of the community or attempts to be invited into, and ultimately be accepted, by the community. Often it is not known by the community that

FIGURE 8.1 Different roles of the observer in observational research

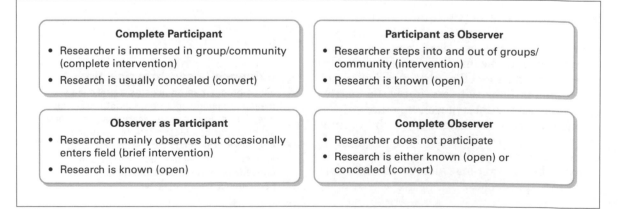

Complete Participant
- Researcher is immersed in group/community (complete intervention)
- Research is usually concealed (convert)

Participant as Observer
- Researcher steps into and out of groups/community (intervention)
- Research is known (open)

Observer as Participant
- Researcher mainly observes but occasionally enters field (brief intervention)
- Research is known (open)

Complete Observer
- Researcher does not participate
- Research is either known (open) or concealed (convert)

the participant observer is a researcher (a form of concealment).

In a *participant-as-observer* role, the researcher is acting as both participant and observer with this openness allowing productive relationships to develop with informants, and also to step in and out of the research environment at will. When an *observer-as-participant*, the researcher's role is made public and the researcher is first an observer with participation a secondary concern. The close relations denoted by a pure participation role, however, are more difficult to establish in this role. As a *complete observer*, a researcher is confined to observations only and offers no interaction with participants. The research may or may not be revealed, but there are major ethical implications for not revealing to people that they are being observed for research purposes and so examples, not just in nursing, are rare. Sometimes, it may be planned that participants are informed instead after the research has been conducted, but this is still usually not an adequate premise for ethical approval to be gained for such a study.

Research in brief

Walsh (2006) utilises a mixture of both observer-as-participant and complete observer (depending on whether he was dealing with colleagues or clients), in his ethnographic study of a free-standing birth centre. In the first instance, he would find himself informally chatting to the women and families and making field-tape recordings. In the other instance (complete observer), as he was not employed by the birth centre, he simply 'hung out there, shadowing the staff as they went about their daily work' (pp 229–30).

A further aspect of observation is in the positioning approach that the observer adopts. These are classified as single, multiple and mobile (Casey 2006). In single positioning, the observer occupies one location only. They are less likely to distract or be distracted. Multiple positioning allows the observer to move to different locations and view events from different angles/perspectives. Mobile positioning is needed in situations where the observer must follow participants as they go about daily activities.

TT Tutorial trigger 6

Devise an observation schedule for observing chronically ill children on a paediatric ward. What type of observer/participant role/s would you employ? What might you expect to observe? Following this, observe your tutorial group and do a similar exercise — but for investigating something to do with your group, such as peer interaction and relationships.

Benefits of observation

Mulhall (2003) suggests that observation has several advantages for qualitative research. These being: capturing data in more natural circumstances, capturing the whole social setting and context of the environment in which people function, and informing about influences of the immediate physical environment. Depending on the observation method used there is opportunity to interact with participants, while gaining rich data and perspectives based on values and experiences. Where the researcher is also a participant, observation allows them to reflect on and evaluate their own perspectives about their experiences in the field. In this case, researchers can choose to either step back from or be immersed in situations. Observation also enables consideration of social and organisational practices, as well as of the research endeavour itself. Therefore, such as with critical paradigm research and through communicative practices and reflection, both the researcher and participants collaboratively discern an 'absolute truth' of the culture investigated (Manias & Street 2001).

Limitations of observation

If researching from an objectivist stance, it is necessary to be aware of Mulhall's (2003) caution that observation is more prone to subjective interpretation by the researcher than is usually the case with interview data. Field notes are often written up following the observation event, potentially adding to the subjectivity of data. However, neither of these aspects would be a primary concern if working in, for instance, a constructivist paradigm of research. For example, Manias and Street (2001) state in their study, that researcher/participant subjectivity was an important and positive aspect of observation.

Mulhall (2003) also points to the incidence of the Hawthorne effect (reactivity) in observational research methods. This effect is a well-known phenomenon whereby people who know that they are being researched (particularly when observed) tend to behave in different ways than they would normally — either to appease the researcher or to present themselves in a different, and perceivably more positive, light (see Chapter 12 for a more detailed account of this phenomenon). To avoid participant reactivity altogether, the research and researcher would need to be concealed, which presents its own set of ethical dilemmas, as identified earlier.

Other types of data collection

Although most qualitative studies use interviews or observations for the collection of data, other data collection methods are also applied — either singularly or in tandem. Qualitative research questionnaires can be used where a list of open-ended questions elicit qualitative data. Journals can be written by participants about experiences, decision-making, or whatever is the focus of the study, with the journaling usually occurring soon after the event or the experience. Amongst new forms of evolving data collection is the 'think-aloud' technique. This is where participants record reflective thoughts, decision-making processes, or impressions about events and incidents, into say a hand-held audio-recorder. This occurs in a study of patients where they are making self-management decisions about their diabetes (Thorne & Paterson 2001).

A long-used method of data collection is utilising a form of systematic searching, for stored or displayed items of relevance (indirect data), that can later be analysed. The search may be for items of historical information (e.g. archival material, minutes of meetings, biographies, personal and organisational diaries, letters and personal documents). For instance, Kirby (2004) used government reports and professional journals to investigate nursing recruitment crises in the 1930s and 1940s; to compare how this impacted on the foundations of nursing research from 1950 to the 1970s. Such sources provide historical and contextual dimensions, either to back up observations and interviews, or to provide data

in its own right. In the Chaboyer et al. (2004) benchmarking project, for embedding evidence-based practice into a nursing curriculum, data were drawn directly from official university documents. Similarly, Leibbrandt et al. (2005) examined the curriculum documents of 26 Australian universities to produce data for the construction of a national curriculum evaluation framework.

The systematic search process may also be used for indirect data that present as a range of literary and artistic media, including paintings, literature and photography. In this context, some qualitative researchers also ask participants to create collages, take photographs, or do other artistic renditions pertinent to the research focus of a study. For example, Turner (2005) investigated hope, from the perspective of ten young Australian people, asking them to take photographs that reflected their experiences and interpretations of hope.

Using multiple data collection methods

More and more nurse and midwifery researchers are conducting research using mixed-method/triangulation research (see Chapter 15). One form of methodological triangulation is where the researcher uses different methods for collecting data within the same study. For

Research in brief

Williams and Irurita (2004) report on their grounded theory study to investigate Western Australian patients' perspectives of therapeutic and non-therapeutic interpersonal interactions. Three types of data collection methods were utilised. Forty patients were interviewed individually; 78 hours of participant observation field notes accompanied this, and patient-related documentation was also reviewed for data retrieval. Emotional comfort and emotional control emerged in the findings as the main factors that either inhibited or enhanced therapeutic relationships. Emotional comfort was found to be related to level of security, level of knowing and level of personal value.

instance, Henderson (2003) details a grounded theory study where she uses interviews and participant observation to investigate power imbalances between nurses and patients in Western Australia. Ray and Street (2005) use interviews and an innovative technique, called ecomapping, to explore the dynamic nature of social networks from the perspective of Australian motor-neurone disease sufferers. Ecomapping is a form of observational technique that maps and tracks relationships, social networks and support over time, and offers a visual schematic representation of identified connections.

When have enough data been collected?

This situation can occur in different ways in qualitative research. The researcher may just 'feel' that they have enough information at hand or, conversely, the emerging data becomes repetitive or uncovers nothing new. If this is the case, then researchers continue collecting data until data saturation, redundancy of data or 'theoretical saturation' is achieved (see Chapter 9). There is some controversy though as to whether it is really possible to achieve true data redundancy or saturation, as further interviews always have the potential to uncover something new or unexpected. Therefore, the point at which this situation seems to occur will vary with each study and cannot be predicted. However, once the researcher is reasonably satisfied that this point has been achieved, data collection can then cease and the researcher can move on to the next stage in the research process — data analysis. Sometimes, it is the actual number of the population sample that will determine to what extent, and when, data collection can cease.

Point to ponder

▶ Close attention is needed when selecting data collection methods for a research study. Without effective data collection strategies, the collected data will be flawed — as will the findings and conclusions of the whole study.

Summary

With qualitative research, sampling methods and methods of collecting data are an integral and closely related part of the study design (see Chapter 2). A number of different options are available which, in turn, will determine the nature and approach of the research to be undertaken; for instance, different types of fields of observation linked with different types of ethnographical studies. Careful attention to detail is required with both sampling and data collection processes. Flaws in either are likely to severely affect overall study outcomes. The effectiveness of these processes profoundly impact on the next stage of any qualitative research study: that of data analysis. Qualitative data analysis is the focus of the next chapter.

KEY POINTS

- Qualitative research employs a wide range of methods and techniques for both sampling from the appropriate population and for collecting required data from the sample. The four main types of sampling used in qualitative research are termed convenience sampling, purposive sampling, snowball sampling and theoretical sampling. Qualitative research usually employs either/both interviews or observation to collect data from sample populations — with face-to-face in-depth interviews being the most common method.

- As with all research methods, qualitative interview and observation methods have specific processes and each has both its strengths and limitations.

- Interviews and observation are not the only data collection options available to the qualitative researcher. Qualitative questionnaires, journaling by participants, 'think-aloud' techniques, systematic searches of stored or displayed items of interest, and requesting artistic renditions by participants, are all examples of other methods of data collection.

Learning activities

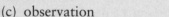

1. In sampling, the inclusion criteria indicate:
   (a) characteristics or properties of the chosen sample that the researcher would not want them to possess
   (b) characteristics or properties of the chosen sample that the researcher would most want them to possess
   (c) characteristics or properties of the sample that the researcher would find most attractive
   (d) characteristics or properties of the chosen sample that the researcher would find least attractive.

2. Which group of participants below would represent a judgment sample:
   (a) all the people working in a hospital
   (b) specialist nurses recommending other specialist nurses
   (c) specialist nurses working in intensive care
   (d) all inpatients in a hospital.

3. When sampling methods are applied to data already collected, this is called:
   (a) data sampling
   (b) information sampling
   (c) theoretical sampling
   (d) non-theoretical sampling.

4. What is the most common method used for collecting qualitative data:
   (a) questionnaire
   (b) interview
   (c) observation
   (d) survey.

5. When interviewing, starting off with simple and broad questions to help ease the participant into the process is referred to as:
   (a) nurturing
   (b) channelling
   (c) funnelling
   (d) easing.

6. Observational methods can employ which of the following approaches:
   (a) in-place participant; participant-as-observer; observer-as-participant; and absolute observer
   (b) complete participant; participant-as-observer; observer-as-participant; and complete observer
   (c) absolute participant; participant-as-observer; observer-as-participant; and in-place observer
   (d) complete participant; in-place observer; in-place participant; and complete observer.

7. Observation techniques are most commonly used in:
   (a) phenomenology
   (b) grounded theory
   (c) historical research
   (d) ethnography.

8. A qualitative researcher knows that it is not useful to collect any further data:
   (a) when they sense that this is the case
   (b) when the participants say that they have nothing more to say
   (c) when data saturation/redundancy of data is reached
   (d) when data overload is reached.

9. A form of methodological triangulation applies when:
   (a) participants are mixed up
   (b) different methods for collecting data are employed in the same study
   (c) different methods for collecting data are employed in different studies
   (d) the data collection methods are mixed up.

10. The Hawthorne effect, in observational research, is when:
    (a) participants behave in different ways than they would normally
    (b) participants are observed when the research is concealed from them
    (c) the researcher becomes totally integrated into the community being researched
    (d) there is more than one observer and observations are integrated for objectivity.

Additional resources

Borbasi S, Jackson D, Wilkes L 2005 Fieldwork in nursing research: positions, practicalities and predicaments. *Journal of Advanced Nursing* 51:493–501

Jamieson L, Williams L M 2003 Focus group methodology: explanatory notes for the novice nurse researcher. *Contemporary Nurse* 14:217

McLafferty I 2004 Focus group interviews as a data collecting strategy. *Journal of Advanced Nursing* 48:187–94

Patton M Q 2002 *Qualitative evaluation and research methods*, 3rd edn. Sage Publications, Newbury Park, California

Wimpenny P, Gass J 2000 Interviewing in phenomenology and grounded theory: is there a difference? *Journal of Advanced Nursing* 31:1485–92

References

Allen J, Fabri A M 2005 An evaluation of a community aged care nurse practitioner service. *Journal of Clinical Nursing* 14:1202–9

Annells M 2006 Impact of flatus incontinence on people with a bowel ostomy: a hermeneutic phenomenology. *Journal of Wound, Ostomy, and Continence Nursing* 33:518–24

Banning M 2005 Conceptions of evidence, evidence-based medicine, evidence-based practice and their use in nursing: independent nurse prescribers' views. *Journal of Clinical Nursing* 14:411–17

Borbasi S, Jackson D, Wilkes L 2005 Fieldwork in nursing research: positions, practicalities and predicaments. *Journal of Advanced Nursing* 51:493–501

Casey D 2006 Choosing an appropriate method of data collection. *Nurse researcher* 13:75–92

Chaboyer W, Willman A, Johnson P, et al. 2004 Embedding evidence-based practice in a nursing curriculum: a benchmarking project. *Nurse Education in Practice* 4:216–23

Cheek J, Ballantyne A, Roder-Allen G 2005 Factors influencing the decision of older people living in independent units to enter the acute care system. *International Journal of Older People Nursing in association with Journal of Clinical Nursing* 14(3a):24–33

Crowe M, O'Malley J, Gordon S. 2001 Meeting the needs of consumers in the community: a working partnership in mental health in New Zealand. *Journal of Advanced Nursing* 35:88–96

Fenwick J, Hauck Y, Downie J, et al. 2005 The childbirth expectations of a self-selected cohort of Western Australian women. *Midwifery* 21:23–35

French B 2005 Evaluating research for use in practice: what criteria do specialist nurses use? *Journal of Advanced Nursing* 50:235–43

Henderson S 2003 Power imbalance between nurses and patients: a potential inhibitor of partnership in care. *Journal of Clinical Nursing* 12:501–8

Higginbottom G M A 2004 Sampling issues in qualitative research. *Nurse Researcher* 12:7–12

Hylton J A 2005 Relearning how to learn: Enrolled nurse transition to degree at a New Zealand rural satellite campus. *Nurse Education Today* 25:519–26

Jackson D, Mannix J 2004 Giving voice to the burden of blame: a feminist study of mothers' experiences of mother blaming. *International Journal of Nursing Practice* 10:150–8

Kirby S 2004 A historical perspective on the contrasting experiences of nurses as research subjects and research activists. *International Journal of Nursing Practice* 10:272–9

Lane P, McKenna H, Ryan A, et al. 2001 Focus group methodology. *Nurse Researcher* 8:45–59

Leibbrandt L, Brown D, White J 2005 National comparative curriculum evaluation of baccalaureate nursing degrees: a framework for the practice based professions. *Nurse Education Today* 25:418–42

Leung S, Arthur D G, Martinson I 2005 Stress in women with postpartum depression: a phenomenological study. *Journal of Advanced Nursing* 51:353–60

Madsen W 2005 Early 20th century untrained nursing staff in the Rockhampton district: a necessary evil? *Journal of Advanced Nursing* 51:307–13

Manias E, Aitken R, Dunning T 2005 Graduate nurses' communication with health professionals when managing patients' medications. *Journal of Clinical Nursing* 14:354–62

Manias E, Street A 2001 Rethinking ethnography: reconstructing nursing relationships. *Journal of Advanced Nursing* 33:234–42

Mulhall A 2003 In the field: notes on observation in qualitative research. *Journal of Advanced Nursing* 41:306–13

Newton J M, McKenna L (in press) The transitional journey through the graduate year: a focus group study. *International Journal of Nursing Studies*

Overcash J A 2004 Narrative research: a viable methodology for clinical nursing. *Nursing Forum* 39:15–22

Patton M Q 2002 Qualitative evaluation and research methods, 3rd edn. Sage Publications, Newbury Park, California

Price B 2002 Laddered questions and qualitative data research interviews. *Journal of Advanced Nursing* 37:273–81

Ray R A, Street A F 2005 Ecomapping: an innovative research tool for nurses. *Journal of Advanced Nursing* 50:545–52

Streeton R, Cooke M, Campbell J 2004 Researching the researchers: using a snowball technique. *Nurse Researcher* 12:35–46

Thorne S, Paterson B 2001 Health care professional support for self-care management in chronic illness: insights from diabetes research. *Patient Education Counselling* 42:81–90

Tuckett A 2004 Qualitative research sampling: the very real complexities. *Nurse Researcher* 12:47–61

Turner S 2005 Hope seen through the eyes of 10 Australian young people. *Journal of Advanced Nursing* 52:508–17

Walsh D J 2006 'Nesting' and 'Matresence' as distinctive features of a free-standing birth centre in the UK. *Midwifery* 22:228–39

Williams A M, Irurita V F 2004 Therapeutic and non-therapeutic interpersonal actions: the patient's perspective. *Journal of Clinical Nursing* 13:806–15

Wynaden D, Chapman R, Orb A, et al. 2005 Factors that influence Asian communities' access to mental health care. *International Journal of Mental Health Nursing* 14:88–95

Zeitz K 2005 Nursing observation during the first 24 hours after a surgical procedure: what do we do? *Journal of Clinical Nursing* 14:334–43

Answers

TT Tutorial trigger 1

You may want to consider a number of issues, such as level of care given by carer, the carers understanding of cancer, the type of cancer, cancer survivability, and issues of gender. The above might or might not be important considerations. Carers that do not have close contact with or do not understand the nature and possible course or outcome of their relative's cancer may not offer the in-depth and rich perspective that a researcher requires. Male and female carers may offer different perspectives — which a researcher might want to either investigate or avoid. Decisions like this will determine if the sample will need to be mixed or single gender.

TT Tutorial trigger 2

Sampling method	Sample examples
Convenience/ opportunistic	All of the nursing staff on a particular ward. All of the clients who are currently on that ward.
Purposive/ judgment	All/some of the senior nursing staff on a particular ward. All/some of the clients who are known to have received client-centred care.
Snowball	Nursing staff on a ward who might know of other staff, on other wards, that deliver client-centred care. Clients on a ward who may know of other clients/relatives/friends who have received client-centred care.
Theoretical	Nursing staff on a ward that may do a procedure differently to other nurses, as suggested to be relevant from interpretation of previously collected data. Clients on a ward who are from a specific cultural group to explore emerging understandings about cultural aspects of responding to a nursing intervention, as suggested to be relevant from interpretation of previously collected data.

It is useful to note in the examples offered that there is no 'best' method to use and a variety of different ways to explore similar topics, both from the client's or health professional's perspective. As with most research methods and processes, it is what is most appropriate for the task at hand and what best suits the qualitative research method being used that is important.

TT Tutorial trigger 3

For inclusion/exclusion criteria, you may want to consider issues such as the types of catheter used, the time that the catheter is in situ, the setting (hospital or home), condition of patient, the condition that the patient has, gender, age ranges and cognitive ability. Again, each of these issues may have no particular bearing on what it is that a researcher wishes to explore in terms of overall perception and experience. Alternatively, it may be important that the researcher desires the feedback that is perceived to be common to quite a specific type of population.

TT Tutorial trigger 4

- How comfortable/uncomfortable is the catheter?
- Any worries/fears about having a catheter?
- Are they embarrassed about having a catheter?
- Do they know why the catheter is in place?
- Do they think that the catheter is helping them?
- What do they hope is the outcome of having a catheter in place?

TT Tutorial trigger 5

- Warm, open and comfortable environment.
- Well-lit, secure, quiet and private environment.
- Non-threatening environment — preferably in the client's 'normal' environment.
- Avoid 'sterile' environments — introduce personalised items.
- Minimum use of gadgets and technology — organised environment.
- Researcher dressed/presented appropriately.

TT Tutorial trigger 6

- How the child behaves generally — during periods of worsening/improving health.
- How the child interacts with health professionals.
- How the child interacts with their parents, siblings etc.
- How the child interacts with peers who are also inpatients.
- How the child is stimulated/educated during his/her stay.

Learning activities

1. b	**2.** c	**3.** c	**4.** b
5. c	**6.** b	**7.** d	**8.** c
9. b	**10.** a		

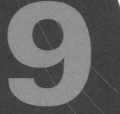

Chapter 9

Analysing data in qualitative research

MERILYN ANNELLS AND DEAN WHITEHEAD

KEY TERMS

categorisation and
    conceptualisation
coding
conceptual ordering
explanatory schema
qualitative data analysis
thematic analysis
trustworthiness

Learning outcomes

After reading this chapter, you should be able to:

- explain the difference between informal and formal interpretation of qualitative data
- recognise the major styles of qualitative data analysis
- describe common processes involved with coding qualitative data
- clarify the difference between categorisation and conceptualisation of qualitative data
- state the broad options about how to organise qualitative data and manage qualitative data analysis, with appreciation for the potential facilitative role of computer programs
- denote the contribution of memoing, diagramming and writing for qualitative data analysis
- examine a report of a qualitative study and understand the presentation of results
- identify strategies used by qualitative researchers to enhance trustworthiness of a study.

Introduction

When the term 'data analysis' is used in regard to qualitative research, what is meant is that data collected are formally interpreted. Qualitative data analysis is deliberate, considered and systematic. It is both a science and a craft. The researcher needs to apply skills in abstraction alongside logical and conceptual thinking. At all times, the research study question is kept in mind and only that focus is sought to be illuminated (see Chapter 5). Analysing qualitative data requires considerable time and planning but is worth the effort, as the product can be both extremely informative for nurses and midwives — and very useful for patients.

This chapter firstly discusses nine key issues relevant to analysing data in qualitative research. Then two major styles for analysis of qualitative data, as commonly used by researchers of nursing issues, are presented: 'fracturing, grouping and gluing' and 'circling and parking'. In addition, mention is made briefly of some other styles that can be applied, such as 'letter-boxing', 'magnifying glass' and 'layering and comparing'. Finally, there is discussion about how it can be known if the results of data analysis are appropriate (trustworthy) and also about ways of reporting and disseminating results.

Key issues regarding analysis of qualitative data

When is qualitative data analysis performed?

Unlike in quantitative research, when data are analysed in a separate stage after data collection, in qualitative research there are essentially three strategies for the timing of analysis.

1. Firstly, after data collection is complete, the complete set of data is focused upon. That is, data analysis is a separate step in the research process following data collection. This is common, for instance, with phenomenological research (see Chapter 7). Advantages are:
   - being able to gain a 'sense' of the whole data set through reading and re-reading several times before commencing formal analysis; this can be particularly useful in hermeneutic approaches (for examining the whole in light of the parts and the parts in light of the whole — see Chapter 7)
   - the most feasible option when access to sample or research duration is limited, either through time or geographical constraints, as with Arthur et al.'s (2006) Philippines-sited research of a primary healthcare curriculum within a school of nursing.

2. Secondly, when data analysis occurs simultaneously with data collection. For this possible strategy, some data are collected then analysed, more data are collected and analysed, and so on. This is often termed 'constant comparative data analysis'. How much data are collected before and in between analysis can vary. It may be one interview or a few, it may be one episode of observation or several, and it may be one document or many. The advantages are:
   - *guidance for sampling*: identifying attributes of the item of interest (e.g. which participant or what item) that would be most useful from which (or about which) to next collect data as informed by growing understandings or gaps in understanding obtained through analysis of previous data
   - *guidance for the next collection of data*: for instance, new or different questions might best be used for the next interview to target new areas of interest, beginning understandings, or gaps in understanding.

   For instance, this simultaneous process of data collection and data analysis was used by Lam et al.'s (2005) Hong Kong-based study, researching Chinese women's decision-making about breast cancer treatment.

3. Thirdly, when the data collection and analysis are 'staged'. This option may

especially occur with method triangulation research designs (see Chapter 15). In this case, if one type of data collection, such as interviewing, is completed then the interview data are analysed before the next type of data collection, such as a questionnaire. The advantage is:

– *guidance for moving onto another stage of data collection*: for instance, using analysed interview results to inform what documents need to be accessed.

O'Brien et al. (2003) used staged data collection and analysis in New Zealand when developing and trialling mental nursing clinical indicators with a bicultural focus. This research had four stages including qualitative dimensions. Stage one used focus groups, stage two conducted a Delphi survey, in stage three a pilot study was completed, and this led to a national field study in stage four. The results of each stage informed the design of the next stage.

TT Tutorial trigger 1

• Why is it, do you think, that constant comparative data analysis has become so popular?
• In what type of situations when participants are patients, might researchers find it necessary to collect data first, then later do data analysis?
• When wanting to develop a quantitative survey questionnaire to send to a sample of nurses or midwives, how can a first stage of interviewing assist questionnaire development — and hence require analysis of the interview data before developing the questionnaire?

What does the research approach require of qualitative analysis?

Data analysis processes are not standardised across qualitative research approaches. However, with most specific approaches (e.g. phenomenology, grounded theory) there are guidelines for data analysis in relevant literature that can be selected and followed. This provides choice. For instance, in grounded theory method there are classic analysis guidelines, a modification of those and variations thereof (see Chapter 7). In phenomenology, there are many guidelines but no set process. Therefore, suggestions are often selected from the suggestions of phenomenologists, but it is also acceptable for the researcher to formulate their own analysis process. Another example is descriptive, exploratory qualitative research (see Chapter 7), where researchers often select aspects of analysis processes from a range of qualitative approaches. What is chosen is at the discretion of the researcher as they see fit for the task at hand, although some specific analysis process suggestions are being recommended for this format (e.g. Thorne et al. 1997).

What needs to be produced?

Closely allied with consideration of the qualitative research approach being applied, is the need to consider what should be the research product's function. If this is a theory for implementation in practice, then data analysis requires adequate breadth and depth in its process. This will help to move beyond description and conceptual ordering in order to look for an explanatory schema. For example, Huang (2005), in a Taiwanese context, aimed to develop a theory about the management of the fear of falling by older people, for use by nurses when assisting older people to prevent falls. The applied extensive and finite analysis process facilitated identification of possible cause-and-effect linkages.

If the function of a qualitative study is to identify possible factors relevant to a clinical situation, so that the clinician can assess for those factors, then a list of concepts carefully derived from the study are descriptively grouped hierarchically, according to similarities. This is needed with descriptive, exploratory qualitative research, such as Manias et al.'s (2005) Australian study about graduate nurses managing patients' medications, where a list of such concepts are identified. However, quite different data analysis processes need to be applied if the study's function is to increase empathetic understanding of the clinician about a patient's experience. This type of research usually provides 'themes' that are explained fully, and often written in narrative, like a story. Therefore, in this case, data analysis process needs to focus on theme identification. This was done for the study of the experience of loss in the day-to-day life of fathers in rural Australia, in relation to their chronically ill children (Peck & Lillibridge 2003).

Research in brief

Buultjens and Liamputtong (in press), in their Victoria-based midwifery study, use a qualitative exploratory research design to examine women's experiences of depression following childbirth. The identified concepts relate to broad themes of 'the birth of the baby: the experience of hospital stay', 'perceptions of causes and experiences of postnatal depression' and 'women's perceived social support'.

Evidence-based practice tip

Consider carefully when seeking qualitative evidence about a practice area, what sort of evidence is needed and for what function in your practice. For example: Do you need a theory with an explanatory scheme to guide intervention selection? If so, then search for grounded theory studies; Do you need themes about a lived experience for increased understanding of that experience? If so, then seek phenomenological studies.

Solo or group effort?

Qualitative data analysis can be done by just one researcher as with Lee's (2005) Taiwanese study of nurses' concerns about using computerised nursing care planning systems. Alternatively, it can involve more than one researcher — as with Fenwick et al.'s (2005) research of the childbirth expectations of Australian women. There is a point of view that collective analysis (by a number of people) of qualitative data is more likely, than solo data analysis, to produce results that are refined. This is not necessarily automatic, but is based on the assumption that multiple perspectives are more likely to lead to a group consensus about what is relevant in data and how to conceptualise those relevant aspects. It is assumed that this will, in some way, either be more 'accurate' or a 'more rich construction'. A singular subjectivity, therefore, is more likely to produce a single-reality perspective than a more likely multiple perspective, potentially arising from a collective cross-referencing process. Where a single reality does emerge from a team of researchers, this can assist in claiming that consensus has been reached and trustworthiness achieved.

When group effort data analysis is conducted, several potential strategies exist, such as those listed below.

- One researcher or more will do the analysis then provide the results to the other research team members who will view those results prior to or during their analysis of data. This might be done separately or collectively, with further communication and negotiation, until consensus is achieved. For example, Chaboyer et al.'s (2005) case study of the impact of an intensive care unit liaison nurse in an Australian hospital or McLeod et al.'s (2003) study of the midwife's role in facilitating smoking-related behaviour change during pregnancy.
- The researchers will do the analysis separately then confer until consensus is reached. For example, McKain et al. (2005) when exploring patients' needs for information on arrival at a rehabilitation unit in Australia.
- The researchers will meet and conduct the analysis collectively until consensus is reached. For example, the New Zealand study by Huntington and Gilmour (2005) that explores women's perceptions of living with endometriosis or Erlandsson and Fagerberg's (2005) study of mothers' lived experiences of co-care and post-care after birth.

Points to ponder

▶ Doing qualitative data analysis as a team requires valuing the opinions of others and skilful negotiation as consensus is sought, but this may be quite a challenge.

▶ It is often considered that seven people is the maximum number to meet when a decision needs to be made. This could possibly have implications for the maximum size of a qualitative research study team.

How to fit with the way data were recorded

As explained in Chapter 8, qualitative research data can be recorded in various ways, such as audio or video recording, field notes and photographs. Usually audio recordings are transcribed into a written (typed) form, as also may occur with video recordings. Works of art, photographs and documents, as data, may not be recorded and interpretation may be directly of that item. Therefore, data analyses processes need to be appropriate. For instance, just doing line-by-line analysis of a transcribed video recording would not be enough, as non-verbal body language data would be lost, whereas this would suffice in transcribing an audio recording.

Using a 'theoretical lens'

When analysing qualitative data, if the study has a pre-chosen theoretical framework (e.g. symbolic interactionism — see grounded theory in Chapter 7) or if the researcher has a theoretical stance intrinsic to the purpose of the study (e.g. in feminist research — see Chapter 2), then data may be viewed and analysed through a metaphorical 'theoretical lens'. This means that aspects of the theory may guide the researcher as to what is considered most relevant in the data. Either this or their conceptualisation of data will be according to explanations and ideas offered by the theory. The trend is, however, not to purposefully use a theoretical lens.

Subsidiary processes to data analysis

Depending on the qualitative research approach used, there may be subsidiary processes to data analysis, such as the writing of different types of memos. For example, coding memos (recording why a concept label was applied to a section of data), theoretical memos (thoughts about possible connections between interpreted concepts, writing the storyline emerging through analysis recording explanatory hypotheses), operational notes (directing modification of questions for following interviews, theoretical sampling requirements, and possible literature to be read), and also sub-varieties of these. Wilkins (2006) in her grounded theory study, exploring the support needs of first-time mothers, uses theoretical memos to aid the uncovering of relationships between concepts and categories.

Another subsidiary process may be the drawing of a series of diagrams that map a

growing understanding about the research focus. This can be very helpful when trying to work out possible links between concepts during conceptualisation and conceptual ordering. Often diagrams are useful to develop an explanatory schema if aiming to produce a theory. There may be a final diagram that can be presented with the written results of a study, such as provided by Chui et al. (2005) to explain the longitudinal representation of *yin* and *yang* forces in relation to four modes of the struggle of Chinese-Australian patients against advancing cancer.

Managing data analysis

Huge amounts of data can be collected. Not only can this represent a storage and filing challenge, but it can be problematic to record the analysis process, re-analysis, linkages between analyses and determinant data and sorting of analyses for conceptual ordering. Added to this, there is the dilemma of ensuring that memos are easily accessible with systematic recording proximal to relevant data.

As in the past, these days, a range of paper-based strategies are possible when trying to sort and connect different interpreted concepts. For instance, different coloured cards, index files or labelling stickers can have the concepts or memos written onto them and then sorted flexibly into different patterns or hierarchies, by pinning to a large noticeboard or placing on a tabletop. Single or multiple systems like these can be used, although a key message is to keep things as simple and accessible as possible. Qualitative researchers can be creative in the way that they manage their data as they are not confined to only some of the methods mentioned here.

As computers became more common, a range of word processing files compiled in some logical order began to be used and this strategy remains in use today by some researchers. This is the case with Liu et al. (2006), in China, who chose a system of multiple 'Word' documents for managing data analysis, when exploring the meaning of caring from the perspective of cancer patients. To further aid this process, over recent decades, a number of computer software programs have been designed and refined to facilitate organisation of qualitative research data and the management of data analysis — with increasingly 'user-friendly' interfaces. These programs do not do the actual analysis, although automatic word or phrase search capability is usually available. The researcher is still required to perform the data analysis through intellectual effort. Rather, what these computer programs facilitate is storage of data in multiple recorded forms (including aural, visual, video and word forms) within a large capacity project file — with sub-files where:

- on the screen, labels for concepts interpreted from data can be recorded next to data
- linkages are recorded with relationships able to be created and displayed both visually and flexibly
- hierarchies of conceptual ordering can be developed, diagrammed, recorded and re-formed if necessary; re-analyses are facilitated
- memos can be recorded and linked to data or to analyses
- tables, pictures and images can be imported
- data security is maintained
- quantitative data analyses can be connected to qualitative data analyses (see Chapter 14)
- analyses by different people can be merged as well as different projects merged
- navigation around the project file and sub-files is relatively easy.

The data analysis process and some subsidiary processes can be conducted while sitting at a computer with print-outs of any section of the project file possible. The most frequently used of the available programs in this era is NVivo7 (http://www.qsrinternational.com). For example, a version of NVivo was used productively by Lam et al. (2005) to manage data analysis for a study in Hong Kong of women's decision-making about breast cancer treatment options. A still-popular predecessor of the NVivo program is the Non-numerical Unstructured Data Indexing Search and Theorising (NUD*IST) tool. Furber and Thomson (2006), in their study on midwives identifying 'deviant' baby feeding practices of women, use NUD*IST version 4, to store and manage their qualitative data during analysis.

TT Tutorial trigger 2

What might be the disadvantages of using a computer program for qualitative research to organise data and manage data collection? Perhaps viewing the NVivo website (noted above) may help you to understand what such a program can offer and entail regarding use.

The importance of writing qualitative data analysis results

In quantitative research, data analysis is completed before writing the results into a report. Contrastingly, in qualitative research studies, data analysis may recommence and continue when the 'results' are being written into a report. During the writing, incongruence in aspects of categorisation or conceptualisation may become discernible or a further interpretive insight of relevance may occur. Therefore, writing may provide additional illumination until meaning is (or seems) complete. With some qualitative research approaches, such as phenomenology, writing and rewriting are considered essential supplementation of the reading and reflection for thematic analysis.

'Fracturing, grouping and gluing' style of qualitative data analysis

This is the most common style of qualitative data analysis. The major analysis strategy in this style is that of coding, which is when data are:

- fractured (divided into labelled abstract bits called codes)
- categorised (codes are grouped into a tentative category, like with like, and the tentative category is labelled)
- integrated or linked 'glued' together) through conceptualisation of grouped data into a hierarchy of definite categories and sub-categories.

Codes should also be defined — sometimes called the 'attributes' of a code.

The overall aim is the description and conceptual ordering of aspects of data relevant to the research study question (see Chapter 5). However, if theory development is the aim, then the linkage (gluing) may continue one step further to develop an explanatory schema. This style of analysis may be free-form or follow set directions.

Free-form analysis

The qualitative researcher may decide to code data without following any specific instructions. This can be acceptable with some qualitative research approaches such as descriptive exploratory research. For written forms of data, usually after having read the whole transcript at least once (but not necessarily so), the two basic choices for the researcher regarding the fracturing part of the coding are:

1. To line-by-line code — carefully examining words, phrases or sentences to check if those data are relevant to the overall research question. If so, the bit of data is abstracted into another word or words (codes) that are an interpretation from insights arising. Sometimes the words in the data are abstract enough and cannot be improved upon. In this case the words are recorded as 'in vivo' codes. Some lines will not have relevant data for abstraction.

2. Scanning paragraphs for units of meaning — relevant to answering the research question and then abstracting into a descriptive word or words (codes). There may be several abstractions per paragraph or perhaps none. Coding involves studying the paragraph, interpreting what is relevant in the paragraph (with regard to the research question) and then writing a code for that interpretation (e.g. hunger). Thus, the item is 'fractured' into an interpreted unit or units that are expressed in a word or words (code/s).

The next step gathers the abstracted, fractured codes into logical groupings (categorisation). This may commence quite early in data analysis, or may only be done after all data have been fractured into codes. The groupings, which are usually tentative with modifications made as analysis continues, are labelled appropriately to signify the interpretation represented in some (but varying) ways, by the codes so grouped. Labels can be changed to give improved meaning. Groups may be abandoned as codes are placed into new groupings. Groupings can be 'collapsed'

together. For maximum clarity, the aim is to have as few groupings as possible.

The third step of stating linkages (relationships), through conceptualisation, is usually a matter of placing (gluing) the groupings into various hierarchies — termed categories and sub-categories. A category will tend to have multiple sub-categories. This is known as *conceptual ordering*. As explained by Morse and Richards (2002), a concept is a mental image that is a higher level abstract construct than a category. A category is simply a putting together of a number of abstracted elements of data into a like-set (group). Sometimes there may be more than two levels in the hierarchy with the third level often referred to as properties of the sub-categories. That is, there will be categories, then sub-categories and then properties of sub-categories. Analysing for conceptual ordering may be a separate step done after grouping codes has been finalised, but usually conceptual ordering has already commenced earlier.

It is possible that all three processes (fracturing, grouping and gluing) are cyclic and the researcher moves back and forth doing these, rather than them being discrete steps. Overall, tentative linkages will be explored, where cutting down to the least number of categories possible is an over-arching aim. When the researcher's carefully considered opinion is that qualitative data have been 'fractured, grouped and glued' satisfactorily, data analysis will cease.

Sometimes the free-form style will be chosen after considering ways in which other qualitative researchers have conducted data analysis. It may be a unique combination of techniques, such as for the analysis conducted in Chaboyer et al.'s (2005) case study of ward nurses' perceptions of the impact of an intensive care unit liaison nurse in Queensland, Australia. A unique feature of this study is that, although 'fracturing, grouping and gluing' was used, a selection of individual transcripts was analysed first — then cross-comparisons made with remaining transcripts.

TT Tutorial trigger 3

Group exercise: each person in the tutorial writes a paragraph explaining the reasons for the latest visit to a family member (can be hypothetical), leaving a large margin on the right-hand side of the paragraph. That paragraph is swapped with another person's paragraph. Analysis of this data is done solo — keeping the possible descriptive exploratory research question in mind, 'What are the motivating reasons for visiting a family member?'. Do line-by-line fracturing and abstraction of relevant data, placing the labelled codes proximal to data in the wide margin. Collectively as a tutorial group, share the codes generated, listing on a whiteboard or similar. Next, collectively place like-codes into groups (categorisation), giving each group an appropriate label.

Following directions

Some research approaches stipulate what type of coding should be conducted and how this is to be done. For instance, in classic grounded theory method (see Chapter 7), two forms of coding, 'open coding' and 'theoretical coding', are required. Open coding (involving fracturing data and some grouping) is looking for underlying meaning, uniformity or pattern in and across data — with the researcher remaining 'open' to possibilities and not trying to fit data to preconceived notions and ideas. Theoretical coding (a form of gluing) involves connecting concepts that have arisen from open coding. The connections between concepts 'emerge' as relationships between categories, sub-categories and their properties are analysed. These classic directions for data analysis are used by Chui et al. (2005), while studying the responses to advanced cancer of Chinese-Australians.

With the grounded theory method, other sets of guidelines can direct a different way to do

> ### Research in brief
>
> O'Haire and Blackford (2005) applied data analysis processes from grounded theory method to analyse interview data from nine nurses, regarding nurses' negotiation of parental participation in care within a paediatric cardiac/renal unit in an Australian city. Constant comparative data analysis was used with open and axial coding applied. Selective coding then identified the core category of 'moral agency'. The five related concepts were integrated to be: the child's best interests, disputes about care and expectations, which could result in either moral distress or provision of coping mechanisms and strategies. The study did not formulate an explanatory schema.

> ### Research in brief
>
> Wilkins (2006) also applied data analysis processes from grounded theory method to analyse interview data from eight primiparous women aged between 20 and 39 years who had given birth normally at term to healthy babies. Open coding revealed recurring concepts such as 'self-doubt', 'unprepared' and 'huge learning curve'. Axial coding enabled the researchers to uncover relationships between the developing categories — such as the relationship between 'expert to novice' and 'perceiving expertise'. Selective coding revealed the core category of 'doing it right'. Three other related concepts emerged as 'losing touch', 'restoring balance' and 'falling into place'.

coding. For instance, following open coding, axial coding can occur where relationships between categories and sub-categories are developed and analysed (termed 'axial' because coding occurs around the axis of a category), thereby linking categories and/or sub-categories at the level of properties and also dimensions (Strauss & Corbin 1998). Additionally, a form of theoretical coding is possible that is termed 'selective coding'. This delimits and refines integrated categories, along the dimensional level, to be glued for formation of a theory with 'validated' relationships among concepts, including selection and refinement of a core category (Strauss & Corbin 1998). However, data analysis may continue even in the writing-up stage, as potentially rough corners of the theory are identified and polished, but always as derived from data which are re-analysed. Hence, the grounded theory, as an explanatory schema (one step further than conceptual ordering), is considered to be satisfactorily resultant from a set process of 'fracturing, grouping and gluing'.

'Circling and parking' style of analysis

The second style of qualitative data analysis, circling and parking, treats the data set as a mass of information that can be best understood by not fracturing it into small abstracted sections. Rather, the optimal analysis process is the gaining of understanding about the overall discernible themes in the data set. These themes can only be ascertained or constructed appropriately (through thematic analysis), by having a 'feel' for the overall meaning of the whole set of data. A theme is more pervasive than a category, being something that 'runs right through data and is not necessarily confined to specific segments of text' (Morse & Richards 2002 p 121). Therefore, it is necessary to circle around the data set, getting to know it well, and at times parking in proximity to some data for close scrutiny. This is before circling some more, parking some more, and so on, until meaning-making is satisfactorily complete. Data analysis is iterative; moving to and fro, rather than in linear steps. Although it can be applied to various qualitative research approaches, this style of data analysis is particularly useful for some specific approaches, like phenomenology. The researcher may use this style 'free-form', or else follow directions suggested by others.

Research in brief

Geanellos (2005) studied nurse unfriendliness by in-depth interviewing of 12 ex-patients. The research design was hermeneutic phenomenology and data analysis interpreted that the overall impact of nursing unfriendliness on patient wellbeing was the undermining of self-efficacy. Two meta-themes were identified, the nature and the consequences of nurse unfriendliness, which arose from key statements that became the basis for other themes evident throughout the data set. Data analysis was a process of 'circling and parking' and involved reduction, integration, aggregation and reflection.

Free-form analysis

A multitude of possibilities exist for free-form 'circling and parking'. The researcher may plan a data analysis process that seems suitable to them and then apply that process according to plan; for example, Huntington and Gilmour's (2005) application of a free-form thematic analysis style to formally interpret transcribed interview data, for their New Zealand-sited qualitative study that

explored women's perceptions of living with endometriosis. Buultjens and Liamputtong's (in press) study, on women's experiences of depression after childbirth, does the same. The plan may be varied if deemed to be necessary when engaged in data analysis.

Alternatively, the researcher may choose to start data analysis with no plan except perhaps to have some general principles — such as the hermeneutical imperative to 'look at the parts in light of the whole and the whole in light of the parts' (see Chapter 7). This style of analysis was encouraged by the phenomenologist Munhall when she posed, 'What if every step we took in a study under the rubric of phenomenology was guided by responses to the flow of material?' (Munhall 1994 p 170). What is meant here is that the data analysis process could be suggested by engagement with the data set and evolve from an increased understanding of the data set. This is what Annells (2006) chose to do for an Australian hermeneutic phenomenology study of the experience of flatus incontinence by people with bowel ostomies. The intention was to analyse the data set of video-recorded in-depth interviews (non-transcribed) by being immersed in the data and remaining open to intuitive construction. Freedom about process and style was guided by flow of interpretation.

In Annells' (2006) study, firstly all videotapes were watched in one sitting and informal reflection on data occurred over a month. Then a period of intense focusing commenced. The first video-recording was viewed with an artist's sketch pad and pencil handy. Rewinding occurred frequently as impressions were jotted onto paper. General situations and experiences were divided from specific examples of impact. Arrows and lines joined or separated bits and pieces of the writing and diagramming. When the tape was finished, 'dot point' summaries were written, concerning ways in which flatus had impacted on the person and about possible meanings. Then the whole tape was watched again, but this time while sitting back and not writing. After this, sitting and thinking (reflecting) about the content of the video occurred before writing tentative overall meanings. A similar process was repeated for the other videotapes. Memoing, thinking and writing continued intensely as videotapes or segments of a videotape were re-watched. Through rewriting, the interpretation of possible meanings was refined. The stories of participants varied, but themes of meaning threaded through the stories. Through this process of engagement with the data set, by 'circling and parking', possible meanings of the phenomenon coalesced. A list of themes resulted that were encompassed within a creative synthesis (as a semi-fictionalised short story), which was the product of the study.

Following directions

There are directions suggested by others that can be followed with a 'circling and parking' style. For instance, the suggestions of Colaizzi (1978) regarding seven aspects of data analysis are often used. Giorgi's (1997) steps of data analysis are also commonly used in nursing studies (see Chapter 7, under 'Phenomenology'). After reading data thoroughly, statements relevant to the research topic are 'extracted' and then interpreted meanings of those statements are produced. This is done for each interview transcript and, later, whilst contemplating the whole data set. Interpreted meanings of the extracted statements plus overall themes are compiled, with these themes combined into descriptions of the topic. The last action is to reflect the themes back onto data to check that the analysis has actually produced a description representative of the collective experiences therein. Hence, considerable circling of the data set and parking at various points are evident.

Research in brief

The qualitative data analysis directions suggested by Colaizzi (1978) were used by Namasivayam et al. (2005) to focus phenomenologically on Western Australian nurses' lived experience of the challenges of caring for families of the terminally ill. Four major themes were produced: walking a journey together, dealing with intense emotions, working as a team, and balancing the dimension of care.

TT Tutorial trigger 4

Group exercise: in pre planning for a tutorial, three volunteers from the group each write (prior to the tutorial) a paragraph about the experience of being woken at night by a violent thunderstorm, with

emphasis upon feelings, reactions and other key elements of the experience. Copies of these paragraphs should be provided for each person in the tutorial and each paragraph should be read aloud by someone in the tutorial, then in small groups, Colaizzi's (1978) suggestions for data analysis should be attempted with the data set (three paragraphs).

Other styles of analysing qualitative data

A search through journals that report nursing and midwifery research results informs readers that, apart from the two major styles for analysing qualitative data as discussed so far, there are a number of other styles that can also be applied, some of which are:

'Letter-boxing' style

It is possible to start qualitative data analysis with a predetermined list of codes (abstractions that are labelled) and then search for examples of data that can be interpreted into these codes. This style is like 'letter-boxing', where an interpretive container pre-exists as a code into which relevant sections of data can be slotted. With some forms of 'content analysis' this style may be required, especially when there are many data sources so that a number of people are needed to do the analysis (multiple coders). Usually the codes are initially developed from either a range of pertinent opinions, previously reported research, or as suggested by experts. Possibly the interview questions (or observation guidelines) have been designed to focus on each separate code. The codes may also already be grouped into categories that pre-date analysis. An example of 'letter-boxing' data analysis style is in the research of Annells and Koch (2002) on older Australians' experience of seeking solutions to constipation, whereby a mass of qualitative data was analysed according to preconceptualised codes (each the focus of an interview question) originating from a pilot study.

'Magnifying glass' style of qualitative data analysis

Sometimes the narrative data that are the focus of qualitative research are subject to minute scrutiny, as if being looked at through a 'magnifying glass' — searching for a multiple of different aspects (related or not related to each other), in order to answer the research study question. One qualitative research approach especially (discourse analysis) requires this 'magnifying glass' style. This style of analysis may focus overall on content, structure, communication strategies, terms used, types and function of language, thematic structure, the construction of social relations, and reality representation in text.

Research in brief

Fowler and Lee (2004) analysed for multiple aspects, such as constructions, tensions, gaps, absences and contradictions, when conducting a discourse analysis of interview-generated text regarding the first-time experience of being a mother in Australia. Disclosed were the complex and often contradictory processes of maternal learning that need to be understood for effective action by nurses and midwives when that care is required.

'Layering and comparing'

It might be necessary to conduct qualitative data analysis in a 'layering and comparing' style, as required with the culturally focused research approach of ethnography (see Chapter 7). Here a layer of first-level description and a second layer of thick description are necessary, followed by comparison of the results from those layers with, for instance, knowledge already in pertinent literature about that culture. Although ethnographic data analysis can be a flexible process, first-level description usually requires an orientation to the setting that may require a number of strategies. These strategies include compiling lists of interpreted observations, charting interpreted relationships and power structures, and analysing discernible routines through some form of coding. The codes are then usually combined into a narrative form of description, although lists or even items such as photographs may be incorporated. The layer of 'thick description' requires

analysis for theoretical insights and may use strategies such as writing and synthesising summaries of interview, observation and diary data, and extraction of key characteristics pertaining to the culture being researched. For supplementation, there may also be a collection and analysis of quantitative data. Strategies for comparison may include application of a series of relevant comparative questions. The flexibility, that is often a feature of the 'layering and comparison' style of qualitative data analysis, is evident within Bland's (2004) critical ethnography of residential aged-care in New Zealand.

T_T Tutorial trigger 5

- What is probably the primary disadvantage of using a 'letter-boxing' style of qualitative data analysis?
- Apart from interview data, what other forms of written texts can be analysed if using a discourse analysis approach for qualitative research?
- If studying the culture in a neonatal intensive care unit, would constant comparative data analysis be potentially more productive or less productive than analysis when all data are collected?

Trustworthiness

There is no one agreed way yet amongst qualitative researchers about how to ensure, or evaluate, the 'rightness/correctness' of the results of a qualitative research study — often termed 'trustworthiness', which is the equivalent of the term 'rigour' for quantitative research. There are multiple opinions in this regard. At present, there seems to be six broad options (positions) about what should be the criteria for trustworthiness, with studies variously selecting one of these positions for making the claim of trustworthiness.

Position 1 — methodological criteria

This position emphasises procedural precision and champions various notions about how to ensure objectivity, internal and external validity, and reliability — these being the traditional aspects for rigour in quantitative research. This is a fading position as understanding has increased that qualitative research is a very different genre of research, for which these criteria are not now suitable.

Position 2 — parallel methodological criteria

Accepting that qualitative research requires unique trustworthiness criteria, this popular position advocates for any criteria to have a parallel relationship to traditional methodological criteria. The most persistent, commonly applied criteria suggested within this position are the four criteria listed with explanations in Table 9.1, a compilation based on criteria initially suggested by Guba and Lincoln (1989). The parallel relationships with traditional methodological criteria are: credibility with internal validity, auditability (dependability) with reliability, fittingness (transferabilty) with external validity, and confirmability with objectivity.

TABLE 9.1 Criteria for judging trustworthiness: credibility, auditability, fittingness and confirmability

Criteria	Criteria characteristic
Credibility	Truth of findings as judged by participants and others within the discipline.
Auditability	Accountability as judged by the adequacy of information leading the reader from the research question and raw data through various steps of analysis to the interpretation of findings.
Fittingness	Faithfulness to everyday reality of the participants, described in enough detail so that others in the discipline can evaluate importance for their own practice, research and theory development.
Confirmability	Findings that reflect implementation of credibility, auditability and fittingness standards.

Position 3 — multiple criteria

Intrinsic to this position is that there should be various lists of criteria for qualitative research trustworthiness, one list per qualitative research approach (e.g. for grounded theory method) or for a research function (e.g. for critical inquiry). Suggestions exist for some qualitative research approaches as to what

these criteria should be. However, various forms of these suggestions are available for some approaches, such as in regard to grounded theory method. So this position is not yet achieved — although quite popular.

Position 4 — fresh and universal criteria

This is a yearning for, and a pursuit of, generic criteria unique to qualitative research (all approaches), these criteria being viewed as yet to be identified and agreed on, although there have been numerous suggestions as to what the criteria should be. For instance, Morse and Richards (2002) offer a number of suggested generic criteria as grouped under the headings of: asking the right question, ensuring an appropriate design, making trustworthy data, verification or completion, and solid theory-building if that is an aim.

Position 5 — each study develops suitable, justified criteria

Growing in popularity, for example as advocated by Rolfe (2006), is the flexibility for researchers to stipulate their own list of criteria for trustworthiness of a study — justifying the choice not only possibly because of the qualitative research approach used, but perhaps also on other grounds, such as philosophical, ethical and political reasons.

Some common criteria selected are:

- *An audit (decision trail)*, where care is taken to record via memos and other means the decisions made, particularly regarding design planning, sampling, data collection methods and analysis decisions — so that a trail of decisions can supposedly be discerned as 'evidence' for trustworthiness of the study by the reader.
- *Member (participant) checking*, where some researchers may seek to claim trustworthiness of analysis by checking the descriptions, categories, concepts or theory produced with the participants for approval and acceptance. However, there can be problems with this. Participants

rarely think abstractly and conceptually about aspects of their life reported to or observed by researchers, and there may be some power differential and/or status difference between the researchers. This may open up a tendency to consciously or subconsciously consider the interpretations offered for perusal as probably 'correct'.

- *Peer analysis checking*, where using peers to check either the acceptability of data analysis or of the research process per se, can be claimed as a trustworthiness measure. This may be sought during the life of the study (e.g. using a supposedly independent peer coder, or using a panel of peers who are 'expert' to evaluate emerging interpretations or application of the research approach) or claimed post-study — when a manuscript reporting results is double blind reviewed via a peer-review journal accepting the manuscript for publication.

Position 6 — no criteria necessary

Although only barely evident so far, there is a type of post-modern position (see Chapter 2) that rejects completely the need for criteria to be selected or stated by a researcher in regard to trustworthiness of a qualitative research study or its product. Part of the rationale for this position is that all qualitative research involves (positively and productively) a subjective construction whereby that reality is relative. For this reason, qualitative research can never be truly 'generalisable'. Rather, the research and its reported product is accepted or rejected by the reader of the report or user of the product according to their own subjective criteria. Where 'absolute truth' is required, therefore, as an outcome of research, qualitative methods should be avoided.

Reporting and disseminating results

The common target audience for nursing and midwifery-related qualitative research results is, unsurprisingly, primarily nurses and midwives. It can, however, include members of other healthcare disciplines, other agencies, patients or their carers, and sometimes members of the general public. Results can be reported in many forms, such as a (technical) report, book, monograph, journal or magazine article, abstracts, pamphlets, online resources, conference paper or poster, seminar or colloquia presentations, guest-speaking engagements, media interviews, or creative works, as discussed later (see Chapter 21).

TT Tutorial trigger 6

What could be the main disadvantage of reporting qualitative research by:
- conference paper
- book
- journal article
- media interview?

Generally the context of the research is made explicit and all necessary design and process elements stated. Unlike with quantitative research, it is acceptable for findings and discussion about the findings to be integrated, but not necessarily so. Usually segments of data (e.g. direct quotes from participants or parts of field notes) are integrated into reported results. As per any research report, limitations, implications and recommendations need to be offered, and in addition, trustworthiness criteria applied should be listed and justified. However, it is essential to write the results to 'grab' the reader, sustain interest, and to give the best representation possible. It is acceptable to use the 'first person' when writing the report (see Chapter 21). The style of presenting results is

---

Points to ponder

▶ Qualitative research is increasingly being accepted as 'evidence' for use in health research. However, because there is not always agreed criteria on how it should be evaluated, the trustworthiness of qualitative studies, and the judicious selection of results to use in practice, needs careful consideration.

▶ With the lack of clarity as to what trustworthiness criteria should be used for qualitative research, success may be hampered in regard to applying for competitive research funds — when in competition with quantitative studies.

somewhat governed by the research approach that was applied, but variability is often possible within certain parameters. Options may include the following.

- *Sequential presentation of concepts*
  This may either be done completely by descriptive and explanatory narrative following an ordered sequence of concepts or may be supplemented by a list or lists of categories and sub-categories, perhaps presented as tables or within an appendix. In the narrative, at appropriate points, there are usually embedded samples of illuminative data.

- *A flow of themes*
  Thematic analysis results tend to be written as a flowing narrative. A list of the themes may be provided prior to the narrative commencing. Headings may or may not be used in the narrative when a different theme is being written about. Examples of illustrative data (e.g. quotes from participants) are also presented.

- *Multiple forms of presentation*
  With some research approaches, such as grounded theory, the results can be presented in multiple forms that may include combinations of either diagramming, tables of hierarchical concepts, a succinct 'storyline' and a necessary detailed narrative text (also with embedded illustrative data).

- *A creative synthesis or representation*
  Becoming more acceptable, but certainly not yet universally embraced, are types of creative synthesis or representation of results. Possible choices include poems, 'fictionalised' or 'semi-fictionalised' novels or short stories, performance renditions (e.g. plays, monologues, movies, dance), visual art (e.g. painting, montage, sculpture, photographs, series of cartoons) or auditory art (e.g. song, orchestral

arrangement). These creative representations can be very effective for empathy-raising and can be readily accepted by clinicians depending on accessibility and how discernible are the key understandings of the qualitative research results in the presentation.

> ● **Evidence-based practice tip**
> When seeking evidence about a practice focus that might have been researched qualitatively (e.g. how to assist parents grieving after a still-birth of a baby), a literature search can be done for separate studies with published reports, but also for any meta-syntheses published that report as a synthesis the results of multiple qualitative studies with this focus.

Summary

The science and craft of qualitative data analysis is in flux but evolving, as qualitative research is in relatively early days of development compared to quantitative research. Data analysis styles are numerous, although some are more common than others. A degree of flexibility exists, although stipulated directions are available for many qualitative research approaches. Also in this era, there are a range of positions regarding how to ensure or evaluate the trustworthiness of qualitative research studies and results, plus varying ways in which to report the results. Nevertheless, qualitative research relevant to nursing and midwifery practice is increasing in amount and continues to offer a wealth of understandings that can be directly or indirectly applied to enhance care delivery. In line with this, the continuing growth of mixed-method research (see Chapter 15) further cements the future of qualitative research. The next few decades should ensure a maturing of this form of nursing research in line with advancements in method and associated issues, regarding qualitative research across disciplines.

KEY POINTS

- Qualitative data analysis is a formal, systematic process of interpretation, where the most common style of qualitative data analysis involves 'fracturing, grouping and gluing' with associated abstractions of data via 'coding' that incorporates description, categorisation and conceptualisation.

- There are a variety of other qualitative data analysis styles, sometimes linked to specific research approaches like content analysis, discourse analysis and ethnography.

- It is possible to follow specific directions regarding styles of qualitative data analysis, as is often offered by methodologists regarding qualitative research approaches, or to have flexibility by using the style free-form.

- The reporting and dissemination of qualitative research results can be presented in various forms.

Learning activities

1. Qualitative data analysis:
   (a) commences with the start of formal interpretation of data
   (b) commences with the start of informal interpretation of data
   (c) can commence with either the start of informal or formal interpretation of data
   (d) commences at the completion of informal and formal interpretation of data.

2. Constant comparative data analysis involves:
   (a) collection of all data then analysis of that data
   (b) sequential segments of data collection and data analysis
   (c) analysis of data during the collection of data
   (d) cyclic collection of data by one method, then analysis of that data, collection of data by another method, then analysis of that data, and so on.

3. Specific qualitative research approaches (e.g. grounded theory method):
   (a) always have one set of analysis processes that must be followed
   (b) may or may not have a set of analysis processes that can be followed
   (c) do not ever have any analysis processes that can be followed
   (d) rely solely on free-form research processes.

4. Coding:
   (a) does not incorporate abstraction of data
   (b) only sometimes incorporates abstraction of data
   (c) incorporates abstraction of data only when relevant
   (d) always incorporates abstraction of data.

5. Coding:
   (a) must involve preselected codes
   (b) must never involve preselected codes
   (c) may involve preselected codes
   (d) must involve preselected and non-preselected codes.

6. Memos, as a subsidiary process of qualitative data analysis:
   (a) are written communications between researcher and participants
   (b) are transcriptions of interview data
   (c) are transcriptions of field notes
   (d) are notes written to yourself as the researcher.

7. Conceptual ordering is:
   (a) the hierarchical placement and/or linkage of categories and possibly sub-categories
   (b) the placing of like-codes into groups
   (c) the initial fracturing and abstraction of data
   (d) the explication of an explanatory schema.

8. Categorisation is:
   (a) the hierarchical placement and/or linkage of categories and possibly sub-categories
   (b) the placement of like-codes into groups
   (c) the initial fracturing and abstraction of data
   (d) the explication of an explanatory schema.

9. Trustworthiness of qualitative research requires:
   (a) always fulfilling parallel methodological criteria to quantitative research criteria for rigour
   (b) always fulfilling the same methodological criteria as for quantitative research rigour
   (c) always justifying in a report what methodological criteria have been applied
   (d) always using the criteria directed by the qualitative research approach.

10. Meta-synthesis of qualitative research results is:
    (a) the integration of results from multiple studies with a similar focus where concepts or themes are comparable
    (b) fusing creatively together the major findings of a qualitative research study
    (c) the process of thematic analysis for phenomenology
    (d) merging the results of individual analyses of data by multiple researchers in a study.

Additional resources

Association for Qualitative Research — international organisation that aims to further the practice and study of qualitative research. Online. Available: http://www.latrobe.edu.au/aqr/

Grounded Theory Institute — focuses on facilitating classic grounded theory method. Online. Available: http://www.groundedtheory.com

QSR International — for information about the qualitative data analysis management computer program, NVivo7. Online. Available: http://www.qsrinternational.com

Rapport F 2004 *New qualitative methodologies in health and social care research*. Routledge, London

Sandelowski M, Barrosa J 2003 Classifying the findings in qualitative research. *Qualitative Health Research* 13:905–23

Thorne S, Jensen L, Kearney M, Noblit G, Sandelowski M 2004 Qualitative metasynthesis: reflections on methodological orientation and ideological agenda. *Qualitative Health Research* 14:1342–65

References

Annells M 2006 Impact of flatus incontinence on people with a bowel ostomy: a hermeneutic phenomenology. *Journal of Wound, Ostomy, and Continence Nursing* 33:518–24

Annells M, Koch T 2002 Older people seeking solutions to constipation: the laxative mire. *Journal of Clinical Nursing* 11:603–12

Arthur D, Drury J, Sy-Sinda M T, et al. 2006 A primary health care curriculum in action: the lived experience of primary health care nurses in a school of nursing in the Philippines: a phenomenological study. *International Journal of Nursing Studies* 43:107–12

Bland M 2004 All the comforts of home? A critical ethnography of residential aged care in New Zealand. *Nursing Praxis in New Zealand* 20:57–8

Buultjens M, Liamputtong P 2007 When giving life starts to take the life out of you: women's experiences of depression after childbirth. *Midwifery* 23:177–91

Chaboyer W, Gillespie B, Foster M, et al. 2005 The impact of an ICU liaison nurse: a case study of ward nurses' perceptions. *Journal of Clinical Nursing* 14:766–75

Chui Y-Y, Donoghue J, Chenoweth, L 2005 Responses to advanced cancer: Chinese-Australians. *Journal of Advanced Nursing* 52:498–507

Colaizzi P 1978 Psychological research as the phenomenologist views it. In: Valle R, King M (eds) *Existential Phenomenological Alternatives for Psychology*. Oxford University Press, New York, pp 48–71

Erlandsson K, Fagerberg I 2005 Mothers' lived experiences of co-care and post-care after birth, and their strong desire to be close to their baby. *Midwifery* 21:131–8

Fenwick J, Hauck Y, Downie J, et al. 2005 The childbirth expectations of a self-selected cohort of Western Australian women. *Midwifery* 21:23–35

Fowler C, Lee A 2004 Re-writing motherhood: researching women's experiences of learning to mother for the first time. *Australian Journal of Advanced Nursing* 22:39–44

Furber C M, Thomson A M 2006 'Breaking the rules' in baby-feeding practice in the UK: deviance and good practice? *Midwifery* 22:365–76

Geanellos R 2005 Undermining self-efficacy: the consequence of nurse unfriendliness on client well-being. *Collegian* 12:9–14

Giorgi A 1997 The theoretical practice and evaluation of the phenomenological method as a qualitative research procedure. *Journal of Phenomenological Psychology* 28:235–60

Guba E, Lincoln Y 1989 *Fourth generation evaluation.* Sage, London

Huang T-T 2005 Managing fear of falling: *Taiwanese elders' perspective* 42:743–50

Huntington A, Gilmour J 2005 A life shaped by pain: women and endometriosis. *Journal of Clinical Nursing* 14(9):1124–32

Lam W, Fielding R, Chan M, et al. 2005 Gambling with your life: The process of breast cancer treatment decision making in Chinese women. *Psycho-Oncology* 14:1–15

Lee T-T 2005 Nurses' concerns about using information systems: analysis of comments on a computerised nursing care plan system in Taiwan. *Journal of Clinical Nursing* 14:344–53

Liu J-E, Mok E, Wong T 2006 caring in nursing: investigating the meaning of caring from the perspective of cancer patients in Beijing, China. *Journal of Clinical Nursing* 15:188–96

McKain S, Henderson A, Kuys S, et al. 2005 Exploration of patients' needs for information on arrival at a geriatric and rehabilitation unit. *Journal of Clinical Nursing* 14:704–10

McLeod D, Benn C, Pullon S, et al. 2003 The midwive's role in facilitating smoking behaviour change during pregnancy. *Midwifery* 19:285–97

Manias E, Aitkin R, Dunning T 2005 Graduate nurses' communication with health professionals when managing patients' medications. *Journal of Clinical Nursing* 14:354–62

Morse J, Richards L 2002 *Read me first for a user's guide to qualitative methods.* Sage, Thousand Oaks, California

Munhall P 1994 *Revisioning phenomenology: Nursing and health science research.* The League for Nursing Press, New York

Namasivayam P, Orb A, O'Connor M 2005 The challenges of caring for families of the terminally ill: nurses' lived experience. *Contemporary Nurse* 19:169–80

O'Brien A P, O'Brien A J, Hardy D, et al. 2003 The New Zealand development and trial of mental health nursing clinical indicators — a bicultural study. *International Journal of Nursing Studies* 40:853–61

O'Haire S, Blackford J 2005 Nurses' moral agency in negotiating parental participation in care. *International Journal of Nursing Practice* 11:250–6

Peck B, Lillibridge J 2003 Rural fathers' experiences of loss in day-to-day life with chronically ill children. *Australian Journal of Advanced Nursing* 21:21–7

Rolfe G 2006 Validity, trustworthiness and rigour: quality and the idea of qualitative research. *Journal of Advanced Nursing* 53:304–10

Strauss A, Corbin J 1998 *Basics of Qualitative Research: Techniques and Procedures for Developing Grounded Theory,* 2nd edn. Sage, Thousand Oaks, California

Thorne S, Kirkham S, McDonald-Emes J 1997 Interpretive description: a noncategorial qualitative alternative for developing nursing knowledge. *Research in Nursing & Health* 20:169–77

Wilkins C 2006 A qualitative study exploring the support needs of first-time mothers on their journey towards intuitive parenting. *Midwifery* 22:169–80

Answers

TT Tutorial trigger 1

- Some possible reasons why constant comparative data analysis has become popular are: it helps to collect relevant data as following each bit of data analysis, adjustment can be made to questions asked (if interviewing), or to the type of data being collected, or regarding method of data collection — to enhance the possibility of having a relevant set of data overall. This is closer to how we interpret (informally) things in everyday life where a growing picture and developing understandings are the norm, so we are used to this. There is an inclination to be informally interpreting all the way through data collection, so by rendering this as formal interpretation (data analysis) between segments of data collection, those insights are not lost. It is less daunting for the researcher to be doing bits of data analysis than to be faced with a mass of qualitative data to be analysed after data collection is complete. To ensure that 'saturation' has occurred (nothing new of significance is being gathered) and to know when data collection should be ceased etc.

- Relevant situations may include: access to a group of patients at one point of time is finite (e.g. soldiers from a battalion who have sustained injury from an incident); the site for the research where the patient(s) is(are) distant from your home and you cannot stay there for a long period of time; the site for the research has only permitted you access to patients for a limited period of time; the patients are experiencing a short-term event or situation that you need to observe (e.g. attending a health education program) etc.

- Qualitative research that is descriptive exploratory is useful for variable identification. To ensure that variables chosen as items in a quantitative survey questionnaire are well grounded, it may be preferable to derive those from interviews of people who can provide relevant information rather than relying solely on derivation from literature or the opinion of so-called experts in the substantive area. Therefore, the interviews would need to be analysed prior to designing the questionnaire.

TT Tutorial trigger 2

Disadvantages of using a computer program for qualitative research data organisation and management may include: over-reliance on the program for word or phrase searches rather than doing a visual search of data with careful coding technique. Fracturing of data when a 'circling and parking' style of data analysis is more appropriate — including losing sight or 'feel' for the whole data set. The temptation is to move prematurely into conceptualisation when categorisation is actually required (e.g. through setting up code hierarchies prematurely). Considerable time and energy are required for entering codes. Considerable resources are required for training in using the program, maintaining the computer, buying the program and updates, and technical support etc.

TT Tutorial triggers 3 and 4

Group exercises not requiring suggested answers.

TT Tutorial trigger 5

- Probably the primary disadvantage of using a 'letter-boxing' style of qualitative data is trying to fit all interpretations into a finite list of predetermined codes when perhaps there is lack of fit.

- Other forms of written texts that can be analysed if using a discourse analysis approach for qualitative research might include: media reports; historical documents such as minutes of meetings; published articles; memo, letter and email communication etc.
- If studying the culture in a neonatal intensive care or midwifery unit, constant comparative data analysis would potentially be more productive than analysis when all data are collected. This is best because data to illuminate increasingly complex and deep layers of meaning would only be sought when the researcher considered that sufficient analysis had occurred at the previous level (e.g. basic description). Other acceptable answers are also possible.

TT Tutorial trigger 6

Although various answers would be acceptable, probably the main disadvantage of reporting qualitative research by the ways listed would be:

- conference paper — restricted audience of only those in attendance, which can be quite small for some concurrent sessions
- book — unlikely to be identified by the common method for a literature search by using databases such as CINAHL, MIDIRS or MEDLINE
- journal article — difficult to condense qualitative research results into the confining word restrictions for submitted manuscripts (e.g. 3000 to 5000 words)
- media interview — the journalist can pick and choose what to include in the media reports and may miss (or even misconstrue) salient aspects of the results.

Learning activities

1. a	**2.** b	**3.** b	**4.** d
5. c	**6.** d	**7.** a	**8.** b
9. c	**10.** a		

10

Common quantitative methods

DOUG ELLIOTT AND DAVID THOMPSON

KEY TERMS

control

experimental designs

explanatory (independent) variable

manipulation

observational designs

outcome (dependent) variable

quasi-experimental designs

randomisation

Learning outcomes

After reading this chapter, you should be able to:

- describe the overall purpose of quantitative designs
- distinguish the differences between experimental, quasi-experimental and non-experimental designs
- list the criteria necessary for inferring cause-and-effect relationships
- apply critical review criteria to evaluate the findings of selected quantitative studies.

Introduction

Quantitative research refers to studies where the variables of interest are measurable and the results are quantifiable and coded as numerical data. These approaches are often referred to as scientific or empirical methods, as they depict reality as something that is objective and external to the researcher. This chapter provides an overview of the meaning, purpose and issues related to quantitative research designs, and presents the common approaches used to answer a variety of nursing and midwifery questions. Related issues such as sampling, data collection, assessment of measuring instruments and data analysis are discussed in Chapters 11–14. The focus is on providing research consumers with the information to critically evaluate quantitative studies.

As illustrated in Table 10.1, there are three major categories of designs along the quantitative continuum: observational, quasi-experimental and experimental. Each category includes a range of designs. Choice of a design relates to the research question or hypothesis, the amount of control a researcher can have, and study feasibility.

Concepts underpinning quantitative research

The empirical paradigm that informs quantitative research designs emphasises 'objective' observation, accuracy and control — elements originating from scientific investigations in laboratory settings. Medicine in particular, but also other disciplines such as nursing and midwifery, has followed this tradition when undertaking quantitative research. Figure 10.1 illustrates the focus on variables and relationships for each type of quantitative design.

The term 'design' implies the organisation of research components into a coherent and systematic plan, and represents the major distinctive approach chosen for the specific purpose of answering an explicit research question. The question or aims and objectives

TABLE 10.1 Continuum of quantitative research designs

	Design	Sub-types	Features
Increasing control & ability to assign causality	Observational	Descriptive	Describes variables
		Correlational	Examines relationships between variables
		Cross-sectional	Examines variables and relationships at one time point
		Retrospective	Re-traces participants with an outcome backwards to a possible exposure
		Case-control	Cases matched to controls
		Cohort	Follows participants from exposure to outcome
		Longitudinal	Repeated measurements of participants over time
	Quasi-experimental	Time-series	Manipulation (intervention)
		Non-equivalent control group	Manipulation + Control
	Experimental	After-only experimental	No measurement prior to intervention
		Randomised controlled trial	Control & Manipulation + Random assignment to groups
		Cluster-randomised controlled trial	Groups of participants (not individuals) are randomised

FIGURE 10.1 Examining variables in quantitative designs

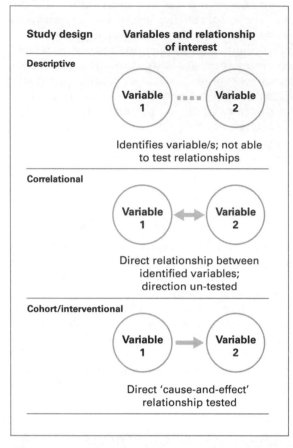

Study design — **Variables and relationship of interest**

Descriptive

Variable 1 ···· Variable 2

Identifies variable/s; not able to test relationships

Correlational

Variable 1 ⟷ Variable 2

Direct relationship between identified variables; direction un-tested

Cohort/interventional

Variable 1 → Variable 2

Direct 'cause-and-effect' relationship tested

influence and guide the choice of design. To make an informed choice about which design will best answer the research question, and for a consumer to understand the implications and the use of research, a clear understanding of designs is important. On this basis alone, clinicians can begin to determine whether a paper describing a research study could be of value in informing their practice (Greenhalgh 1997).

Important elements in quantitative research include objectivity in the conceptualisation of the problem, operational definition, accuracy, feasibility, control of the experimental environment, hypothesis testing, replication, internal validity and external validity. Selection of a particular design gives a researcher more or less control over these elements, particularly three major concepts:

1. control
2. randomisation
3. manipulation.

Control

Control is the presence of constants in a study, including controlling for extraneous variables, using comparison groups and implementing an explicit study protocol so that all participants are involved in the same way. In experimental research the comparison group is the control group (that receives the usual care or treatment), rather than the innovative experimental group under investigation. In some longitudinal, or cross-over, research designs participants act as their own controls.

The strength and rigour of a quantitative design relates to controlling the effects of any extraneous variables that may cause bias (threats to internal validity, such as selection, history and maturation) and influence the study findings. These variables can be either antecedent or intervening. An antecedent (preceding) variable occurs before the study commences but may affect the outcome variable of interest and influence findings (e.g. age, gender, socio-economic status or pre-existing health status could affect outcomes such as recovery time and ability to integrate healthcare behaviours). Similarly, an intervening (mediating) variable is not part of the study design, but occurs during the course of the study and may influence the outcome variable (e.g. a change in the model of clinical care during a longitudinal study). Threats to 'internal validity' are discussed further in Chapter 12.

Randomisation

Randomisation (random assignment) to study groups is designed to ensure that groups or participants are similar on the variables of interest, so that differences in the outcome variable can be attributed to the intervention. If possible, participants are distributed to either the experimental or control group on a purely random, or chance, basis. Each participant therefore has an equal and known probability of being assigned to any group. If randomisation is not possible, the design is quasi-experimental. Random assignment may be done individually or by groups, with a variety of approaches available — coin toss, a table of random numbers, computerised random number generation (see Box 10.1).

Randomisation assumes that important intervening variables are then equally distributed

BOX 10.1 Excerpts from experimental studies of random assignment to study groups

> 'Using a computer-generated random number table, all eligible clients ... were randomly allocated to the control or intervention group.' (Edwards et al. 2005 p 171)
>
> 'The randomisation sequence was generated from a statistical table of random numbers and concealed in sequentially numbered, opaque sealed envelopes.' (Fernandez & Griffiths 2005 p 17)
>
> 'Participants were randomly assigned ... by toss of a coin as we had no access to a centralized random process, and assignments were then sealed in opaque envelopes ahead of time.' (Horn & Chaboyer 2003 p 464)
>
> 'Using a random number table, a schedule of group allocation was prepared for each surgeon.' (Middleton et al. 2005 pp 251, 253)

Research in brief

This randomised controlled trial examined the effect of a post-discharge nurse-led co-ordinated care intervention for 133 patients following carotid endarterectomy surgery. Equivalent study groups at baseline were noted — 'There were no statistically significant differences between the [intervention] ... group and the control group [for] ... age, [sex] ... and level of education. There were ... more symptomatic patients in the control group (70%) than in the [intervention] ... group (55%)' (Middleton et al. 2005 p 254).

The characteristics examined included relevant clinical (presence and type of symptoms prior to surgery, past history, level of artery stenosis) and common demographic variables (age, sex, level of education); it was concluded the two study groups were comparable although some differences were evident. The authors used appropriate statistical tests to examine the equivalence of the groups (χ^2 for categorical variables).

between the groups. Studies should therefore report how groups actually compared on important variables prior to any intervention (see 'Research in brief' opposite).

Evidence-based practice tip

• Random assignment is the random allocation of consenting participants to the intervention or control group of an experimental study.
• Random sampling is a process of selecting a representative group of participants from the population of interest.

Manipulation

Manipulation is relevant only in interventional (experimental or quasi-experimental) studies, not observational designs. A researcher manipulates the causal or 'explanatory (independent) variable' by introducing a 'treatment' or 'intervention'. The intervention (treatment) group receives manipulation of the explanatory variable, while the control group does not. The intervention might be a treatment, a teaching plan or a medication. The effect of this manipulation is measured to determine the effect of the intervention. Studies using true experimental designs in clinical settings are called randomised controlled trials (RCTs), reflecting the high level of control imposed and the importance of randomisation in gain

ing evidence for causation (discussed later in this chapter). A study protocol or procedure ensures that all participants in the intervention group receive similar treatment, and assists the reader in understanding the nature of the experimental treatment.

The three broad categories of observational, quasi-experimental and experimental designs are discussed below.

Observational designs

Observational (non-experimental) designs are used when a researcher wishes to construct a picture of a phenomenon or explore events, people or situations, as they naturally occur in the environment. The aim is therefore to observe and identify variables of interest and explore relationships between those variables. These designs are used when:

• there is little information or research about the topic of interest
• the phenomena of interest are not amenable to experimental designs (e.g. when ethical considerations do not allow a 'treatment' to be denied to a control group).

Observational designs work from a clear, concise problem statement based within an appropriate theoretical framework. Although a researcher does not actively manipulate an intervention variable in this design, the concepts of control and rigour are still important and should be evident to the reader. Demographic data are collected to describe the sample of participants, such as age, gender, income level, ethnicity, occupation and educational level. Reporting this information assists a reader in considering the generalisability of the study and the potential application of the findings to their own practice setting. The common types of observational designs are discussed below, noting their advantages and disadvantages, and using examples from published clinical research to illustrate features of specific designs.

Descriptive/exploratory studies

Descriptive studies use a variety of approaches to measure the variable/s of interest, including observation or questioning of participants via a questionnaire or interview. Direct observation of study participants from a quantitative perspective involves only limited or no interaction with participants. Observers can use a pre-identified classification system to categorise observations or document free-text 'field notes' (see Chapter 12 for further discussion of participant observation).

A survey is another common type of observational design (using either a questionnaire or interview) that enables collection of information about the characteristics of particular individuals, groups, institutions or situations, or about the frequency of a phenomenon's occurrence, particularly when little is known within the positivist paradigm. Variables of interest commonly investigate participants' knowledge, beliefs or attitudes about a particular topic or concept. The terms 'exploratory', 'descriptive' and 'survey' are used to describe this study design. Note that the study purpose is only to relate one variable to another. Relationships between variables or the direction of an effect cannot be tested. There are both advantages and disadvantages to consider when undertaking survey research (see Table 10.2). Importantly, descriptive studies cannot make comparisons between groups or determine causality.

TABLE 10.2 Advantages and disadvantages of survey studies

Advantages	Disadvantages
A lot of information can be obtained from a large population in an economical manner.	Large-scale surveys can be time-consuming and costly.
Accurate if sample is representative of the population of interest.	Information tends to be brief and superficial, with breadth rather than depth of data the outcome.
	Requires expertise in a variety of research areas (e.g. sampling techniques, questionnaire construction, interviewing, data analysis), to produce a reliable and valid study.

Correlational studies

An extension of descriptive research is to explore the relationships between variables that provide a deeper insight into the phenomenon of interest. Correlational studies enable examination of the relationship between pairs of variables, as well as a comparison between groups. A researcher uses this design to quantify the strength of the relationship between variables (i.e. as one variable changes, does a related change occur in the other variable?). For example, a cross-sectional mixed-methods study examined medication knowledge and self-management in a sample of 30 participants with type 2 diabetes attending an outpatient clinic. One of the findings was, 'Education level was associated with greater likelihood of reporting hypoglycaemic episodes ($r = 0.22$, $p = 0.24$)' (Dunning & Manias 2005 p 11). A correlation between two variables — diabetes education and reporting hypoglycaemic events — was examined, although the association (Pearson's r statistic) was weak (0.22; theoretical range 0–1.0) and not statistically significant ($p > 0.05$). See Chapter 14 for explanation of correlation data analysis.

Correlation designs cannot however test a 'cause-and-effect' relationship (i.e. whether a change in one variable causes a measurable change in another variable). When reading a correlational study, identify the variables and the relationship being tested, and consider whether the implied relationship is consistent with the conceptual framework and research question being asked. A common misuse of a correlational design is a researcher's attempt to conclude that a causal relationship exists between the study variables. Despite this limitation, the design is useful — clinical practice applicability relates to the study question and feasibility. The advantages and disadvantages of correlational studies are listed in Table 10.3.

TABLE 10.3 Advantages and disadvantages of correlational studies

Advantages	Disadvantages
Increased flexibility to investigate relationships among variables.	Unable to determine a causal relationship between variables because of the lack of manipulation, control and randomisation.
Efficient and effective method of collecting a large amount of data about an issue of interest.	No random sampling possible with pre-existing groups — the ability to generalise is therefore decreased.
Provides a framework for exploring the relationship between variables that are not able to be manipulated.	Unable to manipulate the variables of interest.
A foundation for potential, future interventional studies.	

Cross-sectional studies

Surveys that measure data at one point in time (i.e. data are collected on only one occasion with the same participants rather than on the same participants at several points in time) are called cross-sectional studies. These studies are categorised as either 'descriptive' or 'analytic'. Importantly, cross-sectional analytic (CSA) studies use inferential statistics to infer a causal relationship between two or more variables of interest.

To examine calcium intake and beliefs and knowledge about osteoporosis in a community sample of 265 young Taiwanese women, a cross-sectional design was used with a mailed questionnaire. Respondents had low calcium intake, but felt that osteoporosis was not serious and prevention was difficult. Correlation and regression (inferential) analyses demonstrated seven factors (e.g. knowledge, number of children, self-rated health) that accounted for 32% of the differences (variance) in calcium intake by participants, leading to a conclusion that '… calcium intake is a combined function of cognitive and social factors.' (Chang 2006 p 25). This design was appropriate to measure the variables of interest in a broad sample at one point in time. It was not clear how participants were approached and selected (potential for selection bias), and the response rate was only 17% (potential for non-representative sample). The use of inferential statistics was appropriate and demonstrated links between certain knowledge and social factors, and calcium intake in this sample.

A limitation of this design is that the outcome of interest and the causal factor are measured simultaneously. The lack of time as a factor therefore provides only weak evidence of causality. In contrast, a longitudinal study which followed a group of people for a period of time during a series of studies would provide more strength of causality (see later in this section).

Retrospective studies

The aim of a retrospective study is to link present outcomes to some past events. The design is also called 'ex-post facto' (favoured by social scientists), or comparative, and is similar to a case-control study (see below). In a retrospective audit of hospital records, 110 patients who suffered an in-hospital fall were matched by casemix and length of stay with a sample of patients who did not fall. Records were examined for predictor variables (e.g. biochemistry levels). Significant differences were noted between the two groups for age, confusion state 24 hours prior to the fall, and abnormal serum alkaline phosphatase levels. (O'Hagen & O'Connell 2005). The authors noted the limitations of this design, although other limitations were evident; for example, assessment of confusion was not specified. A case-control design, with controls matched for age, gender and admission date, and the use of correlation and regression analyses would have provided greater confidence in the associations noted.

Case-control studies

A case-control study is an epidemiological approach which examines participants on the basis of a study outcome (clinical characteristic, condition or disease) that is or is not present (e.g. lung cancer; heart disease). The study direction is retrospective, from the study outcome backwards to the cause or the exposure. Individuals with the outcome of interest are the 'cases'. Cases are matched with 'controls', a sample of people who come from the same 'study base' (similar to the cases for characteristics such as age, gender or clinical procedure), but do not have the outcome of interest. There are commonly multiple controls matched to each case (2–3 : 1). Detailed past histories, particularly in relation to possible risk factors (exposure), are examined from both groups to see if the cases have been more exposed to the suspected causative factor variable than the controls.

Research in brief

This case-control study examined the association between kava use and ischaemic heart disease (IHD) in Aboriginal communities in Arnhem Land, Australia. '... cases comprised 83 people admitted to hospital ... with a diagnosis of IHD ... Up to four randomly selected controls (n = 302) were matched with each case for age, sex, and home locality ... a further 20 people with no record of hospital admission [who] died ... were matched with 75 controls' (Clough et al. 2004 p 140). Although there was no clear evidence of an association between kava use and IHD, a non-significant tendency of a 50% increase in risk of IHD was noted (Odds ratio [OR] = 1.51; 95% confidence interval [CI] = 0.75 – 3.05), suggesting more research is required to examine possible associations (Clough et al. 2004).

This study base was well defined, with multiple 'controls' per 'case'. A larger sample size (perhaps involving participants with diagnosed IHD who were not admitted to hospital) may have improved the precision of the noted 50% increase in risk (an OR of 95% CI that includes 1.00 denotes a non-significant finding).

Selection bias may exist if the cases are not from a well-defined study base (in time and place). A critical reader therefore needs to cautiously evaluate the conclusions drawn in relation to measurement error. Advantages are similar to those of a correlational design, but a higher level of control is possible. Disadvantages include an inability to draw a causal linkage between the two variables (an alternative hypothesis may cause the relationship), and finding naturally occurring groups of participants who are similar in all respects except for their exposure to the variable of interest is very difficult.

Cohort studies

A cohort study is an epidemiological approach where the direction is from the exposure to the outcome, or cause to effect. Commonly, a researcher studies the development of a particular health outcome or disease state. Participants are selected from a population known to be free of the health outcome under study, and then classified according to whether they have one or more explanatory variables hypothetically related to the outcome. These participants (referred to as the cohort), are then studied over a time period ranging from months to years, to determine who develops the outcome of interest. The incidence of the study outcome is observed in relation to exposure to possible causes/risk factors (Grimes & Schulz 2002).

For example, the classic Nurses' Health Study is one of the largest cohort studies of risk factors for major chronic diseases in women. In 1976 over 120 000 married registered nurses aged 30–55 were initially enrolled in the study (Belanger et al. 1978) and the cohort continues to be followed (Colditz & Hankinson 2005), examining a wide range of issues including diet, menopause and breast cancer. At the time of writing, contemporary articles continue to be published from follow-up assessments — over 70 articles were identified using Medline from 1978–2006 — (see the Nurses' Health Study website in 'Additional resources' at the end of this chapter). Similarly, the Framingham heart study examined the effect of blood pressure, cholesterol levels, smoking, exercise and other variables, on the development of coronary artery disease in a cohort of healthy men, at specified intervals over a period of years (e.g. Margolis et al. 1974; Peeters et al. 2002).

Cohort designs can be used to examine relationships both retrospectively and prospectively. Prospective (longitudinal) studies explore hypothesised causes, differences or relationships, and move forward in time to the presumed effect. A disadvantage of this design is the time period and high costs involved, as there may be a considerable time lag between time of exposure and the subsequent study outcome. This may be partly overcome in an historical cohort study if some of the data of individuals exposed in the past are available for use.

Longitudinal studies

In contrast to a cross-sectional design, longitudinal studies collect data from the same group of participants at different points in time (repeated measures). By collecting data from each participant at certain intervals, a longitudinal perspective of the outcome variable is possible. The advantages and disadvantages of a longitudinal design are listed in Table 10.4. An example of this design is a study that assessed dietary fat intake in a sample of 239 women admitted to hospital with an acute myocardial infarction (AMI) or for coronary artery bypass graft

TABLE 10.4 Advantages and disadvantages of longitudinal studies

Advantages	Disadvantages
Each participant is followed separately and therefore acts as her or his own control.	Long duration of data collection — costly in terms of time, effort and resources.
Both relationships and differences can be explored between variables.	Threats to internal validity include 'testing' and 'mortality' (loss to follow-up), and the influence of confounding variables.
Changes in the variables of interest are assessed over time; early trends in data can be investigated at a subsequent measurement.	Social desirability bias is possible (participants respond in a way they believe is congruent with the researchers' expectations) — 'Hawthorne effect'.

(CABG) surgery, using repeated measures (in hospital 2, 4 and 12 months post-event). A valid questionnaire assessed dietary fat intake. Self-reports reflected a significant decrease in dietary fat intake at 2 months, then it increased over the next 10 months; at 12 months scores were still significantly lower than baseline (Murphy et al. 2006). This observational longitudinal design was appropriate for the study aims. Some loss to follow-up was evident, with limitations in generalisability noted by the authors.

> **Point to ponder**
> ▶ When assessing the appropriateness of a cross-sectional study compared to a longitudinal study, first examine the purpose of the study in relation to the design.

Causality in observational designs

As noted in this section, observational designs are often limited in their ability to determine 'causality' — where one variable influences another in a cause-and-effect relationship. Historically, only experimental research has been able to support the concept of causality. There are, however, many instances in clinical research where experimental studies cannot be conducted because of ethical or practical reasons. To overcome this limitation, several statistical analytical techniques are available to explain relationships among variables and establish causal links. These 'causal modelling' analyses (also termed 'causal analysis', 'path analysis', 'Linear Structural Relation Analysis [LISREL]', and 'structural equation modelling [SEM]') are introduced in Chapter 14 and discussed further in other specialty statistics texts (see 'Additional resources' at the end of this chapter).

Quasi-experimental designs

Quasi-experiments are designs where a researcher manipulates an experimental treatment (intervention; explanatory variable) but some characteristic of a 'true' experiment is lacking — either control or randomisation. Both designs test cause-and-effect relationships, but the lack of control and/or randomisation in quasi-experimental designs threatens the study's internal validity and weakens any causal inference. Many different quasi-experimental designs exist; the common types are discussed here (see Figure 10.2).

Suppose a researcher is interested in the effects of a new cardiac education program on the physical and psycho-social outcome of patients newly diagnosed with acute coronary syndrome. A researcher could randomly assign participants to either the group receiving the new program or the group receiving the usual program, but for any number of practical reasons, that design is not possible. One difficulty is when patients on the same clinical unit have to receive both experimental and control interventions, without any overlap. The potential for participant 'contamination' needs to be considered by the researcher — how to stop participants receiving or adopting the 'wrong' intervention. The choices are to abandon the experiment, or conduct a quasi-experimental study. With the latter, a researcher can find a similar clinical unit that has not introduced the new educational program and study the newly diagnosed cardiac patients who are admitted as the comparison (control) group.

> ● **Evidence-based practice tip**
> 'Study contamination' occurs when participants allocated to a specific study group receive the alternate intervention.

There is no random assignment of patients by the researcher in this situation — therefore a quasi-experimental design. There are however a range of potential threats to validity when interpreting the results of quasi-experimental studies (see Table 10.5).

Non-equivalent control group studies

This design is the quasi-experimental version of a 'true experimental' design, except participants are unable to be randomised to study groups because of practical or feasibility issues (see Figure 10.2, A). Despite the lack of randomisation, this design is commonly used in clinical research as it is relatively

FIGURE 10.2 Comparison of quasi-experimental designs

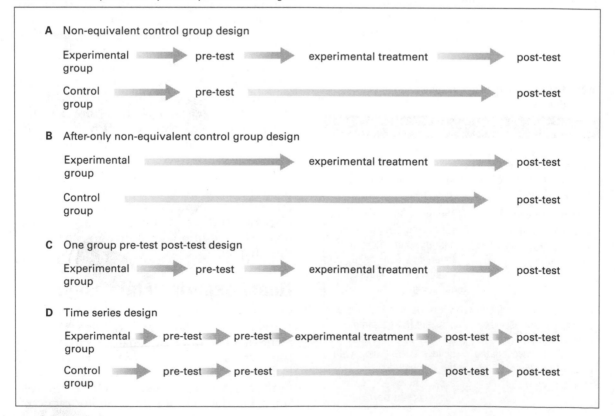

TABLE 10.5 Advantages and disadvantages of quasi-experimental studies

Advantages	Disadvantages
Practical, feasible and able to be generalised.	Need to rule out any plausible alternative explanations for the findings — control by design or statistical analysis.
May be the only design to evaluate some hypotheses, particularly in clinical settings.	Unable to make clear cause-and-effect inferences.
More adaptable to the real-world practice setting than controlled experimental designs.	

robust to threats to internal validity. Collection of data at 'pre-test' (measurement prior to the intervention) allows comparison of the two groups before the intervention is introduced, and any differences between groups can also be controlled during data analysis. This feature strengthens the influence of the intervention, and minimises any effects of extraneous variables.

Research in brief

A quasi-experimental study examined the effects of a back-pain reducing intervention in pregnant women attending antenatal clinics in South Korea. Participants in one clinic were offered an educational and exercise intervention, while another clinic served as the control. Measures of back pain, functional limitation and anxiety were assessment at baseline, and 6 and 12 weeks after the intervention. The intervention group had significantly lower back pain at 12 weeks (4.2 vs 5.7; 0–10 scale), but no differences were detected for functional limitations and anxiety (Shim et al. 2007). This design was used to prevent study contamination. Measuring instruments were established as reliable and valid. The sample size was small (n = 56) and from one hospital site, therefore generalisability was limited.

After-only non-equivalent control group studies

Suppose a clinical researcher did not measure specific characteristics of participants before the introduction of a new intervention, but later decided that it would be useful to have data demonstrating the effect of the program. Perhaps a health service manager asked for these data to determine whether the extra cost of a new teaching program was justified. The study that could be conducted would be the after-only non-equivalent control group design, shown in Figure 10.2, B. This design minimises 'testing effects' (completing a pre-test can effect the post-test scores), but assumes that the two groups are equivalent before the intervention is introduced.

Point to ponder

▶ Check that two non-randomly assigned groups are comparable on important characteristics at the beginning of the study.

In the previous example of a teaching program for patients with newly diagnosed cardiovascular disease, measuring the participants' motivation after the teaching program would not tell us whether their motivation levels differed before they received the program, or whether the teaching program motivated individuals to learn more about their health problem. Therefore a researcher's conclusion that the teaching program improved physical status and psycho-social outcome would be subject to the alternative conclusion that the results were an effect of pre-existing motivations (selection effect) in combination with greater learning in those more motivated (selection–maturation interaction). See Chapter 12 for further description of these threats to study validity.

One group pre-test–post-test studies

This design is used when only one group is available for studying the effects of an intervention (see Figure 10.2, C). The lack of randomisation and a control group limit the internal validity and generalisability of any findings. A one group pre-test–post-test design was used to evaluate a 1–day training program for 40 nurses on managing violent behaviours in a regional Australian emergency department. The questionnaire examined incidence of aggression experienced, confidence in managing behaviour, and attitudes of participants, using a pre-test 2 months prior and post-test 3 months after the training day. The training raised awareness for participants in '… managing aggressive behaviour and improving their attitudes towards potentially violent patients' (Deans 2004 p 17).

Attempting to include a control group in this environment would have led to study contamination, but limited generalisability. There was minimal description of the training program. The measuring instrument was previously developed by the researcher; acceptable reliability was reported but validity was not discussed. The sample was small and in one site only; these limitations were noted by the author.

Before–after design

Sometimes researchers use a 'before–after' design to test the effects of an introduced intervention, when participants are different individuals before the intervention than after the intervention. For example, a study examined the effects of a clinical pathway for inpatients with chronic lung disease. Patients on the clinical pathway (n = 88) demonstrated a non-significant decrease in length of stay (LOS) — 6.7 vs 7.6 days (13% decrease), and a significantly lower level of anxiety at hospital discharge when compared to the standard care group (n = 90). The two groups were equivalent on other clinical outcomes (Santamaria et al. 2004). Although labelled a 'cohort' design, this study examined patient outcomes before and after an intervention (the clinical pathway) was introduced. Sample size was calculated on a 15% decrease in LOS difference. The authors noted the limitation of the study design, but also the practical reasons why an RCT was not possible.

τ τ Tutorial trigger 1

Given the information in the 'before–after design' section, describe the reasons why an RCT design was not possible in the study (Santamaria et al. 2004).

Time-series studies

Another approach when only one group is available, is to study that group over a longer period, using a time-series design (illustrated in Figure 10.2, D). To rule out alternative explanations for the findings of a one-group pre-test–post-test design, the variable/s of interest are measured over a longer period while introducing the intervention at some time during the data collection period.

An example of this design is an Australian study that explored the shelf-life of clinical items sterilised using three different methods in a hospital's Central Sterilising Supply Department. Assessment of continued sterility was undertaken every 3 months for 2 years. No contamination of stock was noted for any method, while the material costs were substantially lower for laminate when compared to single or double linen and paper wraps (Barrett et al. 2003). This design was appropriate for the aims of the study; control of the quasi-experiment was evident, including compliance with Australian Standards for sterility. Sterility was maintained while demonstrating considerable resource savings.

Even with the absence of a control group, the number of data collection points minimises threats to validity such as 'history' effects. However, 'testing' is a threat to validity with this design because measures are repeated so many times. Why alternative explanations for the findings in a quasi-experimental study are not plausible should be discussed by the researcher. In some cases, clinical or practical knowledge of the problem and patient population can suggest that a particular explanation is not plausible. Nonetheless it is important to replicate studies to support any causal inferences developed through quasi-experimental designs.

Experimental designs

An experiment is a scientific investigation that involves observation and data collection according to explicit criteria and protocol. Experimental designs have all three identifying properties: randomisation, control, and manipulation. These designs are used to test 'cause-and-effect relationships' between an intervention (treatment) and an outcome, and minimise or control any alternative explanations (threats to validity) for the study findings (Thompson 2004). To infer causality requires:

- the explanatory (causal) and outcome (effect) variables must be associated with each other
- the 'cause' to precede the 'effect'
- that the relationship is not able to be explained by another (extraneous) variable/s.

Experiments can be classified by setting. While 'field' experiments such as a randomised controlled trial and 'laboratory' experiments share the same design characteristics and properties, they are conducted in fundamentally different environments. Laboratory experiments take place in an artificial setting created specifically for the purpose of research, enabling almost complete control by a researcher. Field experiments, however, occur in a real, existing social setting such as a hospital unit, clinic or community where the phenomenon of interest actually occurs.

Conducting an experimental study is difficult, as all relevant variables need to be identified and then controlled, manipulated or measured. Unlike the physical sciences, nursing and midwifery researchers continue to identify important complex concepts and relationships that are the province of our disciplines. Other designs may therefore be more appropriate to answer certain questions, unless the above requirements for variables can be met.

While most experiments in nursing and midwifery are field experiments and control is such an important element, it is common that a researcher cannot control contamination. Conversely, studies conducted in the laboratory are by nature 'artificial', and therefore not 'real-world'. Although laboratory experiments have stronger internal validity than field-work studies, their weakness is with external validity. When reading research reports, it is important to consider the setting of the experiment and what impact this may have on the study findings.

There are several different experimental designs, each based on the classic 'true experiment' presented in Figure 10.3, A. Participants are randomly assigned to the control or experimental group(s), with the treatment given only to those in the experimental group.

The outcome variable is measured in both groups as a pre-test and post-test (before and after the intervention is introduced).

When reviewing experimental (or quasi-experimental) studies, the prime focus is on assessing the validity of the findings. Did the intervention (explanatory variable) cause the desired effect on the outcome variable? Validity of the findings and conclusion depend on how well the researcher has controlled other variables that may also explain any change in the outcome variables. Although random assignment and control in the classic experimental design minimise the effects of many threats to internal validity, it is not perfect in practice as some threats are difficult to control. In particular, 'mortality' effects (a threat to internal validity) may be a problem for studies with long follow-up periods, as participants tend to drop out because of the burden over an extended period of time (called 'loss to follow-up'). There may be important differences between participants who withdraw and those who complete the study; these differences may explain the study findings, not the intervention. Guidelines for reporting experimental studies have been developed by the CONSORT (consolidated standards of reporting trials) group for reporting these types of threats (Moher et al. 2001; see 'Additional resources' at the end of this chapter). This issue is discussed in more detail in Chapter 20.

T_T Tutorial trigger 2

The group assignment for your research subject is to critique an assigned quantitative study. To proceed, you must first decide on the design to be used: you think it is an ex-post facto design; the others in the group think it is an experimental design because it has several explicit hypotheses. How would you convince them that you are correct?

Randomised controlled trials

A randomised controlled trial (RCT) is the clinical equivalent of a true experiment, and is the 'gold standard' for testing cause-and-effect relationships in clinical research (Thompson 2004). As illustrated in Figure 10.3, A, participants are randomly assigned to the experimental and control groups, so that any pre-intervention differences (antecedent variables) are measured and/or controlled. These pre-test measures or observations provide a baseline

FIGURE 10.3 Comparison of experimental designs

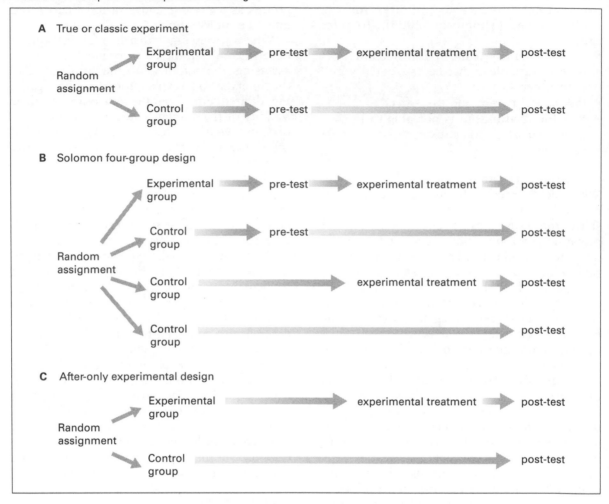

score for verifying similar characteristics between control and treatment groups, and therefore the effect of the intervention. The intervention is then introduced to the 'treatment' group and the outcome variable is again measured to see whether it has changed. The control group gets no experimental treatment but is also measured for comparison with the experimental group. The difference between the two groups at post-test reflects whether a causal link actually exists between the explanatory and outcome variables (see the 'Research in brief' p 169).

The effect of a continuity of midwifery care model on women's experiences was also examined using an RCT design (Homer et al. 2002). Participants were randomised to a midwifery care model (n = 325) or usual care (n = 332). A small team of midwives provided antenatal, intrapartum and postpartum care

as the intervention. A mailed questionnaire at 8–10 weeks post-delivery examined women's preferences for care, level of knowledge, continuity of care and sense of personal control during labour. Overall, the midwifery care model was associated with more positive experiences when compared with standard care. Importantly, during labour women had a higher sense of control and a more positive birthing experience when they knew their midwife.

Solomon four-group design

A more complex experimental design used to minimise the effect of repeated 'testing' (a threat to internal validity) is the Solomon four-group design. This design has two groups identical to those used in the classic experimental design, but two further groups, an experimental after–only

Research in brief

This RCT examined the effect of a post-discharge nurse-led co-ordinated care intervention for 133 patients following carotid endarterectomy surgery. The intervention included phone follow-up with participants at 2, 6 and 12 weeks post-surgery, mailed information about stroke risk factors, and liaison with the participant's GP for targeted support. The intervention group demonstrated statistically significant knowledge on stroke warning signs, improved lifestyle changes and diet modification, when compared to the control group (Middleton et al. 2005).

The design was appropriate and rigorous, with the allocation of participants to groups conducted according to the CONSORT guidelines. The intervention was well described, and measurements targeted this specific clinical cohort for health status, physical activity, lifestyle and risk factors.

group and a control after–only group are also included. As Figure 10.3, B illustrates, all four groups have randomly assigned participants. Addition of the last two groups helps to rule out 'testing' threats that the pre-test groups may experience. This design enables evaluation of the effect of the pre-test on the post-test. A limitation however is the need for a larger sample size when compared to a two-group design. In contemporary research, this design is not common in nursing or midwifery.

Research in brief

In a health promotion study, this design was used to examine the effect of a 'measurement intervention' of physical activity on 635 patients from 29 Dutch general practices (van Sluijs et al. 2006). Participants completed a questionnaire on their current physical activity (the intervention), and then a 6-month follow-up. The findings demonstrated a positive effect of the interventional measurement on participants' physical activity behaviour, possibly triggered by an increased awareness of their health status.

After-only design

Another alternative design is the after-only design (or post-test-only control group), shown in Figure 10.3, C. This design is composed of two randomly assigned groups, but neither group is measured at pre-test. The process of randomly assigning participants to groups is assumed to be sufficient to ensure a lack of bias in determining whether the treatment created significant differences between the two groups. This design is particularly useful when testing effects are expected to be a major problem and the number of available participants is too limited to use a Solomon four-group design.

Point to ponder

▶ Experimental studies are not the most commonly used designs in nursing or midwifery research. Experimentation assumes that all of the relevant variables involved in a phenomenon have been identified and are measurable. For many areas of nursing and midwifery this is not the case, and descriptive or exploratory studies need to be completed before experimental interventions can be applied to a clinical issue.

Cluster-randomised controlled trials

A cluster-randomised controlled trial (c-RCT) uses coherent groups or clusters of individuals, such as wards (Priestley et al. 2004), hospitals (e.g. Hillman et al. 2005), or general practices (e.g. Fletcher et al. 2004), as the random allocation unit, not individuals. All individuals in the group allocated to the intervention then receive the experimental treatment, eliminating the potential for study contamination. These studies are, however, expensive to conduct as the 'cluster' is the unit of analysis and any variance within the group works against any intervention effect (Flynn et al. 2002) (see 'Research in brief' p 170 and 'Additional resources' at the end of this chapter).

Chapter 16 discusses the critical review process, which is directed towards evaluating the appropriateness of the study design in relation to factors such as the research

Research in brief

This cluster-randomised controlled trial examined the effects of a medical emergency team (MET) system on the composite outcome measure (cardiac arrest, unexpected death, unplanned ICU admission) in 23 Australian hospitals. This design was used in preference to an RCT to avoid contamination across study groups within individual hospitals. The intervention resulted in a non-significant decrease in the incidence of events (5.3 vs 5.9/1000 hospital admissions) (Hillman et al. 2005).

This was a rigorously designed and highly resourced study, but there was still 'contamination' of the control sites with pseudo-MET responses occurring in the 'control' sites. The actual event rate was lower than the hypothesised rate, and the study was therefore under-powered. A suitably powered study may not be feasible or fundable.

BOX 10.2 Criteria for evaluating quantitative designs

1. What design was used in the study (observational, quasi-experimental or experimental)?
2. Which specific type of the above design was used in the study, and was it appropriate?
3. Was the design appropriate for the research problem and data collection methods?
4. Was the problem examining a cause-and-effect relationship?
5. Were the common threats to the validity of findings for this design addressed?
6. Was the design suited to the study setting?
7. Were the limitations of the design adequately discussed?
8. Were there other limitations related to the design that you identified but they were not discussed?
9. For observational designs, did the report go beyond the parameters of this design, and infer cause-and-effect relationships between variables?
10. For experimental designs, how were randomisation, control and manipulation applied?
11. What were the plausible alternative explanations for findings, and were they discussed and discounted?
12. Are the findings able to be generalised to other practice settings and the larger population of interest?

problem, theoretical framework, hypothesis, methods and data analysis, and interpretation. The overall purpose of reviewing studies is to assess the validity of findings and to determine whether these findings are worth incorporating into your professional practice and/or as the evidence base for current institutional clinical practices. Criteria for the review of quantitative designs relate to how well any potential biases in the methods have been addressed (see Box 10.2).

The most important question to ask as you read experimental studies is, 'What else could have happened to explain the findings?' This question of potential alternative explanations will be addressed by a well-written report, which will systematically review potential threats to the validity of the findings. You must then decide if the author's explanations are clear and logical.

Summary

Quantitative research methods enable a researcher to manipulate numerical data to answer specific research questions and draw inferences from their findings. Observational (non-experimental) designs are used to construct a picture or description of events as they naturally occur, but cannot establish cause-and-effect relationships between variables. Quasi-experimental designs are frequently used in clinical research to test cause-and-effect relationships, as there are times when experimental designs are impractical or unethical to conduct within that setting. True experiments are characterised by control of extraneous variables, manipulation of the explanatory variable and to randomly assign participants to study groups.

The following four chapters discuss sampling, data collection, measuring instrument assessment and data analysis issues for quantitative research, respectively.

KEY POINTS

- Three main strengths of quantitative approaches are the objectivity, precision and control afforded through design, sampling strategies and analytical tests.

- Experimental and other quantitative designs allow nurses and midwives to justify in a scientific manner the outcomes of their actions and provide the basis for effective high quality and evidence-based clinical practice.

- Extraneous and confounding variables represent a major influence on the interpretation of any quantitative study as they limit the validity of the study and generalisability of the findings; this is particularly evident with observational designs.

- When reviewing experimental studies, check that the author has addressed all of the relevant issues, such as evidence of a representative sample, and minimal and unbiased loss to follow-up.

Learning activities

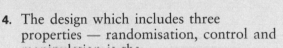

1. Administration of an intervention to one group of participants and not another is an example of:
   i.   homogeneity of participants
   ii. manipulation of the explanatory variable
   iii. an experimental study
   iv. the introduction of bias
   (a) i and ii
   (b) ii and iii
   (c) iii and iv
   (d) i and iv.

2. Why are non-experimental correlation studies used frequently in nursing and midwifery research?
   (a) The findings from this design can be generalised to larger populations.
   (b) The explanatory variable can be easily manipulated in this design.
   (c) Many of the phenomena of clinical interest cannot be manipulated, controlled or randomised.
   (d) This design provides a high level of evidence.

3. The type of design that has two groups identical to the true experimental design plus an experimental after-group and a control after-group is called a:
   (a) time-series design
   (b) Solomon four-group design
   (c) non-equivalent control group design
   (d) after-only experimental design.

4. The design which includes three properties — randomisation, control and manipulation is the:
   (a) true experiment
   (b) Solomon four-group design
   (c) non-equivalent control group design
   (d) quasi-experiment.

5. Identify whether the following studies are experimental or quasi-experimental. Use the abbreviations E for Experimental and Q for Quasi-experimental.
   (a) Fifty teenage mothers are randomly assigned into an experimental parenting support group and a regular support group. Before the program and at the end of the 3-month program, mother–child interaction patterns are compared between the two groups.
   (b) Patients on two separate clinical units are given a patient satisfaction-with-care questionnaire to complete at the end of their first hospital day and on the day of discharge. The patients on one unit receive care directed by a nurse case manager, and the patients on the other unit receive care from the usual rotation of nurses. Patient satisfaction scores are compared.
   (c) Students are randomly assigned to two groups. One group receives an experimental independent study program and the other receives the

usual classroom instruction. Both groups receive the same post-test to evaluate learning.

(d) A study was conducted to compare the effectiveness of a music relaxation program with silent relaxation on lowering blood pressure ratings. Participants were randomly assigned into groups and blood pressures were measured before, during and immediately after the relaxation exercises.

6. Which of the following are means by which control is introduced into the design of a study?
    i. manipulation of the outcome variable
    ii. manipulation of the explanatory variable
    iii. randomisation
    iv. use of control groups.
    (a) i, ii and iii
    (b) ii, iii and iv
    (c) i, iii and iv
    (d) i, ii, iii and iv.

7. Which type of design is the most powerful for examining cause-and-effect relationships?
    (a) randomised controlled trial
    (b) quasi-experimental
    (c) non-equivalent control group
    (d) time series.

8. When data are collected multiple times before and after the introduction of the intervention, the study:
    i. is called a time-series design
    ii. cannot be called a quasi-experimental design
    iii. is a non-equivalent control group design
    iv. may have threats of selection and maturation.
    (a) i and ii
    (b) ii and iii
    (c) iii and iv
    (d) i and iv.

9. In quasi-experimental designs:
    (a) the threats to external validity are numerous
    (b) the level of evidence obtained is II
    (c) one of the characteristics of a true experimental design is lacking

(d) the findings are not as valuable as those of experimental designs

10. What are the potential disadvantages of longitudinal studies?
    i. participant loss due to study attrition
    ii. loss of a control group
    iii. the Hawthorne effect
    iv. superficiality of data
    (a) i and ii
    (b) i and iii
    (c) ii and iii
    (d) i and iv.

Additional resources

Campbell M J, Elbourne D R, Altman D G, for the CONSORT group 2004 The CONSORT statement: extension to cluster randomised trials. *British Medical Journal* 328:702–8

Cook T D, Campbell D T 1979 *Quasi-experimentation: design and analysis issues for field settings*. Rand-McNally, Chicago

Critical Appraisal Skills Program (CASP), UK National Health Service Critical Appraisal Tools — randomised controlled trials; cohort studies; case control studies. Online. Available: http://www.phru.nhs.uk/casp

Fletcher R H, Fletcher S W 2005 *Clinical epidemiology: the essentials* (4th edn). Lippincott Williams & Wilkins, Baltimore

Hanson B P 2006 Designing, conducting and reporting clinical research: a step by step approach. *Injury, International Journal of the Care of the Injured* 37:583–94

Medical Research Council (United Kingdom) 2000 A Framework for Development and Evaluation of RCTs for Complex Interventions to Improve Health. Online. Available: http://www.mrc.ac.uk/pdf-mrc_cpr.pdf

Medical Research Council (United Kingdom) 2002 Cluster randomised trials: methodological and ethical considerations. Online. Available: http:/www.mrc.ac.uk/index/publications/publications_ethics_and-best_practice/pdf-cluster_randomised_trials-link

Moher D, Schulz K F, Altman D G, for the CONSORT Group 2001 The CONSORT statement: revised recommendations for improving the quality of reports of parallel-group randomised trials. *Lancet* 357:1191–4

Munro B H 2005 Statistical methods for health care research (5th edn). Lippincott Williams & Wilkins, Philadelphia

Nurses' Health Study. Online. Available: http://www.channing.harvard.edu/nhs/index.html

Polivka B J, Nickel J T 1992 Case-control design: an appropriate strategy for nursing research. *Nursing Research* 41:250–3

Weinert C, Burman M 1996 Nurturing longitudinal samples. *West Journal of Nursing Research* 18: 360–4

References

Barrett R, Stevens J, Taranter J 2003 A shelf-life trial: examining the efficacy of event related sterility principles and its implications for nursing practice. *Australian Journal of Advanced Nursing* 21:8–12

Belanger C F, Hennekens C H, Rosner B, et al. 1978 The nurses' health study. *American Journal of Nursing* 78:1039–40

Campbell M J 2004 Extending CONSORT to include cluster trials [editorial]. *British Medical Journal* 328

Chang S-F 2006 A cross-sectional survey of calcium intake in relation to knowledge of osteoporosis and beliefs in young adult women. *International Journal of Nursing Practice* 12:21–7

Closs S J, Cheater F M 1999 Evidence for nursing practice: a clarification of the issues. *Journal of Advanced Nursing* 30:10–17

Clough A R, Wang Z, Bailie R S, et al. 2004 Case-control study of the association between kava use and ischaemic heart disease in Aboriginal communities in eastern Arnhem Land (Northern Territory) *Australian Journal of Epidemiology and Community Health* 58:140 1

Colditz G A, Hankinson S E 2005 Nurses' Health Study: lifestyle and health among women *Nature Reviews. Cancer* 5:388–96

Deans C 2004 The effectiveness of a training program for emergency department nurses in managing violent situations. *Australian Journal of Advanced Nursing* 21:17–22

Dunning T, Manias E 2005 Medication knowledge and self management by people with type 2 diabetes. *Australian Journal of Advanced Nursing* 23:7–13

Edwards H, Courtney M, Finlayson K, et al. 2005 Improved healing rates for chronic venous leg ulcers: pilot study results from a randomized controlled trial of a community nursing intervention. *International Journal of Nursing Practice* 11:169–76

Fernandez R, Griffiths R 2005 A comparison of an evidence-based regime with the standard protocol for monitoring postoperative observation: a randomised controlled trial. *Australian Journal of Advanced Nursing* 23:15–21

Fletcher A E, Ng E S W, Stirling S L, et al. 2004 Population-based multidimensional assessment of older people in UK general practice: a cluster-randomised factorial trial. *Lancet* 364:1667–77

Flynn T N, Whitley E, Peters T J 2002 Recruitment strategies in a cluster randomised trial: cost implications. *Statistics in Medicine* 21:397–405

Greenhalgh T 1997 *How to read a paper: the basics of evidence-based medicine.* BMJ Publishing Group, London

Grimes D A, Schulz K F 2002 Cohort studies: marching towards outcomes. *Lancet* 359:341–5

Hillman K, Chen J, Cretikos M, et al. 2005 Introduction of the medical emergency team (MET) system: a cluster-randomised trial. *Lancet* 365:2091–7

Homer C S E, Davis G K, Cooke M, et al. 2002 Women's experiences of continuity of midwifery care in a randomised controlled trial in Australia. *Midwifery* 18: 102–12

Horn D, Chaboyer W 2003 Gastric feeding in critically ill children: a randomized controlled trial. *American Journal of Critical Care* 12:461–8

Margolis J R, Gillum R F, Feinleib M, et al. 1974 Community surveillance for coronary heart disease: the Framingham Cardiovascular Disease Survey: methods and preliminary results. *American Journal of Epidemiology* 100: 425–36

Middleton S, Donnelly N, Harris J, et al. 2005 Nursing intervention after carotid endarterectomy: a randomized trial of Co-ordinated Care Post-Discharge (CCPD). *Journal of Advanced Nursing* 52:250–61

Moher D, Schulz K F, Altman D G, for the CONSORT Group 2001 The CONSORT statement: revised recommendations for improving the quality of reports of parallel-group randomized trials. *Lancet* 357:1191–4

Mulhall A 2000 The case for a more epidemiologically informed nursing profession. *Nt Research* 5:65–74

Murphy B M, Worcester M U C, Elliott P C, et al. 2006 Change in women's dietary fat intake following an acute cardiac event: extent, predictors and comparison with non-cardiac Australian women and older adults. *European Journal of Cardiovascular Nursing* 5:206–13

O'Hagen C, O'Connell B 2005 The relationship between patient blood pathology values and patient falls in an acute-care setting: a retrospective analysis. *International Journal of Nursing Practice* 11:161–8

Overland J, Yue D K, Mira M 2001 Use of Medicare services related to diabetes care: the impact of rural isolation. *Australian Journal of Rural Health* 9:311–16

Peeters A, Mamun A A, Willekens F, et al. 2002 A cardiovascular life history: a life course analysis of the original Framingham heart study cohort. *European Heart Journal* 23: 458–66

Priestley G, Watson W, Rashidan A, et al. 2004 Introducing critical care outreach: a ward-randomised trial of phased introduction in a general hospital. *Intensive Care Medicine* 30:1398–404

Santamaria N, Conners A-M, Osteraas J, et al. 2004 A prospective cohort study of the effectiveness of clinical pathways for the in-patient management of acute exacerbation of chronic obstructive pulmonary disease. *Collegian* 11:12–16

Shim M-J, Lee Y-S, Oh H-E, et al. 2007 Effects of a back-pain-reducing program during pregnancy for Korean women: a non-equivalent control-group pretest-post test study. *International Journal of Nursing Studies* 44:19–28

Thompson C 2004 Fortuitous phenomena: on complexity, pragmatic randomised controlled trials, and knowledge for evidence-based practice. *Worldviews on Evidence-Based Nursing* 1:9–17

van Sluijs E M F, van Poppol M N M, Twisk J W R, et al. 2006 Physical activity measurements affected participants' behavior in a randomised controlled trial. *Journal of Clinical Epidemiology* 59: 401–11

Answers

TT Tutorial trigger 1

The clinical pathway was introduced into one clinical unit. Although not discussed by the authors, attempting an RCT in one ward (some patients receiving the pathway care while others received 'usual care'), would have resulted in 'study contamination'. The study authors did note that an RCT was not possible because the hospital required that all suitable patients receive treatment via the clinical pathway. Patients with cognitive impairment, inadequate English language skills or end-stage disease were excluded, limiting study generalisability (Santamaria et al. 2004 p 16).

TT Tutorial trigger 2

An ex-post facto (retrospective) design examines whether a current health state or event can be linked to some past event. This relationship can be formatted as an hypothesis. The retrospective design is observational, so participants are not assigned to a study group and no intervention is introduced by the researcher. Randomisation, manipulation (and control) are elements of an experimental design.

Learning activities

1. b   **2.** c   **3.** b   **4.** a
5. (a) E
   (b) Q
   (c) E
   (d) E
6. b   **7.** a   **8.** d
9. c   **10.** b

Sampling in quantitative research

ZEVIA SCHNEIDER AND DOUG ELLIOTT

Learning outcomes

After reading this chapter, you should be able to:

- describe the purpose of sampling
- define element, population, and sample
- describe the various procedures for drawing samples
- describe the types of probability and non-probability sampling
- discuss the factors that influence determination of sample size
- discuss eligibility criteria for sample selection.

KEY TERMS

element
eligibility criteria
exclusion criteria
inclusion criteria
non-probability sampling
population
probability sampling
random selection
randomisation
representative sample
sampling
target population

Introduction

Sampling is a process in which representative units of a population are selected for study in a research investigation. The most common element in nursing and midwifery research is humans, but other elements, such as places and objects, can form the basis of a sample or population. Sampling is a familiar process in everyday life; we gather knowledge, formulate predictions and make decisions based on sampling procedures. For example, a woman and her family may make generalisations about the quality of midwifery care in a hospital, based on their experiences during a 2-day hospital stay for the birth of her child. Nursing and midwifery students may also make generalisations about the quality of care and student support following a single clinical placement in a hospital.

Scientists derive knowledge from samples. Many problems cannot be solved without employing sampling procedures. For example, when testing the effectiveness of a medication for patients with cancer, the drug is administered to a sample of the population for whom it is potentially useful. The scientist must come to some conclusion without administering the drug to every known patient with cancer. But because human lives are at stake, the scientist cannot afford to arrive casually at conclusions that are based on the first dozen patients available for study. The consequences of arriving at erroneous conclusions or making inaccurate generalisations from a small, non-representative sample are much more harmful in scientific investigations than in everyday life. Consequently, research methodologies have expended considerable effort developing sampling theories and procedures that produce accurate and meaningful information. This chapter introduces the basic concepts of sampling applicable to quantitative research studies. (Sampling issues in qualitative research are discussed in Chapter 8.)

● **Evidence-based practice tip**

The foremost criterion in sampling is its representativeness. A representative sample is one whose key characteristics reflect those of the population. If an appropriate sampling strategy is used, then a reasonably accurate understanding of the phenomena of interest in the target population is possible by obtaining data from the study sample.

Sampling concepts

The purpose of sampling from a quantitative perspective is to increase the efficiency of a research study, while maintaining representativeness. There is no easy way to guarantee that a sample is representative without obtaining data about the entire population. As it is difficult and inefficient to access a population, a researcher employs sampling strategies that minimise or control for sampling bias. Samples should therefore be drawn in such a stringent way as to ensure that valid generalisations can be made from the sample to the population. For example, if 70% of the population in a study of child-rearing practices consisted of women and 40% were full-time employees, a representative sample should reflect these characteristics in the same proportions.

A *population* is a well-defined set that has specific characteristics. A population can be composed of people, animals, objects or events. A *sample* is a sub-set of sampling units from a population. An *element* is the most basic unit about which information is collected, and a *sampling unit* is the element or set of elements used for selecting the sample. Buist et al. (2004) compared the psychological and social aspects of the transition to motherhood of primiparous women from two regions in Melbourne, eastern and western. Women were recruited from four antenatal clinics, two in each area. The regions were identified as the sampling units. Examples of possible populations include everyone attending an emergency department in New South Wales during 2006, or all independent midwife practitioners in New Zealand. These examples show that a population can be broadly defined and potentially involve thousands of people or narrowly specified to include only several hundred people. The population criteria are a precise description of the population that enable generalisability of the findings from a quantitative study to similar populations. The population criteria are then reflected in the eligibility criteria of the sample, so that the important characteristics of the population and sample are congruent.

Researchers derive knowledge from using samples, as many clinical problems cannot be solved without employing sampling procedures. A reader of a research report should consider whether the researcher has identified the population descriptors precisely. The population criteria define the *target population*, that is, the group about whom the researcher wants to make generalisations. A target population might include student nurses enrolled in a Bachelor of Nursing program in Victoria. Would this population include both part-time and full-time students? Would it include students who had previously attended another nursing program? Would it include first-, second- and third-year students? Would students from culturally and linguistically diverse (CALD) backgrounds be included? As far as is possible, the researcher must specify the exact criteria used to decide whether a student nurse will be included in, or excluded from, the sample. For example, if a population were defined as Australian-born, full-time, third-year nursing students enrolled in a Bachelor of Nursing program, the sample would be expected to reflect these characteristics. Sometimes it is not feasible because of time constraints, money, personnel and access to use a target population.

Hoffman and Elwin (2004) examined the relationship between critical thinking and confidence in decision-making in new graduate nurses. The target population from which the sample of 83 nurses was recruited was new graduate nurses entering two area health services in Australia, one within a major metropolitan area, the other a regional area health service. An *accessible population*, one that meets the criteria of the study, is often used. For example, instead of including the entire population of registered nurses (RNs) throughout Australia, the sample could include a percentage of RNs from each state/territory using a random sampling strategy to obtain the sample.

Inclusion and exclusion criteria

The population criteria establish the target population — the entire set of participants or cases who are the focus of the study. The study criteria identify the specific characteristics required for participants in the study sample, and are commonly listed in proposals or published papers as inclusion criteria and/or exclusion criteria. Eligibility criteria can be viewed as delimitations or those characteristics that restrict the population to a homogeneous group of participants, such as: gender, age, marital status, socioeconomic status, religion, ethnicity, level of education, age of children, health status and diagnosis (see Table 11.1).

These examples demonstrate the potential differences between the sample actually selected and a larger population. Remember that criteria for inclusion/exclusion in a study are designed to control for any extraneous variability or bias. Each criterion should have a rationale, presumably related to a potential confounding effect on the outcome (dependent) variable. Precise development of the study inclusion and exclusion criteria will improve

TABLE 11.1 Examples of inclusion and exclusion criteria

Author	Edwards et al. 2005	Middleton et al. 2005	Li et al. 2003
Study description	Healing rates for patients with chronic venous leg ulcers.	Short-term impact on patient outcomes of nursing-led coordinated care after discharge following carotid endarterectomy.	Describing Chinese-Australian (Mandarin speaking) mothers' knowledge about and attitudes toward breastfeeding.
Inclusion criteria	A venous ulcer below the knee. Ankle Brachial Pressure Index (ABPI) of >0.8 and <1.3	Having a carotid endarterectomy; agree to sign a consent form and complete a pre-operative questionnaire; and agreement to be randomly assigned to one of two groups.	Born outside Australia; speak Mandarin; given birth to at least one live child, living in Perth, and aged less than 60 years.
Exclusion criteria	Clients who had diabetes mellitus; had ulcers of non-venous origin; were too immobile to be transported to Leg Club (i.e. unable to sit up in a wheelchair for 1–2 hours).	Could not give informed consent; insufficient level of English to complete a self-administered questionnaire; those having emergency operations.	

the precision of the study and strength of evidence for generalisability. A confounding (confusing) or false relationship exists when findings incorrectly show an association between two or more study variables. Adequate design and statistical control should prevent such a problem occurring (see 'Study validity' in Chapter 12).

Sample size and power analysis

For quantitative research, particularly interventional studies where an effect is being measured, the sample size is determined prior to study commencement. A number of factors influence the proposed sample size, including the design, need for generalisability, the proposed effect of any intervention, feasibility and costs. Generally, a larger sample size has more chance of demonstrating an effect, although this may be costly. A pilot study can be conducted to determine an appropriate sample size (see Chapter 20).

Power analysis is a mathematical strategy used to determine the correct size of a sample so that accurate inferences can be made about the true relationship between the study variables. Power is the product of sample size and the effect of the study intervention. A

study suitably 'powered' provides confidence in interpreting the findings; statistically, this reflects the ability of a statistical test to reject a null hypothesis that is false (Cohen 1988).

Research in brief

The effects of a needs-based education program for family carers with a relative in an intensive care unit were examined (Chien et al. 2006). Power calculations based on two previous studies indicated that a sample of 64 participants (i.e. 32 family carers in each group) was required (both before and after intervention). The intervention was a needs-based educational program for family carers based on their identified needs; for example, need for information, assurance and support. This sample was sufficiently large enough to detect a significant difference of a large effect size on anxiety reduction between the treatment and control groups at a 5% significance level with a power of 80% including an average attrition rate of 10%. Limitations are small sample size and non-probability sampling. A convenience sample was used which may have affected the homogeneity of the two groups.

(See Chapter 14 for a more detailed discussion of power analysis.)

> **Points to ponder**
>
> ▶ In what way are inclusion and exclusion criteria important in delineating the composition of the sample?
>
> ▶ How may criteria influence the research consumer's interpretation of the study's outcomes?

Types of samples

Sampling strategies are generally grouped into two categories: non-probability sampling and probability sampling (see Table 11.2). In non-probability sampling, elements are chosen by non-random methods; there is no way of checking that each sampling element has been included in the sample. In contrast, probability sampling uses some form of random selection when choosing the sample units and therefore minimises bias and enables generalisability of the findings. This more rigorous sampling strategy is more likely to result in a representative sample; an important consideration in quantitative research.

Non-probability sampling

As noted in Chapter 8, this sampling approach is most appropriate for qualitative research, as well as small exploratory quantitative studies. Non-probability samples are useful when information on the total population is unknown or unavailable. The non-probability sampling strategy is less rigorous than the probability strategy and tends to produce less accurate and less representative samples, thus limiting the ability of the researcher to make generalisations about the findings at a population level. The three major types of non-probability sampling are: convenience, quota and purposive.

TABLE 11.2 Summary of sampling strategies

Sampling strategy	Ease of drawing sample	Risk of bias	Representativenesss of sample
Non-probability			
Convenience	Very easy	Greater than any other sampling strategy	Because samples tend to be self-selecting, representativeness is questionable
Quota	Relatively easy	Contains unknown source of bias that affects external validity	Builds in some representativeness by using knowledge about the population of interest
Purposive	Relatively easy	Bias increases with greater heterogeneity of the population; conscious bias is also a danger	Very limited ability to generalise because sample is handpicked
Probability			
Simple random	Laborious	Low	Maximised; probability of non-representativeness decreases with increased sample size
Stratified random	Time-consuming	Low	Enhanced
Cluster	Less time-consuming than simple or stratified	Subject to more sampling errors than simple or stratified	Less representative than simple or stratified
Systematic	More convenient and efficient than simple, stratified or cluster sampling	Bias in the form of non randomness can be inadvertently introduced	Less representative if bias occurs as a result of coincidental non-randomness

Convenience sampling

Convenience sampling (also called incidental sampling or accidental sampling) uses the most readily accessible persons or objects as study participants. Jenkins and Elliott (2004) investigated levels of stressors and burnout of qualified and unqualified nursing staff. A convenience sample of 93 nursing staff from eleven acute adult mental health wards was obtained. Only 93 of a total of 240 questionnaires were returned completed (a response rate of 39%). An issue to consider is whether the respondents were representative of the target population. The use of a convenience sample and self-selection limits generalisation and unrepresentative findings. Another convenience sample was used in a study exploring self-reported changes in coronary risk factors by patients 3 to 9 months following coronary artery angioplasty. A questionnaire was sent to 560 self-selected patients undergoing angioplasty within a 6-month period in two major metropolitan hospitals in Melbourne (Campbell & Torrance 2005). Two hundred and thirty-four (41.7%) questionnaires were returned. Using a convenience sample and the low response rate may limit generalisation.

Snowballing (network sampling) is an effective convenience sampling strategy used to access samples difficult to locate. This approach uses social networks and the fact that friends or colleagues tend to have common or similar characteristics. Individuals who meet the eligibility criteria are asked to assist in getting in touch with others whom they know also meet the inclusion criteria. A snowball sampling approach was used to obtain a sample of public health nurses for a study to explore the tacit knowledge of public

health nurses in identifying community health problems and developing relevant projects (Yoshioka-Maeda et al. 2006). In addition to snowballing, nine participants were recruited on the basis of information obtained from five representative Japanese public health nursing journals. Findings indicated that all nine public health nurses used similar approaches in identifying community health problems. Limitations of the study concerned the number of participants and recruitment process.

The advantage of a convenience sample is that it may be easier for the researcher to obtain participants. The only concern is obtaining a sufficient number of participants who meet the criteria dictated by the study. The major disadvantage is that the risk of bias is greater than in any other type of sample. The problem of bias exists because convenience samples tend to be self-selecting, and the information obtained comes only from those people who volunteer to participate (e.g. those who chose to return questionnaires sent to them). In this case the following questions must be raised:

• What motivated some of the people to participate and others not to participate?
• What kind of data would have been obtained if non-participants had also responded?
• How representative of the population are the people who did participate?

While recruiting research participants is a problem for many nurse researchers, a variety of recruitment strategies may be used. For example, in a study exploring the labour and childbirth expectations of women, Fenwick et al. (2004) recruited their sample through a newspaper display advertisementplaced in all community newspapers in eight major centres in Western Australia. Prospective participants were invited to contact the midwifery researchers on a toll-free telephone number. A recorded telephone message informed the caller that their call would be returned as soon as possible. The recruitment strategy resulted in a sample of middle-class women (half had a university qualification and earned over AU$60,000 a year), who were not representative of the target population. It is important that inappropriate generalisations are not made from a non-representative sample.

Point to ponder

▶ Consider the method of sample recruitment in the above example and the extent to which sample bias could have affected the findings. What different recruitment strategies could have been used to improve sample representativeness?

Quota sampling

Quota sampling addresses the issue of appropriate representation for each segment of a population. This form of non-probability sampling uses prior knowledge about the population of interest to build some representativeness into the sample. A quota sample accounts for the proportion of various strata in a population. Characteristics chosen to form the strata are selected according to a researcher's judgment based on knowledge of the population and the literature to reflect important differences in the variables of interest; for example, age, gender, religion, ethnicity, medical diagnosis, socioeconomic status, level of completed education or occupation. For example, data in Table 11.3 reveal that 20% of the 5000 nurses in city X are diploma graduates, 40% are certificate qualified and 40% are Bachelor degree graduates. In this case, a researcher would use proportional quota sampling to sample 10% (500 nurses) of a population of 5000. Based on the proportion of each stratum in the population — 100 diploma graduates, 200 certificate qualified graduates and 200 Bachelor degree graduates — the quotas were established for the three strata. Participants who meet the eligibility criteria of the study would be recruited until the quota for each stratum was filled.

As with all non-probability strategies, those who choose to participate may not be typical of the population with regard to the variables being measured. There is no way to assess the biases that may be operating.

Research in brief

In order to test and validate the postpartum stress scale developed for Taiwanese women, Hung (2006) used a proportional stratified quota sampling technique from ten hospitals and six clinics with the highest birth rates. Participants were 505 and 518 postpartum women at each time point respectively. Factor analysis at two points in time identified three attributes of postpartum stress. The Cronbach's alphas at each time point were 0.94 and 0.92 respectively, supporting the postpartum stress scale as a validated instrument.

Evidence-based practice tip

When reviewing a study that used stratified random sampling, determine whether the sample strata appropriately reflect the population of interest, and the stratifying variables are sufficiently homogeneous to ensure a meaningful comparison of differences among strata. Also remember that the quota strategy contains an unknown source of bias that affects external validity.

Purposive sampling

In purposive sampling the researcher's knowledge of the population and its elements are used to handpick cases typical of the population to be included in the sample. A purposive sample can be used to study a highly unusual group, such as those individuals with a rare genetic disease. In another situation a researcher may wish to interview individuals who reflect different ends of the range of a particular characteristic; for example, exploring the psychosocial needs of individuals who are sero-positive for hepatitis C virus but have no symptoms, compared with individuals who have active hepatitis C. Online services can be of great value in helping researchers access and recruit participants for purposive samples.

TABLE 11.3 Number of percentages of students in strata of a quota sample of 5000 graduates of nursing programs in city X

	Diploma graduates	Certified qualified graduates	Bachelor degree graduates
Population	1000 (20%)	2000 (40%)	2000 (40%)
Strata	100	200	200

Research in brief

Arthur et al. (2005) used purposive sampling to recruit five registered nurses, from a college on the island of Negros Oriental, experienced in the provision of primary healthcare (PHC) nursing. The aim of the study was to examine the experiences of nurses working as faculty and providing PHC to their community. The identified limitation of the study was that PHC practice appears to be region specific and unique in the Philippines.

When using a purposive sample in a quantitative study, a researcher assumes that errors of judgment in over-representing and under-representing elements of the population in the sample will tend to balance out. However, there is no objective method for determining the validity of this assumption.

As with any non-probability sample, the ability to generalise is very limited. The following are instances of when a purposive sample may be appropriate:

- effective pre-testing of newly developed instruments with a purposive sample of divergent types of people
- validation of a scale or test with a known-groups technique
- collection of exploratory data from an unusual or highly specific population, particularly when information on the total target population is unknown.

Probability sampling

The primary characteristic of probability sampling is the random selection of elements from the target population. Each element (participant) in the population therefore has an equal and independent chance (probability) of being selected in the sample. As noted previously in Table 11.2, four commonly used probability sampling strategies are simple random, stratified random, cluster and systematic.

Simple random sampling

In simple random sampling, the population elements are identified, and the sample is then selected, using some form of random number generation; for example, via computer software or a table of random numbers (see Figure 11.1). For the latter, consecutive numbers are assigned to units of the population, and a researcher starts at any point on the table of random numbers and reads consecutive numbers in any direction (horizontally, vertically or diagonally). The numbers corresponding with the sampling frame indicate units to be chosen for the sample. This process continues until a sample of the desired size is drawn. For example, if the numbers 76, 16, 46, 5, 93, 41... were randomly selected, then the potential participants corresponding with those numbers would form the sample. In a study designed to assess the effectiveness of a counselling intervention after a traumatic childbirth (Gamble et al. 2005), women (n = 103) were randomly assigned to the intervention (n = 50) or control group (n = 53) using sealed, opaque envelopes containing computer-generated, random allocations.

Research in brief

A study commissioned by the Australian Nursing Council aimed to develop an approach to the maintenance of continuing competence in nursing (Pearson & FitzGerald 2001). The researchers decided to accept a random sample rate of 2% of registered nurses in each state and territory (except the ACT). The researchers contacted 2% (n = 4133) of nurses, but only 1005 responded (24% response rate), resulting in a final sample of <0.5% of the population. A low response rate should have been considered when calculating the sample size so that the final sample would approximate the 2% of all RNs in Australia.

Point to ponder

▶ Random selection of sample participants should not be confused with 'random assignment' (or allocation) to different study groups. Random allocation refers to the assignment of participants to an 'intervention' or 'control' group on a purely random basis, after participants have been enrolled in the study.

FIGURE 11.1 Table of random numbers

40	23	0	29	10	94	17	58	12	85	13	25	80	84	72	74	54	63	55	31
32	98	49	23	74	97	51	42	21	87	48	64	54	38	84	68	14	17	35	48
84	34	84	14	53	65	67	37	2	45	84	21	71	34	10	80	72	27	11	13
86	37	24	89	23	4	44	40	72	81	44	69	25	44	34	34	34	75	50	50
50	58	85	8	22	24	73	20	63	35	60	87	91	92	96	80	19	22	87	24
1	87	43	82	9	31	40	88	33	28	82	73	18	6	48	64	59	45	34	3
21	19	42	76	84	67	29	68	8	66	93	89	96	28	12	14	38	47	52	65
32	66	33	21	81	97	39	76	67	27	97	22	76	89	41	11	91	29	6	66
16	82	42	75	35	42	92	90	77	24	21	8	36	16	5	54	89	51	57	85
74	32	63	65	93	96	18	36	82	72	39	69	37	97	51	17	36	71	38	30
50	94	4	66	17	37	10	53	8	29	67	74	88	38	11	59	60	91	56	17
71	47	81	18	53	98	7	87	29	37	22	93	13	6	95	7	95	71	14	6
71	93	48	16	33	19	46	21	60	44	52	91	52	58	10	9	41	31	35	18
20	94	13	99	45	6	53	54	1	25	79	28	1	48	36	26	68	37	59	7
75	22	69	56	62	40	64	45	40	99	94	14	98	84	22	38	24	87	43	71
16	87	41	0	88	83	11	37	71	78	22	39	43	37	75	84	84	11	55	58
92	90	80	2	30	37	85	55	56	50	3	71	24	13	62	74	82	44	90	32
96	89	31	32	37	45	70	67	80	55	58	9	55	60	61	55	86	44	27	77
38	29	36	94	65	39	56	29	29	65	88	13	71	38	71	8	81	66	31	44
20	6	61	66	90	13	70	60	92	53	87	49	34	42	14	47	75	33	26	9
63	44	94	21	14	13	41	80	39	72	29	3	25	89	44	88	13	49	18	58
13	32	93	90	31	75	86	95	18	51	61	59	84	95	67	54	40	30	29	63
26	35	48	01	19	24	36	36	76	16	46	5	93	41	97	46	79	54	95	49
89	74	96	95	94	69	31	60	16	69	76	42	28	71	69	34	46	55	20	42
50	39	28	64	20	68	60	33	92	82	61	70	5	68	95	88	12	85	18	94
55	86	5	96	87	69	75	93	54	79	0	57	45	8	86	59	25	21	9	29
75	35	1	2	86	62	70	83	85	13	97	37	13	73	16	38	36	23	54	11
74	50	1	77	87	92	68	87	57	36	17	47	0	97	78	72	72	45	54	51
34	24	35	13	26	42	22	75	47	2	34	87	15	50	65	27	5	72	28	68
73	33	42	65	91	24	44	84	71	55	70	1	27	30	8	61	65	61	18	92
7	55	12	6	61	17	23	95	91	58	60	30	35	61	34	27	75	44	35	64
10	94	18	4	3	19	21	37	28	55	76	25	10	29	80	64	8	81	20	32
20	48	92	87	95	58	57	73	42	1	12	81	94	85	63	97	24	19	93	51
81	10	92	49	70	15	76	4	36	92	62	99	78	32	86	74	43	22	98	46
66	67	82	94	67	75	16	88	84	98	0	52	37	0	43	9	0	51	2	62
64	92	36	11	3	52	44	65	45	67	97	86	92	2	50	5	93	66	73	40
36	29	98	46	88	23	28	44	8	71	69	43	53	16	87	21	56	23	37	24
15	11	82	30	59	94	23	30	40	25	87	26	24	30	44	53	33	65	72	55
89	57	49	79	83	80	42	46	11	93	38	24	15	80	97	18	61	12	13	42
23	36	65	9	64	26	93	37	26	44	42	17	45	68	27	77	74	56	49	34
9	93	90	61	45	40	75	85	64	66	36	89	72	43	99	90	92	10	10	85
53	94	30	31	62	92	82	30	94	56	40	4	50	53	9	74	87	2	36	36
18	69	77	38	89	78	30	68	71	92	22	93	91	74	52	1	97	69	71	42
50	20	76	36	6	20	75	56	36	5	14	70	9	78	23	33	91	33	25	72
30	46	1	10	16	72	69	26	94	39	80	36	36	68	92	74	22	74	41	42
59	47	7	92	77	55	2	12	5	24	0	30	25	62	83	36	92	96	36	75
93	22	3	20	82	44	16	69	98	72	30	57	77	15	90	29	32	38	3	48
9	55	27	41	40	94	77	14	54	10	25	75	1	74	72	15	69	80	33	58
70	8	3	5	46	89	28	86	40	6	25	40	81	26	63	97	87	48	26	41
19	6	89	31	80	60	13	89	17	69	38	93	58	55	54	69	74	33	8	55

The advantages of simple random sampling are:

- the sample selection is not subject to the conscious biases of the researcher
- the representativeness of the sample in relation to the population characteristics is maximised
- the differences in the characteristics of the sample and the population are purely a function of chance
- the probability of choosing a non-representative sample decreases as the size of the sample increases.

TT **Tutorial trigger 1**

One thousand adults were seen by nurse practitioners in the emergency department of hospital X. You have been asked to send a patient satisfaction questionnaire to this group, and have been advised that a sample of 200 patients is adequate. How would you go about selecting a simple random sample from the group of 1000?

● **Evidence-based practice tip**

Despite using a carefully controlled sampling procedure to minimise any bias or error, there is still no guarantee that a sample will be representative of the population. Factors such as sample heterogeneity and participant drop-out may affect representativeness.

The major disadvantage of this approach is that it is a time-consuming and inefficient method for obtaining a random sample. Consider the task of listing all RNs in Australia. It may be impossible to obtain an accurate or complete listing of every element in the population. Or imagine attempting to obtain a list of all drownings in Queensland for the year 2006. It may be the case that although drowning may have been the cause of death, another cause, such as cardiac arrest or respiratory failure, appears on the death certificate. It would be difficult to estimate how many elements of the target population would be eliminated from consideration. The issue of bias would definitely be a factor, and a reader must be cautious about generalisations from reported findings, even when random sampling is used, if the target population has been difficult or impossible to list completely.

Stratified random sampling

Stratified random sampling divides the population into 'strata' or sub-groups that are homogeneous (composed of similar or identical elements). An appropriate number of elements from each sub-set are randomly selected on the basis of their proportion in the population to maintain representativeness in the sample. The population is stratified according to any number of attributes (e.g. age, gender, ethnicity, religion, socioeconomic status or level of education). The variables selected to make up the strata should be adaptable to homogeneous sub-sets for the attributes being studied. This approach is equivalent

FIGURE 11.2 Participant selection using a proportional stratified random sampling strategy

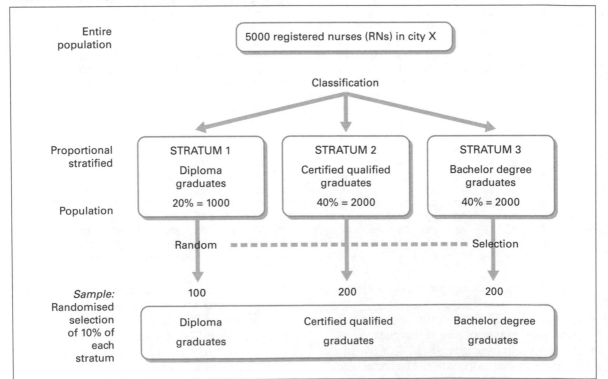

to quota sampling (see Table 11.3), using random sampling. Figure 11.2 provides an example that illustrates proportional stratified random sampling.

Stratified random sampling was used in a study investigating the general population regarding the preferences and use of 'advance directives' in Japan (Akabayashi et al. 2003). A self-administered questionnaire was sent via mail to a stratified random sample of 560 residents listed in one residential district (n = 165 567) of Tokyo. The list was divided by town and contained all residents in alphabetical order. Fourteen towns were first randomly chosen from 69 towns. Participants were then randomly selected from each of the 14 areas based on population size of each town (sampling rate 1/60). The total sampling rate was 1/300.

Cluster sampling

Cluster sampling (multi-stage sampling) involves successive random sampling of units (clusters) that progress from large to small and meet sample eligibility criteria. The first stage sampling unit consists of large units or clusters. The second stage sampling unit consists of smaller units or clusters and so on. When multi-stage sampling is used for large national surveys, such as those carried out by the Australian Bureau of Statistics, states are used as the first stage sampling unit, cities, suburbs and street blocks as the second stage sampling unit and then households as the third stage sampling unit. Sampling units or clusters can be selected by simple random or stratified random sampling methods.

Research in brief

A sample of patients who had undergone carotid artery surgery was used to test a co-ordinated nurse-led post-discharge intervention (Middleton et al. 2005). The first stage sampling unit was vascular surgeons in NSW. Of the 56 eligible surgeons, 30 agreed to participate (first stage sampling unit), although only 20 performed any carotid surgery during the recruitment period. The second stage sampling unit was all patients with those surgeons who had the surgical procedure.

Suppose that the surgeons described in the 'Research in brief' opposite were grouped into four strata according to size (number of carotid surgical procedures performed per year): (1) 1–10; (2) 11–20; (3) 21–30; and (4) more than 30. Hypothetically, each stratum was composed of the following proportions of the population: 1: 30%; 2: 25%; 3: 30%; 4: 15%. This means that either a simple random or a proportional stratified sampling strategy could be used to randomly select surgeons that would proportionately represent the population of vascular surgeons in NSW.

The main advantage of cluster sampling as noted in Table 11.2, is that it is more economical in terms of time and money than other types of probability sampling, particularly when the population is large and geographically dispersed or when a sampling frame of the elements is not available. Two major disadvantages however are:

1. more sampling errors tend to occur than with simple random or stratified random sampling
2. statistical analysis from cluster samples is complex.

TT Tutorial trigger 2

Your research group wants to obtain a sample of final year midwifery students enrolled in the Bachelor of Midwifery program in three universities to determine their perceptions of their knowledge and competency in drug calculation. What sampling strategies would you employ to recruit the participants? What might the inclusion/exclusion criteria be for your study?

Systematic sampling

Systematic sampling involves the selection of cases drawn from a population list at fixed intervals ('k'). Systematic sampling might be used to sample every 'kth' person presenting to the emergency department (ED) during the winter months, or hospitalised with a diagnosis of traumatic brain injury in 2006. When systematic sampling is used, the population is narrowly defined (e.g. all people presenting to the ED) for the sample to be considered a probability sample. Systematic sampling can also sometimes represent a non-probability strategy. If people aged over 80 years old were sampled systematically on entering the ED, the resulting sample would not be a probability sample as not every person aged over 80 would have a chance of being selected (only those who were acutely ill).

Systematic sampling strategies can be designed to fulfil the requirements of a probability sample. First, the listing of the population (sampling frame) must be random in relation to the variable of interest. Suppose participants were selected from every tenth hospital bed for a study on patient satisfaction with nursing care. Every tenth bed happens to be a single room in the hospital where the study is being conducted. It is possible that the responses of patients in single rooms with regard to satisfaction might be different from those of patients in shared rooms. Because of the non-random arrangement of the rooms, bias may have been introduced. Second, the first element or member of the sample must be selected randomly. In this case the researcher, who has a population list or sampling frame, divides the population (N) by the size of the desired sample (n) to obtain the sampling interval width (k). The sampling interval is the standard distance between the elements chosen for the sample. To select a sample of 50 patients from a population of 500, the sampling interval would be: k = 500/50 = 10.

Essentially, every tenth case on the patient list would be sampled. Once the sampling interval has been determined, a table of random numbers (e.g. Figure 11.1) is used to obtain a starting point for the selection of the 50 participants. If the population size is 500 and a sample size of 50 is desired, a number between 1 and 500 is randomly selected as the starting point. In this instance, if the first number is 51, the patient corresponding to numbers 51, 61, 71... would be included in the sample of 50. Another recommended approach is to randomly select the first element from within the first sampling interval. If the sampling interval is 5, a number between 1 and 5 would be selected as the random starting point. For example, if the number 3 is randomly chosen, and keeping in mind the sampling interval of 5, the next elements selected would correspond to the numbers 8, 13, 18 and so on until the sample was obtained.

To determine the construct validity of published competency standards as a tool for assessing the clinical practice of specialist level critical care nurses in Australia, Fisher et al. (2005) used a systematic sampling technique to identify participants from the ACCCN membership database and establish a representative sample of 1000 Australian critical care nurses.

TT Tutorial trigger 3

You want to find out what second-year student nurses enrolled in the Bachelor of Nursing program in three universities in Victoria think about their 6-week placements in medical wards. Your lecturer suggests you use a simple random sampling strategy. How would you go about choosing the sample?

● **Evidence-based practice tip**

An appropriate systematic sampling plan maximises the efficiency of a research study, increases the accuracy and meaningfulness of the findings, and enhances the generalisability of the findings from the sample to the population. Systematic sampling can satisfy the requirements of a probability sample.

Systematic and simple random sampling are essentially the same procedure. The advantage of systematic sampling is that the results are obtained in a more convenient and efficient manner (see Table 11.2). The disadvantage is that bias in the form of non-randomness can be introduced inadvertently. This may occur if the population list is arranged so that a certain type of element is listed at intervals that coincide with the sampling interval. For example, if every tenth nursing student on a population list of all types of nursing students in Queensland was a Graduate Diploma of Nursing student and the sampling interval was ten, Graduate Diploma of Nursing students would be over-represented in the sample. Cyclical fluctuations are also a factor. Consider a list of students using the university library each day. A biased sample will probably result if every seventh day is chosen as the sampling interval, because perhaps fewer and different students study in the library on Sundays. It is important to know whether a satisfactory random selection procedure was carried out. If randomisation were not used, the systematic sampling may be a non-probability quota sample. In this case the implications related to interpretation and generalisability are altered.

Summary

Sampling is a process through which a researcher selects participants from the population for study. The purpose of sampling from a quantitative perspective is to obtain a sample which is representative of the population. The study criteria define specific characteristics of participants called inclusion and/or exclusion criteria which are designed to control for bias. There are two categories of sampling strategies: non-probability sampling and probability sampling. Non-probability sampling strategies are: convenience, quota and purposive. This method of sampling is less rigorous and accurate than probability sampling. Probability sampling refers to the random selection of participants from the target population and aims to ensure that each participant in the population has an equal chance of being selected in the sample. The probability sampling strategies are: simple random, stratified random, cluster and systematic.

KEY POINTS

- Sampling is a process that selects representative units of a population for study. Researchers sample representative segments of the population because it is rarely feasible or necessary to sample entire populations of interest to obtain accurate and meaningful information.
- Types of non-probability sampling are: convenience, quota and purposive sampling.
- Criteria for drawing a sample vary according to the sampling strategy. Systematic organisation of the sampling procedure minimises bias.
- An appropriate systematic sampling plan will maximise the efficiency of a research study. It will increase the accuracy and meaningfulness of the findings and enhance the generalisability of the findings from the sample to the population.

- Simple random sampling is the basic technique of probability sampling.
- Probability sampling uses some form of random selection when choosing the sample units and therefore minimises bias and enables generalisability of the findings.
- Non-probability sampling tends to produce less accurate and less representative samples.
- A representative sample is one whose key characteristics closely approximate those of the population.
- Power analysis is a mathematical strategy used to determine the correct size of a sample so that accurate inferences can be made about the true relationship between the study variables.
- Non-probability samples are useful when the total population is unknown or unavailable.

Learning activities

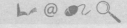

1. The purpose of sampling is to:
   (a) make predictions about the study
   (b) generalise the findings to the population
   (c) increase the efficiency of a research study
   (d) test the effectiveness of a drug.

2. Eligibility criteria reflect the:
   (a) randomness of a sample
   (b) population criteria
   (c) number of participants in a study
   (d) diagnosis of the participant in a study.

3. The population criteria establish the:
   (a) way a sample is drawn
   (b) representative of a sample
   (c) number of participants in a study
   (d) target population.

4. A convenience sample:
   (a) allows generalisability of the findings to the population
   (b) gives everyone an opportunity to participate in a study
   (c) is made up of the most readily available and accessible persons
   (d) is made up of people who enjoy being part of a research study.

5. Sample size is determined:
   (a) immediately upon starting the study
   (b) after the study has started
   (c) once the consent forms have been signed
   (d) prior to commencement of the study.

6. The primary characteristic of probability sampling is:
   (a) the random selection of elements from the population
   (b) the opportunity to generalise the findings of the study to the population
   (c) to select participants who meet the criteria of the study
   (d) to prevent bias in the sample.

7. Stratified random sampling divides the population into strata that are:
   (a) heterogeneous
   (b) homogeneous
   (c) purposefully chosen for the study
   (d) different for each age group.

8. The study criteria identify:
   (a) the group of people who want to participate in the study
   (b) the target population
   (c) all the participants who are the focus of the study
   (d) the specific characteristics required for participants.

9. Criteria for inclusion/exclusion in a study are designed to:
   (a) control for any bias or extraneous variability
   (b) keep the wrong people out of the study
   (c) get the best people into the study

   (d) control for a confounding effect on the dependent variable.

10. Random allocation or assignment:
    (a) allows participants to choose the group they want to join
    (b) divides the participants into groups based on age, gender and education
    (c) participants are randomly assigned to a treatment or control group
    (d) excludes some participants from the study.

Additional resources

Annells M, DeRoche M, Koch T, et al. 2005 A Delphi study of district nursing research priorities in Australia. *Applied Nursing Research* 18:36–43

Dunning T, Manias E 2005 Medication knowledge and self-management by people with type 2 diabetes. *Australian Journal of Advanced Nursing* 23(1):7–13

Maputle M, Mothiba M 2006 Mothers' knowledge of foetal movements monitoring during pregnancy in relation to perinatal outcome. *Health SA Gesondheid* 11(2):13–22

Pascoe T, Foley E, Hutchinson R 2005 The changing face of nurses in Australian general practice. *Australian Journal of Advanced Nursing* 23(1):44–7

Pelletier D, Donoghue J, Duffield C 2005 Understanding the nursing workforce: a longitudinal study of Australian nurses six years after graduate study. *Australian Journal of Advanced Nursing* 23(1):37–42

Seekoe E 2005 Reproductive health needs and the reproductive health behaviour of the youth in Mangaung in the Free State province: a feasibility study. *Curationis* 28(3):20–30

References

Akabayashi A, Slingsby B T, Kai I 2003 Perspectives on advance directives in Japanese society: A population-based questionnaire survey. *MBC Medical Ethics* 4:1–9

Arthur D, Drury J, Sy-Sinda M T, et al. 2005 A primary health care curriculum in action: The lived experience of primary health care nurses in a school of nursing in the Philippines: A phenomenological study. *International Journal of Nursing Studies* 43:107–12

Buist A, Milgrom J, Morse C, et al. 2004 Metropolitan regional differences in primary health care of postnatal depression. *Australian Journal of Advanced Nursing* 21(3):20–7

Campbell M, Torrance C 2005 Coronary Angioplasty: Impact on risk factors and patients' understanding of the severity of their condition. *Australian Journal of Advanced Nursing* 22(4):26–31

Chien W-T, Chiu Y L, Lam L-W, et al. 2006 Effects of a needs-based education programme for family carers with a relative in an intensive care unit: A quasi-experimental study. *International Journal of Nursing Studies* 43:39–50

Cohen J 1988 *Statistical power analysis for the behavioral sciences*, 2nd edn. Lawrence Erlbaum Associates, Hillsdale, NJ

Edwards H, Courtney M, Finlayson K, et al. 2005 Improved healing rates for chronic venous leg ulcers: Pilot study results from a randomized controlled trial of a community nursing intervention. *International Journal of Nursing Practice* 11:169–76

Fenwick J, Hauck Y, Downie J, et al. 2004 The childbirth expectations of a self-selected cohort of Western Australian women. *Midwifery* 21:23–35

Fisher M J, Marshall A P, Kendrick T S 2005 Competency standards for critical care nurses: do they measure up? *Australian Journal of Advanced Nursing* 22(4):32–40

Gamble J, Creedy D, Moyle W, et al. 2005 Effectiveness of a Counseling Intervention after a Traumatic Childbirth: A Randomized Controlled Trial. *Birth* 32(1):11–19

Hoffman K, Elwin C 2004 The relationship between critical thinking and confidence in decision-making. *Australian Journal of Advanced Nursing* 22(1):8–12

Hung C 2006 Revalidation of the postpartum stress scale. *Journal of Clinical Nursing* 15(6):718–25

Jenkins R, Elliott P 2004 Stressors, burnout and social support: nurses in acute mental health settings. *Journal of Advanced Nursing* 48(6):622–31

Li L, Zhang M, Binns C W 2003 Chinese mothers' knowledge and attitudes about breastfeeding in Perth, Western Australia. *Breastfeeding Review* 11(3):13–18

Middleton S, Donnelly N, Harris J, et al. 2005 Nursing intervention after carotid endarterectomy: a randomized trial of Co-ordinated Care Post-Discharge (CCPD). *Journal of Advanced Nursing* 52(3):250–61

Pearson A, FitzGerald M 2001 A survey of nurses' views on indicators for continuing competence in nursing. *Australian Journal of Advanced Nursing* 19(1):20–6

Rodger M, Hills J, Kristjanson L 2004 A Delphi Study on Research Priorities for Emergency Nurses in Western Australia. *Journal of Emergency Nursing* 30:117–25

Yoshioka-Maeda K, Murashima S, Asahara K 2006 Tacit knowledge of public health nurses in identifying community health problems and need for new services: A case study. *International Journal of Nursing Studies* 43:819–26

Answers

TT Tutorial trigger 1

To select a sample of 200 patients from a population of 1000, the sampling interval is: k = 1000/200 = 5. Every 5th patient on the list would be sampled and included in the sample; that is, sent a questionnaire. To obtain a starting point select any number between 200 and 1000, say 420. In this case, if the first number is 420, the patients corresponding to 425, 430, 435, 440 and so on, would be included in the sample of 200.

TT Tutorial trigger 2

1. Establish the number of final-year midwifery students in the three universities in your state/territory. Let us say there is a total of 300 midwifery students currently enrolled in the final year of the program.
2. To ensure that you get a good response you have decided on a sample of 100 students. Your sampling interval is 300/100 = 3. Select a number from 1 to 3, say 3. Using a table of random numbers, the first number is 3, the next 6, 9, 12, 15, and so on until you have selected 100 students.
3. The inclusion criteria might be:
   - only final-year students currently enrolled in the midwifery program at universities A, B and C in your particular state
   - able to read and understand English
   - successfully completed Year 12 in your state's education system
   - successfully completed Year 11 mathematics
   - sign a consent form if included in the study, knowing that they may not be included in the sample
   - the consent form should indicate to the participants that the information obtained will be confidential, that anonymity is ensured, and the freedom to withdraw from the study at any time without penalty.
4. The exclusion criteria would be:
   - inability to read and understand English
   - Year 12 not completed successfully
   - Year 11 mathematics not completed successfully
   - refusal to sign a consent form.

T_T Tutorial trigger 3

1. Establish the number of third-year student nurses at each university.
2. You know that a simple random sample is a probability sampling strategy in which every individual has a chance of being included in the study.
   - The population is all the third-year student nurses in the three universities. (You may like to define the population still further by stating eligibility criteria.)
   - A decision based on power analysis to determine sample size must be made.
   - Let's say the sample size is determined at 200 nurses.
   - Each nurse is assigned a number, and a decision made that every kth nurse will be included in the sample.
   - The required number of nurses (200) is made using a table of random numbers.
   - Having identified the sample, decide on the design, method and approach to obtain the information you require.

Advantages of a simple random sampling strategy:
   - this method aims to ensure that every person in the population has an equal chance of being included in the study and may therefore be considered 'representative' of the wider population of third-year student nurses
   - findings are generalisable to the wider population if sample size is adequate
   - risk of bias is low.

Disadvantages of a simple random sampling strategy:
   - knowledge of the population is required
   - Method of obtaining the sample is laborious and slow (time-consuming).

Learning activities

1. c	**2.** b	**3.** d	**4.** c
5. d	**6.** a	**7.** b	**8.** d
9. a	**10.** c		

Quantitative data collection and study validity

DOUG ELLIOTT AND ZEVIA SCHNEIDER

Learning outcomes

After reading this chapter, you should be able to:

- define the types of data collection methods used in quantitative research
- list the advantages and disadvantages of each of these methods
- explain how internal and external validity can affect the rigour of a study
- critically evaluate the data collection methods used and study validity of published studies.

Introduction

The success of a study primarily depends on the quality of the data collection methods selected. As noted in Chapter 10, the chosen quantitative design guides the selection of a sampling strategy and data collection approach. A logical flow between research question, design and methods should therefore be clear to a reader. The 'methods' section of a research proposal, grant application, report, or published journal article describes the researcher's operational plan for addressing the research question, objective or hypothesis. The 'procedure' (how the data were collected) forms the major component of the methods.

This chapter focuses on data collection and study validity. The common approaches to data collection in nursing and midwifery research include physiological measurement, observation, participant reports using questionnaires or interviews and health records or other documentation. These methods and procedures, used to collect information about participants, are identifiable and repeatable steps that enable the major variables to be studied in a systematic, objective and rigorous manner. The aim is that data collection from a quantitative perspective should not be influenced by an observer or data collector, and that data are collected consistently for each participant in the study. The quality and rigour of this process is important in determining the credibility of the study findings (called 'internal validity'), and the resulting ability to generalise these findings from a representative sample to a larger population (called 'external validity'). Threats to study validity are discussed later in the chapter.

Measuring a variable of interest

As quantitative research focuses on 'empirical measurement', a researcher must first operationally define the variable/s of interest. Determining what types of measurement to use in a particular study is a complex and time-consuming step in study design that begins during the review of the background literature. A review of similar studies will indicate what measuring tools/instruments other researchers have previously used and how they measured the concepts of interest. Crucial to the meaningfulness of the study findings is the evaluation of the most appropriate and available instrument for collecting the data.

Two important and necessary aspects of reviewing the literature are to build on previous knowledge and to place the study in the historical context of that knowledge. As well as an objective and systematic process, measurement of data requires accuracy ('validity') and consistency ('reliability') (discussed in Chapter 13).

Conceptual and operational definitions

Many different approaches are available to collect information about concepts or phenomena of interest to nurses and midwives.

Clinical practice issues requiring study can focus on measurement variables ranging from biological and physical indicators of health (e.g. blood pressure and heart rate) to psychosocial variables, such as anxiety, hope, social support, self-concept or health-related quality of life (Ferrans et al. 2005). An 'operational definition' translates a 'conceptual' definition into a form that is measurable.

For example, a conceptual definition of anxiety might be 'a subjective feeling of apprehension and tension, manifested by physiological arousal and varying patterns of behaviour'. While this definition enables a reader to understand the concept, in this form anxiety cannot be measured in an operational sense. Using an operational definition allows the concept to be measured. For example, an operational definition of anxiety could be 'a subjective feeling of apprehension and tension, as measured by the Depression, Anxiety Stress Scale' (Lovibond & Lovibond 1995).

Types of data collection

The variables of interest are measured using one or a combination of the five common quantitative data collection approaches: physiological, observation, interviews, questionnaires, and records or other documentation. Each method has a specific purpose, as well as certain advantages and disadvantages inherent in its use. A

FIGURE 12.1 Data collection methods decision path

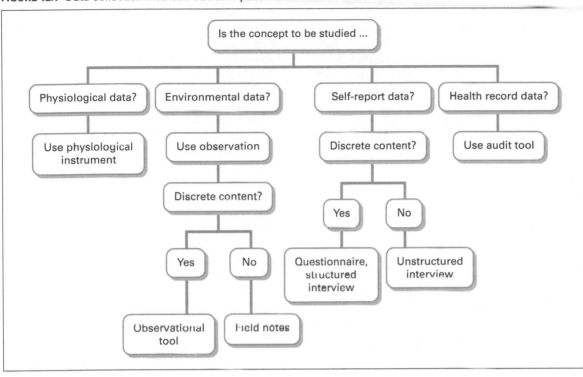

decision path for the selection of data collection methods is illustrated in Figure 12.1.

Physiological or biological measurement

In clinical practice, nurses and midwives collect and document a range of physiological data about patients, often using specialised equipment. Measures can be physiological (e.g. weight, temperature, pulse oximetry, urinalysis); biochemical (e.g. blood glucose level); microbiological (e.g. bacterial cultures); or anatomical (e.g. radiological examinations). Physiological or biological measurement is particularly suited to the study of several types of clinical issues, including examination of the effectiveness of specific practice activities.

The advantages of using physiological data collection methods include their objectivity, precision and sensitivity (ability to detect subtle variations in the measured variable), assuming that calibration and instrument error have been addressed. These methods are generally reliable because unless there is a technical malfunction, two readings of the same instrument taken at the same time are

Research in brief

An experimental study compared the effects of pressure bandaging on complications and comfort in patients undergoing coronary angiography (Botti et al. 1998). One variable measured was haematoma (bruise) size, measured in square centimetres. A standard measurement protocol and measures of inter-rater reliability ensured that all data collectors were rating or measuring haematoma size in the same way for all study participants. To increase reliability of data collected, information sessions for data collectors were conducted throughout the study period. The results showed no difference in bruise size between the bandage and no-bandage groups, however, participants who were not bandaged expressed greater comfort than those with a bandage.

likely to yield similar results (see Chapter 13 for further discussion).

The limitations of physiological measurements include the costs of obtaining specialised knowledge and training of personnel to collect the data reliably, environmental influences, and/or the effect of instrumentation and testing (see 'Internal validity' later in this chapter). For example, the presence of a heart rate monitor may elicit a stress response and make some patients anxious and increase their heart rate, unless suitable information is provided to allay their concerns.

Evidence-based practice tip

Researchers must indicate clearly the processes involved in ascertaining the validity and reliability of any data collection instrument used.

Observation

Some clinical researchers are interested in determining how participants behave in certain conditions. Depending on the aims and questions of a study, a researcher may opt for a quantitative or qualitative observational approach. For example, a researcher may be interested in how children respond to painful stimuli within a clinical context. Children could be asked how painful an experience was, but they may not be able to answer the question or quantify the amount of pain, or they may distort their responses to please the researcher. Conversely, observing a participant may give a more accurate picture of the behaviour than by directly asking the patient.

Although observing patients and the environment is a normal component of clinical practice, research observation using a quantitative approach places emphasis on the objective and systematic nature of the research process. The focus is observing with a trained eye certain specific events identified in a literature review of previous research. To be rigorous, observations must fulfil the following conditions:

- observations are consistent with the study's specific objectives and related scientific concepts and theories
- a standardised and systematic plan for observation and recording of data is used
- all observations are checked and controlled.

Observation is particularly suitable as a data collection method in complex research situations that are best viewed as total entities or difficult to measure in parts, such as studies dealing with clinical practice, social interactions or group processes. This approach may also be the best way to develop an operational

definition for some variables of interest, particularly individual characteristics and conditions, such as traits and symptoms, verbal and non-verbal communication behaviours, activities, skill attainment, or environmental characteristics.

The four basic types of observational roles are distinguished by the amount of involvement by the observer/researcher, and the issues of 'concealment' (of the observation) and 'intervention' (active involvement as a participant in the social situation being studied):

1. complete participant (concealment + intervention)
2. participant as observer (no concealment + complete intervention)
3. observer as participant (no concealment + brief intervention)
4. complete observer (concealment + no intervention).

These types of participant observation were discussed earlier in Chapter 8, as observation is also a common data collection approach in qualitative research.

Point to ponder

▶ Concealment in observational studies is rarely used in clinical research today. Consider the ethical issues regarding informed consent for participants being observed in a study?

A researcher would need to justify why concealment is necessary to their human research ethics committee (HREC). If the researchers can argue that there is no other way to collect the data and the data collection procedure is unlikely to have negative consequences for the participants, the study may be approved. Approval may also be given subject to participants being informed by a 'debriefing session' after the observation period; this would give them the opportunity to refuse to have their data included in the study or to discuss any questions they may have.

Observations may be structured or relatively unstructured. Structured observations use tools, checklists or rating scales to document observed activities or behaviours. The behaviours or events to be observed are specified in advance, and data forms are prepared for documentation. During data collection, the observer watches the participant and documents what they observed on the recording form. An example of structured observation was a study observing the activities of registered nurses using a work sampling technique (Duffield et al. 2005). This study required a design that observed participants in the naturalistic setting; with no interventions or control. Six wards in one Australian hospital were each sampled for two weeks during daytime weekday shifts, with clinical staff observed by trained observers using a previously used and established observational tool. Work sampling (Pelletier & Duffield 2003) was a cost-effective method for determining that senior clinical nurses (CNSs) were spending more time than anticipated on non-direct patient care activities. When observations are undertaken by more than one observer, adequate training to determine inter-rater reliability is required to ensure consistency of the observations.

Point to ponder

▶ 'Being there' is a major strength of participant observation and may be the only way to study a complex variable of interest. A limitation is, however, potential bias of the observations by the presence and/or interaction of the observer.

Observation and documentation using an unstructured approach requires the observer to write free-text field notes of their observations during and/or immediately after the period of observation. From a quantitative perspective, these data are reviewed then coded into categories developed after data collection (post hoc), then analysed for commonalities or differences.

Point to ponder

▶ Observational methods are frequently used in nursing and midwifery research. What are the advantages and disadvantages of using this method of data collection?

Research in brief

A mixed-method study explored interaction between family members and staff in a Swedish intensive care unit. In the observation phase, a researcher '... made non-participating observations ... having no verbal communication with the staff or the family ... Each family was observed on average five times, about 30 to 90 minutes at a time, mostly daytime. Field notes were made of the context and all interactions between family members and staff ... All verbal communication was taped' (Soderstrom et al. 2006 p 709). This 'non-participant observation' technique was appropriate for a quantitative study where the observer did not interact with participants. No observational schedule or instrument was selected prior to data collection. A mixed-method approach allowed for increased depth of understanding through family interviews.

TT Tutorial trigger 1

Assume you are working in the children's ward of the hospital. You are interested in finding out what a parent or parents talk about with their child during the hospital visit. Describe the various types of observation and motivate for which type of observation you think most appropriate for this study.

Interviews

Participants in a study often have information that can only be obtained by asking questions. Interviews can be used in both qualitative and quantitative studies, although the style and process differ. From a quantitative perspective, questions are usually focused and a researcher works from an 'interview schedule'. Questions or items in the schedule may be direct (e.g. asking about a participant's level of pain), or more indirect by using a combination of items to estimate to what degree the respondent has some trait or characteristic (e.g. anxiety). Items may allow open-ended answers or require a response to a series of statements (close-ended).

Interviews are best used when a researcher may need to clarify the task for the respondent or is interested in obtaining sensitive or personal information. Telephone interviews allow a researcher to reach more respondents than face-to-face interviews. Both interviews and questionnaires require participants to report data about their knowledge, attitudes and beliefs, but each approach has unique advantages and disadvantages. Advantages of interviews when compared to questionnaires include:

- the response rate is almost always higher, which limits bias in the sample
- children, some people with disabilities, and those who are unable to write or complete a questionnaire can participate effectively in an interview
- the actual participant responds; if questionnaires are mailed, someone else could supply the responses
- direct two-way communication and a developing rapport may improve the quality and rate of responses to sensitive or intimate information; however, participants may prefer the relative anonymity and indirect nature of a questionnaire about moral, cultural, or ethico–legal issues (e.g. religious beliefs, sexual behaviour, substance use).
- opportunity to clarify questions and observe the participant's non-verbal behaviour.

Questionnaires

Measuring instruments (or tools) are commonly a set of questions (or items) used in a quantitative study to measure the study variable/s. Many questionnaires are available to measure variables that are of interest to nursing and midwifery researchers (see 'Additional resources' at the end of this chapter for examples of books and websites that list instruments). A set of items can be constructed in different forms (see Table 12.1). Questionnaire items should:

- be written so that the intent of the question and the nature of the information sought are clear to the respondent
- ask only one question, be grammatically correct, free of jargon and value-laden terms, and not open to alternative interpretations
- be written at a level of language understandable to respondents.

TABLE 12.1 Forms of measuring instruments

Instrument form	Description
Scale	Individual items are combined to obtain an overall score.
Profile	A comprehensive instrument that assesses different components of a concept within one measurement approach.
Battery	Comparable to a profile with assessment of multiple components, but derived from different original sources.
Index	A single number (total score) derived from various sources and/or list of items.

As for interviews, items used in questionnaires can also be open-ended or close-ended (see Box 12.1). Open-ended items enable participants to respond in their own words, and can be used when the researcher does not know all of the possible alternative responses. Unstructured open-ended response formats therefore allow a greater range of responses to be collected. A technique called content analysis is used to interpret this information. This process uses previously identified categories to group the open-ended responses so that the information can be coded and examined in a numerical form.

Close-ended items use a fixed number of alternative responses, although the format can vary (e.g. fixed response, multi-choice formats, or lists of items where participants rank-order the items) (Considine & Botti 2005). Fixed-response items can be used for questions requiring a dichotomous 'yes' or 'no' response, or when there are categories such as language spoken at home, highest educational level, or employment status. Structured, fixed-response items are best used when the question has a limited number of responses; the participant is asked to choose the response closest to their preferred answer. While fixed-response items have the advantage of simplifying the respondent's task and the researcher's analysis, they may however miss some important information about participants' views regarding the variable/s of interest.

A Likert Scale is an example of a fixed-response format used to determine a participant's

BOX 12.1 Examples of close ended and open-ended questions

Close-ended: Likert-type scale

How satisfied are you with your learning in this current research subject?

1. Very satisfied
2. Moderately satisfied
3. Undecided
4. Moderately dissatisfied
5. Very dissatisfied

To what extent do the following factors contribute to your current level of satisfaction?

	Not at all	Very little	Somewhat	Moderate amount	A great deal
Subject content	1	2	3	4	5
Learning process	1	2	3	4	5
Related readings	1	2	3	4	5
Student activities	1	2	3	4	5
Assessments	1	2	3	4	5

Close-ended

On average, how many clients do you see in the community health centre in a day?

1. 1–4
2. 5–9
3. 10–14
4. 15–19
5. 20 or more

How would you characterise the pace of your midwifery clinic?

1. Too slow
2. Slow
3. About right
4. Busy
5. Too busy

Close-ended: analogue scale (Linear Analogue Anxiety Scale — LAAS)

Mark on the scale below the amount of anxiety you are exeriencing now.

1	2	3	4	5	6	7	8	9	10
No anxiety								Extreme	anxiety

Open-ended

Are there incentives that the Australian College of Critical Care Nurses ought to provide for members that are currently not being offered?

attitude or opinion. For example, lists of statements are provided for the respondents to indicate whether they 'strongly agree', 'agree', 'disagree' or 'strongly disagree'. Likert Scales are commonly constructed as 4, 5, 7 or 10-point scales (Box 12.1 illustrates a 5-point scale). Including a neutral response such as

'neither agree nor disagree' creates an odd point scale, although a neutral category may limit analysis and is difficult to interpret.

Questionnaires are most useful when there is a finite set of questions to be asked and the researcher can be assured of the clarity and specificity of the items. If questionnaires are too long or complicated, they are less likely to be completed; this relates to 'respondent burden'. Advantages of questionnaires compared to interviews include:

- being less expensive to administer
- no researcher being present eliminates interviewer bias
- a larger sample can be accessed to enable increased generalisability of results.

Instruments found during a literature search may be used in original form or adapted for use in a new study (although any modification may alter the instrument's accuracy and validity). If instruments are already available, a researcher obtains permission for their use from the original author or copyright holder (often the publisher of the journal where the instrument or article was first published).

The Medical Outcomes Study Short-Form 36-item (SF-36) is a common clinical research instrument measuring functional status that originated from a larger battery of 149 items (Functioning and Well-Being Profile) developed from questionnaires in the 1970–1980s. The SF-36 examines eight concepts reflecting self-evaluation of physical and mental functions (physical functioning; physical role; bodily pain; general health; vitality; social functioning; emotional role and mental health) (Ware 2000). The instrument was presented in developmental form in 1988 and standard form in 1990. Continued psychometric testing in international and a variety of clinical cohorts enabled development of version 2, as well as related instruments (e.g. SF-12, SF-8) designed for population surveys (see 'Additional resources' at the end of this chapter).

Availability of the internet now offers opportunities for research data to be collected online (Davis et al. 2004) via questionnaires or other methods such as discussion boards or chat rooms (Gallagher 2005).

Records, databases and other documentation

All data collection methods previously discussed illustrate the approaches researchers use to gather new or 'primary' data to study phenomena of interest. Records and other existing documents or data are termed 'secondary' sources, and include hospital records, care plans, clinical databases, and census or population data (see 'Additional resources' at the end of this chapter). These existing data sources can also be used to answer specific primary research questions.

Research in brief

Data from a midwifery/obstetric database were accessed and analysed to examine the effects of a primary health midwifery care model on maternal and neonatal outcomes when compared to standard hospital care in a sample of low-risk women. Women in the midwifery care group had less delivery interventions (fewer episiotomies but higher incidence of perineal tears), and more received narcotics during delivery. Neonates in both groups had similar outcomes (Johnson et al. 2005). This design was used in preference to an RCT, as the researchers supported women's rights to select their care option, and not be randomised to one group or another. Selection bias was noted by the authors as a study limitation — women with high-risk pregnancies or a non-English speaking background were excluded.

With the exponential increase in clinical data collection and storage, use of 'data mining' approaches now enable examination of clinical practice issues (Berger & Berger 2004; Pelletier & Diers 2004). Contemporary data mining involves specific approaches and steps as one element in an emerging discipline called 'knowledge discovery in databases'. Data mining uses specific software to undertake automated processes and algorithms for interrogating the dataset. Either a hypothetic-deductive (hypothesise and test) or inductive (test and hypothesise) approach can be used (Berger & Berger 2004).

TT Tutorial trigger 2

You want to find out what your second-year colleagues in hospital X thought of their recent clinical placement in the medical ward. What kinds of statements (open- and close-ended questions) could you ask? You may also ask the ward clinical staff to provide comments. Design a Likert-type questionnaire to obtain the data.

Using available data has distinct advantages. As the data collection step of the research process is sometimes the most difficult and time-consuming, the use of available records enables significant time-saving. If records have been kept in a similar manner over time, as with clinical databases, analysis of these records allows for the examination of trends over time. Various government privacy acts protect the rights of individuals who may be identified in records. As a result, healthcare institutions may therefore be reluctant to allow researchers access to medical records, unless the information is provided in a format that is de-identified, thus preserving anonymity (Berger & Berger 2004). Current policies on storage of research data in Australia are governed by the National Health & Medical Research Council (NHMRC) (see 'Additional resources' at the end of this chapter).

Data quality is particularly important as a potential bias with existing datasets (Pelletier & Diers 2004), and it may be difficult for a research consumer or primary researcher to uncover these types of subtle biases. Despite these potential limitations, health records and other available data constitute a rich source for study which remains as yet mostly untapped by nurses and midwives (Berger & Berger 2004; Pelletier & Diers 2004).

Study validity

For a study to form the basis of further research, practice and theory development, the findings must be believable and dependable. Two important criteria for evaluating the credibility and dependability of findings are internal validity and external validity.

● **Evidence-based practice tip**
- Internal validity refers to the methodological rigour and quality of a study, where any potential biases are minimised.
- External validity relates to the generalisability of a study's findings to the wider population of interest.

The aim of a researcher is to select a design, sampling approach and data collection method that maximise both internal and external validity. A threat to internal validity can also be a threat to external validity (see Figure 12.2).

FIGURE 12.2 Interacting threats to study validity

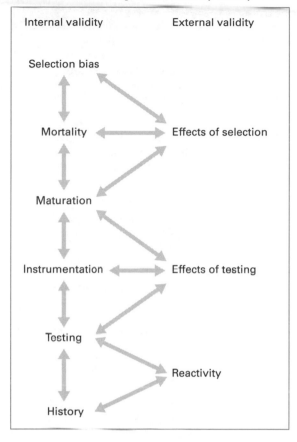

Internal validity

Internal validity relates to whether the intervention (explanatory or independent variable) had a real measurable effect on the outcome (dependent) variable, or whether some 'confounding' variable influenced and jeopardised the results. Confounding of findings occurs when extraneous variables are not controlled in the experimental design. A study therefore has internal validity when all confounding variables have been controlled or minimised (Campbell & Stanley 1966). These threats are considered when planning the design and methods of a study, and before implementing results into practice. Threats to internal validity are most clearly applicable to experimental designs, but these factors should be considered in all quantitative designs (see Table 12.2).

Researchers should report any aspects of participant recruitment and retention that may influence a study's findings, as outlined in the

TABLE 12.2 Description of threats to internal validity

Threat	Description
Selection bias	Study participants need to be a representative sample of the population of interest; problematic where individuals self-select for participation in a study.
Mortality (drop out; loss to follow-up)	Non-response of enrolled participants from the first data collection point (pre-test) to the final data collection point (post test).
Maturation	Developmental, biological or psychological processes of an individual that change over time and may influence the study variable.
Instrumentation	Changes in measurement or observational techniques of the variables that may influence measurement; includes consistency for multiple observers (inter-rater reliability).
Testing	The effect (experience) of taking a pre-test on the score of a post-test.
History	A specific event that may affect the study variable, either within or external to the study setting.

CONSORT statement (Moher et al. 2001). More than one threat may exist in a study depending on the type of study design. Finding a threat to internal validity in a study does not invalidate the results and is usually acknowledged by the investigator in the results or discussion section of the study.

'Selection effects' are an issue where actual study participants do not constitute a representative sample (e.g. when participants self-select for a study). In situations where a random sample cannot be obtained, bias becomes a concern as the study findings may not be able to be generalised to other samples or the population of interest (then also an issue of external validity). For example, a study advertised for a sample of women who were currently pregnant or had birthed within the past 12 months. Although the researchers did not identify selection bias as a potential threat or problem in their findings, it was noted that the resulting sample consisted of middle-class women (in terms of university education and income) (Fenwick et al. 2004 p 32). This sample did not therefore reflect the overall population of interest. To counter selection bias the researcher could randomly assign participants to the intervention or control group.

There are also occasions when, for various reasons, participants withdraw from a study. This 'study mortality' or 'loss to follow-up' may affect the study findings if participants who withdraw are significantly different on the important study variables compared to those remaining. Importantly, the final sample may not still be representative of the original samples of the population of interest (again also affecting external validity).

The natural process of 'maturation' by participants (particularly in a longitudinal study) may also influence their responses to study variables. For example, a study may investigate the relationship between two methods of teaching on the knowledge of self-care for children with a chronic illness. Post-tests of student learning would need to be conducted in a relatively short timeframe after the teaching intervention is completed, to ensure that the findings are not influenced by the maturation of children who are learning new skills rapidly.

'Instrumentation' threats are changes in the measurement of variables or observational techniques that may account for changes in the obtained measurement. For example, if an investigator has several research assistants collecting observational data, all must be trained in a similar manner. If they are not similarly trained, a lack of consistency may occur in their ratings and therefore a major threat to internal validity will occur. In a study of pressure bandaging following coronary angiography (Botti et al. 1998), observers were trained to use the same methods of measuring patients' haematomas and recording data, therefore reducing the risk of instrumentation effects.

When a study uses a pre-test, exposure to the test may prime participants and affect their responses at post-test (Campbell & Stanley 1966). The differences between post-test and pre-test scores may therefore not be a result of the intervention but rather of the experience gained through 'testing'.

'History' refers to an event external to the intervention that occurs between the measurement points. For example, in a study of the effects of a quit smoking program, an event such as the graphic pictures of lip cancer and decayed teeth in external government-sponsored media advertisements may threaten internal validity. In this instance, the researcher would be in some doubt as to which event had a greater influence on participants' responses.

> ● **Evidence-based practice tip**
>
> Internal validity addresses whether the explanatory variable (intervention) really caused a change in the outcome variable, or whether some other factor caused bias and influenced the findings.

External validity

External validity refers to the generalisability of a study's findings to other populations or settings. Factors that may affect external validity are related to the selection of participants, study conditions and types of observations. These factors are termed:

- interaction effect of selection
- reactive effects of being studied
- reactive or interaction effect of testing.

As noted in Figure 12.2, there are inherent links between the factors of selection and testing and those of threats to internal validity. When considered as internal threats, the focus is how they influence the study variables within the study. When assessing them as external threats the focus is in terms of generalisability, or applicability outside the study to other populations and settings. It is important to remember that this path is not exhaustive in describing the type of threats and their interactions.

Effect of selection

Selection relates to the generalisability of study results to other populations, and is influenced by the 'selection bias', 'mortality' and 'maturation' of internal validity threats. An example is when a researcher is unable to obtain the ideal sample population. At times, numbers of available participants may be low or not accessible to a researcher, who may then need to choose a non-probability method of sampling over a probability method.

Reactive effect of testing

Administration of a pre-test in an intervention study may also affect external validity, influencing the generalisability of findings to other clinical situations or populations. Reactivity is influenced by the internal validity effects 'maturation', 'instrumentation' and 'testing'. Suppose a researcher wants to assess changing attitudes towards people with mental illness. To accomplish this, an education program on mental illness is implemented. To test whether the education program changes attitudes towards mental illness, tests are given before and after the education intervention. The pre-test on attitudes, however, may prompt participants to reflect on their attitudes regarding mental illness. The participants' responses on follow-up testing may therefore differ from those of individuals who were given the education program but did not see the pre-test.

Reactive effects of being studied

Reactivity reflects participants' responses to being studied, and is influenced by the internal validity threats 'testing' and 'history'. Participants may respond to a researcher as an extraneous response to being studied, not because of the actual study procedures. This is known as the 'Hawthorne effect', named after Western Electric Corporation's Hawthorne plant (in the United States), where a study of working conditions was conducted. In this classic study, the researchers implemented several different working conditions (e.g. turning up the lights, piping in music loudly or softly, and changing work hours). The researchers noted however that no matter what intervention was introduced, workers' productivity increased. It was therefore concluded that production increased as a result of the workers knowing that they were being studied rather than because of the actual experimental conditions.

> ● **Evidence-based practice tip**
>
> Identification of internal and external threats to validity does not render a study unusable or irrelevant; recognition of the threats allows researchers to build on the research evidence and clinicians to consider which elements of the study can be applied to practice.

BOX 12.2 Criteria for evaluating data collection methods

1. Are all of the data collection instruments clearly identified and described?
2. Is the rationale for their selection given?
3. Is the method used appropriate to the problem being studied?
4. Is the method used appropriate to the clinical situation?
5. Are the data collection procedures similar for all subjects?

Physiological measurement

1. Is the instrument used appropriate and consistent with the research problem?
2. Is a rationale given for why a particular instrument was selected?
3. Is there a provision for evaluating the reliability, validity, responsiveness of the instrument and those who use it?

Observational methods

1. Were the observations performed using the principles of informed consent?
2. How were any observers trained to minimise any bias?
3. Was there an observers' guide?
4. Were the observers required to make inferences about what they observed?
5. Is there any reason to believe that the presence of the observers affected the behaviour of the subjects?

Questionnaires

1. Is the instrument (questionnaire) adequately described to assess whether it addresses the concept of interest?
2. Is there evidence that subjects were able to complete the responses?
3. Is there a clear indication that the subjects understood the questionnaire?
4. Are the majority of the items appropriately close-ended or open-ended?

Records and other available documents or data

1. Are the records used appropriate to the problem being studied?
2. Are the data examined in such a way as to provide new information rather than summarising current information?
3. Is there any indication of selection bias in the available records?

All studies should have clearly identified data collection methods. The conceptual and particularly the operational definitions of all important variables should be presented. The researcher may provide a rationale for the particular method chosen, however, the paper should adequately describe the methods and data collection procedures for the reader. A number of questions can be considered when examining the study procedure (see Box 12.2).

Interviews and questionnaires should be clearly described to allow a reader to decide whether the variables were adequately operationalised to allow measurement. Evaluating the adequacy of measuring instruments is often challenging for research consumers, as the actual instrument used is not always provided in the paper for inspection, and the reader may not feel confident about judging the adequacy of the method without reviewing it. Readers may therefore need to check the reference list of the paper and obtain any other papers that describe or evaluate the instrument/s.

Once you have decided that the data collection method was appropriate to the problem and the procedures were appropriate for the sample studied, the reliability and validity of the instruments themselves need to be considered. These issues are discussed in the following chapter.

Summary

Quantitative designs guide the choice of sampling techniques and data collection methods. Data collection methods include physiological, observational, interviews, questionnaires and records. Important criteria for determining the creditability and dependability of findings are internal validity and external validity. Internal validity (credibility) must be established before considering external validity.

K EY POINTS

- Data collection methods are both objective (data are not influenced by the data collector) and systematic (data are collected in the same way for each study participant).

- Physiological measurements use technical instruments to collect data about patients' physical, or biological status; the advantages of physiological measurements are objectivity, precision and sensitivity.

- Observational methods are used when the variables of interest are events or behaviours; quantitative observation requires preplanning, systematic recording, and controlling observations.

- Interviews and questionnaires are commonly used in nursing and midwifery research; participants report information about themselves, responding to open-ended or close-ended items (questions); the form of the question should be clear to the respondent, free of bias and grammatically correct.

- Records and other data are an important source for research data, and can save considerable time and money when conducting a study. However, data are subject to problems of availability, authenticity and accuracy.

- Internal validity and external validity must be considered within the sampling design and data collection procedures.

Learning activities

1. Data collection in quantitative research must be objective. In other words:
   (a) data must be collected in the same way throughout the study
   (b) the researcher must clearly identify each outcome variable
   (c) data must not be influenced by the people collecting the data
   (d) every variable must be measurable.

2. Which of the following conditions enhance the generalisability of study findings?
   i.   few threats to validity
   ii. small sample size
   iii. random selection of participants
   iv. representative sample.
   (a) i, ii and iii
   (b) i, iii and iv
   (c) ii, iii and iv
   (d) i, ii and iv.

3. One way to determine if the findings from one study can be generalised to the larger population is to:
   (a) determine the Pearson's r coefficient
   (b) calculate the confidence interval
   (c) examine the research findings for bias
   (d) match findings from similar studies that have similar samples.

4. Bias is introduced into a study when:
   (a) sample selection is carried out inconsistently
   (b) eligible individuals do not participate
   (c) probability sampling techniques are used
   (d) the population is homogeneous.

5. Which of the following are ways of controlling extraneous variables?
   i.   randomly selecting participants
   ii. using a homogeneous sample
   iii. manipulating the explanatory variable
   iv. conducting a pilot study.
   (a) i and ii
   (b) ii and iii
   (c) iii and iv
   (d) i and iv.

6. Which of the following would be considered as disadvantages of using observational data collection methods?
   (a) individual bias may interfere with the data collection
   (b) ethical concerns may be increasingly significant to researchers using observational data collection methods

(c) individual judgments and values may influence the perceptions of the observers

(d) all of the above.

7. When might questionnaires be used as an appropriate method of data collection?
   i. when costs are a concern
   ii. when a researcher is interested in obtaining information directly from participants
   iii. when a researcher needs to collect data from a large group of participants that are not easily accessible
   iv. when accuracy is of utmost importance.
   (a) i, ii and iii
   (b) ii, iii and iv
   (c) i, iii and iv
   (d) i, ii, iii and iv.

8. Which of the following is not consistent with a Likert Scale?
   (a) it contains close-ended items
   (b) it contains open-ended items
   (c) it contains lists of statements
   (d) items are evaluated on the amount of agreement.

9. Controlling for extraneous variables and eliminating potential alternative explanations for study findings means eliminating:
   (a) threats to validity
   (b) independent variables
   (c) *a priori* control
   (d) randomisation of participants.

10. Which of the following are most likely operational definitions of variables?
    i. verbalised satisfaction with care received
    ii. health-related quality of life
    iii. pain rated on a scale of 1 to 10
    iv. heart function.
    (a) i and ii
    (b) i and iii
    (c) ii and iii
    (d) i and iv.

Additional resources

Australian Institute of Health and Welfare provides examples of available data. Online. Available: http://www.aihw.gov.au/

Frank-Stromborg M, Olsen S 2004 *Instruments for Clinical Health-Care Research*, 3rd edn. Jones & Bartlett, Boston

Kite K 1999 Participant observation, peripheral observation or a participant observation? *Nurse Researcher* 7(1):45–55

MAPI Research Institute's Quality of Life Instruments Database (QOLID). Online. Available: http://qolid. org: site lists over 800 instruments with information and contact details

National Health & Medical Research Council provides policies on research data storage and protection. Online. Available: http://www.nhmrc.gov.au

Waltz C F, Strickland O L, Lenz E R 2004 *Measurement in Nursing and Health Research*, 3rd edn. Springer, New York

References

Berger A M, Berger C R 2004 Data mining as a tool for research and knowledge development in nursing. *CIN: Computers, Informatics, Nursing* 22:123–31

Botti M, Williamson B, Steen K, et al. 1998 The effect of pressure bandaging on complications and comfort in patients undergoing coronary angiography: a multicenter randomized trial. *Heart & Lung* 27:360–73

Campbell D T, Stanley J C 1966 *Experimental and quasi-experimental designs for research*. Rand-McNally, Chicago

Considine J, Botti M 2005 Design, format, validity and reliability of multiple choice questions for use in nursing research and education. *Collegian* 12:19–24

Davis Kirsch S E, Lewis F M 2004 Using the world-wide web in health-related intervention research: a review of controlled trials. *CIN: Computers, Informatics, Nursing* 22:8–18

Duffield C, Forbes J, Fallon A, et al. 2005 Nursing skill mix and nursing time: the roles of registered nurses and clinical nurse specialists. *Australian Journal of Advanced Nursing* 23:14–21

Fenwick J, Hauck Y, Downie J, et al. 2004 The childbirth expectations of a self-selected cohort of Western Australian women. *Midwifery* 21:23–35

Ferrans C E, Zerwic J J, Wilbur J E, et al. 2005 Conceptual model of health-related quality of life. *Journal of Nursing Scholarship* 37:336–42

Gallagher P 2005 Synchronous computer mediated group discussion. *CIN: Computers, Informatics, Nursing* 23:330–4

Johnson M, Stewart H, Langdon R, et al. 2005 A comparison of the outcomes of partnership caseload midwifery and standard hospital care in low risk mothers. *Australian Journal of Advanced Nursing* 22:21–7

Lovibond P, Lovibond S 1995 The structure of negative emotional states: comparison of the Depression Anxiety Stress Scale (DASS) with the Beck Depression and Anxiety Inventories. *Behavioral Research and Therapy* 33:335–43

Moher D, Schulz K F, Altman D G, for the CONSORT Group 2001 The CONSORT statement: revised recommendations for improving the quality of reports of parallel-group randomized trials. *Lancet* 357:1191–4

Pelletier D, Diers D 2004 Developing data for practice and management: an Australian educational initiative. *CIN: Computers, Informatics, Nursing* 22:197–202

Pelletier D, Duffield C 2003 Work sampling: valuable methodology to define nursing practice patterns. *Nursing & Health Sciences* 5:31–8

Soderstrom I-M, Saveman B-I, Benzein E 2006 Interactions between family members and staff in intensive care units: an observational and interview study. *International Journal of Nursing Studies* 43:707–16

Ware J E, Jnr 2000 SF-36 health survey update. *Spine* 25:3130–9

Answers

TT Tutorial trigger 1

Open-ended questions — examples:
- Briefly comment on the three most enjoyable aspects of your placement.
- Briefly comment on the three least enjoyable aspects of your placement
- Do you have any suggestions to enhance/improve clinical placements in the future?

Learning activities

1. c	**2.** b	**3.** b	**4.** a
5. a	**6.** d	**7.** a	**8.** b
9. a	**10.** b		

TT Tutorial trigger 2

Close-ended Likert-type scale example:

To what extent did the following factors contribute to your enjoyment in your clinical placement on the medical wards?

Contributing factors to your placement enjoyment	A great deal	Moderate amount	Somewhat	Very little
Senior nursing clinicians				
Other nurses				
Interactions with domestic staff				
Interactions with patients				
Medical staff				
Allied health professionals e.g. occupational therapists				
Conferences/discussions about patient care etc with senior nurses				
Opportunity to learn from the environment e.g. nursing and medical procedures				
Responsibility involved in patient care				
Night duty				
Day duty				
General assistance and support from nurses on the ward				

Assessing measuring instruments

DOUG ELLIOTT

KEY TERMS

consistency

equivalence

homogeneity

minimal important
difference

random error

reliability

responsiveness

stability

systematic error
(constant error)

validity

Learning outcomes

After reading this chapter, you should be able to:

- describe how measurement error can affect the findings of a study
- discuss the reasons for testing reliability, validity and responsiveness
- describe the tests of stability, equivalence and homogeneity as they relate to the concept of reliability
- define validity in relation to a measuring instrument
- discuss the approaches used to examine construct validity
- outline the issues related to the measurement of responsiveness
- identify the criteria for evaluating the reliability and validity of measuring instruments
- evaluate the reliability and validity of measuring instruments used in published studies.

Introduction

Being able to accurately and consistently measure concepts of interest is a major focus for nursing and midwifery researchers who use quantitative methods. A measuring instrument is a research tool that enables empirical measurement of the study variables. An instrument can be a questionnaire, survey, observational data sheet, physiological equipment or laboratory test. Any instrument must exhibit appropriate reliability and validity when measuring the concept of interest — that is, consistency and accuracy. If these properties are not present, then any conclusions drawn may be invalid and not advance our understanding of that concept.

This chapter examines the complex issues related to assessment of measuring instruments — also called psychometrics. Instrument testing in clinical research focuses on the major constructs of 'reliability' and 'validity', but should also consider the related concept 'responsiveness'. The common approaches for assessing instrument reliability and validity are explored in relation to how these concepts inform the development, selection and evaluation of measurement tools used in nursing or midwifery research. Demonstrating acceptable levels of reliability and validity in a quantitative study is of crucial importance when:

- using a previously developed instrument with different study participants
- comparing similar instruments that are supposed to measure the same study variable or concept
- constructing a new instrument.

Measurement error

Before discussing reliability, validity and responsiveness in more detail, the theory of measurement error needs some exploration. One important issue to initially consider is to what extent does a measuring instrument display errors when measuring the concept of interest. Ideally, the instrument scores obtained from a sample of participants are consistent and true measures of the behaviours for that population of interest, and therefore an accurate reflection of the real differences between individuals. An observed test score actually consists of the true score plus error (see Figure 13.1). The extent of variability in test scores attributed to error, rather than the true measure of the behaviour or observation of interest, is the error variance. The error component may be either chance (or random) error, or it may be systematic (or constant) error.

If a questionnaire on the knowledge of self-care for patients with continuous ambulatory peritoneal dialysis was given to the same patients several times, the participants would not always give exactly the same response. Some of the variation may be caused by true or systematic differences (e.g. the likelihood of improved scores in a subsequent test). Other differences may however be due to random error (e.g. motivation, boredom, fatigue of

FIGURE 13.1 Components of observed scores

Observed scores	=	True variance	+	Error variance	
Actual score obtained		Consistent, hypothetical stable or true score		*Chance/random error*	*Systematic error*
				• Transient participant factors	• Consistent instrument, participant or environmental factors
				• Instrumentation variations	
				• Transient environment factors	

the respondents). The aim for psychometric researchers is to produce instruments that measure systematic rather than unsystematic (random) changes in scores.

Random error

Chance or random errors are unsystematic in nature and difficult to control. These errors reflect a transient state in a participant within the context of a study. For example, a participant may be anxious about being 'tested', which may then affect their performance in completing the instrument. These perceptions or behaviours that occur at a specific point in time are transient, and are often beyond the awareness or control of a researcher. Random error can also occur with instrumentation; for example, different clinicians assessing blood pressure with the same patient but obtaining different values (inter-observer error); or the same clinician obtaining different blood pressure values on repeated assessment of the same patient when no real change has occurred (intra-observer error).

> ### Point to ponder
> ▶ Being 'tested' may affect different participants in different ways, resulting in random measurement error. This threat to internal validity can also affect external validity (generalisability of the study findings).

Systematic error

Conversely, systematic (constant) error occurs from relatively stable characteristics of the study population, which may also bias their behaviour and/or cause incorrect instrument calibration. This error has a systematic bias influencing participants' responses, and therefore influences instrument validity. Level of education, socio-economic status, social desirability, or other characteristics may influence the validity of an instrument by altering measurement of the 'true' responses in a systematic way. For example, a participant who wants to please a researcher may constantly answer items in a socially desirable way, making the measurement actually inaccurate.

Systematic error also occurs when an instrument is improperly calibrated, such as a set of scales for weighing infants. If the scales were incorrectly calibrated and consistently weighed each infant at 500 g less than their actual body weight, the scale would be reliable (that is, capable of reproducing a stable repeatable measurement), but the results would be incorrect and therefore invalid. Research consumers need to therefore consider how systematic or random measurement errors may occur with different types of instruments.

> ### Point to ponder
> ▶ Validity is concerned with systematic error (accuracy), while reliability is concerned with random error (consistency).

Performance characteristics of an instrument

The psychometric properties of an instrument consist of the major concepts:
* reliability
* validity
* responsiveness.

A research consumer, when reading studies, independently assesses the reliability and validity of the instruments used, to determine the soundness of instrument selection in relation to the constructs being investigated. Reliable and valid measures produce:
* consistent estimates of the relationships between variables, thereby affecting internal validity
* accurate generalisations to the populations being studied, therefore enabling external validity and the ability to apply research findings in clinical practice.

Assessment of the reliability and validity of an instrument is therefore an important skill for a critical reader of nursing or midwifery research to develop. Instrument assessment is a complex process, and a range of resources are available to assist research consumers when evaluating these properties for instruments commonly used in studies (see 'Additional resources' at the end of this chapter). The specific purpose of instrument testing guides the type of analytical test used to establish

FIGURE 13.2 Performance characteristics of a measuring instrument

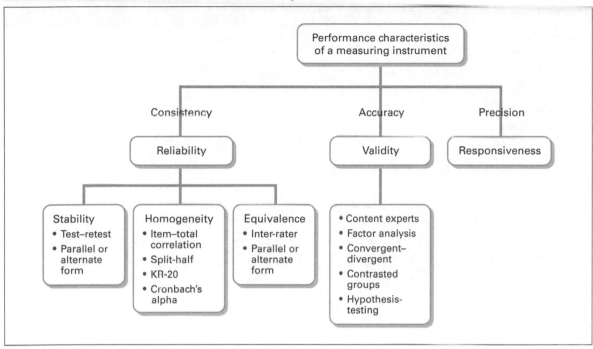

reliability and validity, and the reader needs to be familiar with these purposes and the results obtained from the analyses (see Figure 13.2). The following subsections examine each property separately.

Reliability

Reliable people are those whose behaviour can be relied on to be consistent and predictable. Similarly, reliability of a research instrument is the extent to which the instrument produces the same results on repeated measures. Reliability is therefore concerned with consistency, precision, stability, equivalence and homogeneity. A question to always consider when reading a report of a quantitative study is, 'How reliable is the instrument?' A reliable instrument produces the same results on more than one occasion when measuring a set of behaviours that ordinarily remain relatively constant. Attributes of reliability are concerned with the degree of consistency between scores:
- obtained at two or more independent times of testing (test–retest)
- between different observers (inter-rater)
- between alternate forms of instruments (parallel form).

The test of association between items and/or instruments is commonly expressed as a 'correlation coefficient', ranging from 0–1. This value reflects the relationship between the error variance, true variance and the observed score. When the error variance is low, the reliability coefficient is closer to 1 (commonly >0.7), indicating a reliable instrument. A correlation closer to zero indicates that there is no significant relationship between the two scores. A reliability coefficient of 0.89 indicates that an instrument has little measurement error (the error variance is small). In contrast, a reliability coefficient of 0.49 reflects high error variance (the measurement error is of concern).

Evidence-based practice tip

A reliability (correlation) coefficient of 0.70 or higher reflects a reliable instrument.

When reading a paper, ensure that the method of reliability testing is consistent with the study's aim and the type of measure used. Reliability analysis actually tests three different attributes: stability, homogeneity and equivalence using seven major tests of reliability, depending on the purpose and format of the instruments (see Table 13.1).

TABLE 13.1 Measures to test different attributes of reliability

Attribute	Test	Purpose
Stability Produces the same result on repeated testing	Test–retest reliability	Tests the consistency on repeated measures of the instrument.
	Parallel (alternate form)[1]	Tests the consistency of two versions of an instrument with different items.
Homogeneity All items measure the same concept or characteristic	Item–total correlation	Tests individual items against the total instrument.
	split-half reliability	Tests the consistency of two sub-sets of instrument items.
	KR-20 coefficient	Tests the internal consistency of an instrument with dichotomous response levels.
	Cronbach's α	Tests the internal consistency of an instrument with Likert-type response levels.
Equivalence Same results produced with different observers, or similar/equivalent instruments	Inter-rater reliability	Tests the consistency between two or more observers.
	Parallel or alternate form[1]	Tests consistency between alternate forms of an instrument.

Note 1: This test can examine both the 'stability' and 'equivalence' of an instrument.

The three different attributes of reliability — stability, homogeneity and equivalence; are discussed in the following sub-sections.

Stability

An instrument exhibits stability when the same results are obtained on repeated administration of the instrument. The stability of an instrument to measure a construct consistently over a period of time is an important issue for researchers. It is expected that personality traits or other characteristics remain relatively constant or stable over time. This stability is important when an instrument is used in a repeated-measures longitudinal study. If an intervention (the explanatory variable) is expected to affect the outcome variable, then 'stability' should not be evident, as a measurable effect from the intervention is hypothesised.

When measuring the health status of patients following coronary artery graft surgery over 6 months post-discharge (Elliott et al. 2006), several functional domains measured by the health-related quality of life (HRQOL) instrument 15D (Sintonen 2001) were stable over time — vision, hearing, eating, speech, elimination, mental function and depression (see Figure 13.3). Reported another way, there were no statistically significant differences

for those HRQOL domains when measured repeatedly. This is clinically logical, as those characteristics are stable 'traits' that one would expect to see, even in the presence of an event such as recovery from cardiac surgery.

Also note that these scores are close to the ceiling of the instrument (in this case, '1'), which relates to a limitation of responsiveness (precision) for concepts with small response ranges (i.e. 5-point Likert Scale); this effect can occur at either end of the scale, and is termed the 'floor and ceiling' effect (see the 'Responsiveness' section below for further discussion). Stability has two possible tests: the most common is test–retest; and parallel form.

Test–retest reliability

Test–retest reliability is the administration of the same instrument to the same participants under similar conditions on two or more occasions when true stability of the observed behaviour or characteristic is expected. Scores on repeated testing are compared and expressed as a correlation coefficient, usually 'Pearson's r'. The interval between repeated administrations is variable and depends on the construct being measured, but should be a sufficient timeframe to minimise any bias related to 'testing' (a threat to 'Internal validity'; previously discussed in Chapter 12).

FIGURE 13.3 Mean 15D scores for cardiac surgical patients

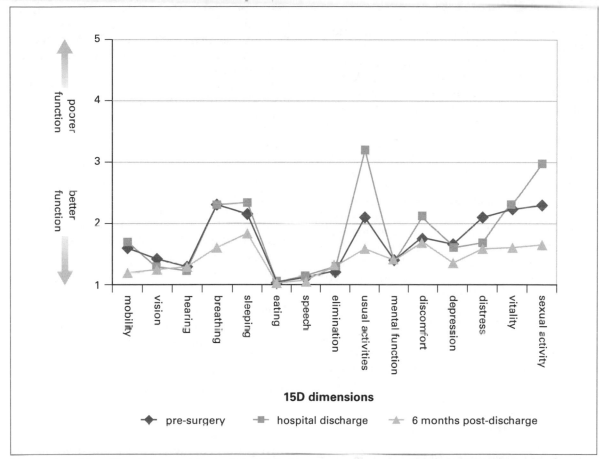

(Source: adapted from Elliott D, Lazarus R, Leeder S R 2006 Health outcomes of patients undergoing cardiac surgery: repeated measures using Short Form-36 and 15 Dimensions of Quality of Life questionnaire. *Heart & Lung* 35:248, used with permission)

A study of attitudes towards patients of 189 psychiatric nurses in Japan used a 30-item self-report instrument, with subscales of 'criticism', 'hostility' and 'positive remarks' (Katsuki et al. 2005). Test–retest scores with 60 participants at 6 weeks demonstrated acceptable reliability for the total instrument, 'criticism' and 'hostility' (r = 0.72, 0.65 and 0.77, respectively), but not 'positive remarks' (r = 0.44). Further testing of the instrument was recommended to confirm the reliability noted in this study.

Parallel form reliability

Parallel (alternate form) reliability is applicable if two comparable forms of the same instrument measuring the same construct exist. Parallel form instruments contain the same types of items that are based on the same domain or construct, but wording of the items is different. It is like test–retest reliability, in that the same individuals are tested within a specific time interval, but it differs because a different form of the same instrument is given to the participants on the second testing.

Development of parallel forms is important if the instrument is intended to measure a variable for which a researcher believes that 'testing' bias will influence a study's internal validity. If alternate forms of an instrument yield a high correlation, then stability is demonstrated. This approach is also used to examine the equivalence between two instruments measuring the same construct. In practice, it is difficult to develop alternate forms of an instrument when considering the many issues required for instrument validity.

Homogeneity

Internal consistency (homogeneity) tests whether the items within the scale/instrument reflect or measure the same construct (concept). That is, items within the scale correlate or are complementary to each other. A uni-dimensional scale is one that measures one construct, while a multidimensional scale measures different but related constructs. For example, the State-Trait Anxiety Inventory (STAI) (Spielberger 1973) is a uni-dimensional scale. In contrast, the Hospital Anxiety and Depression Scale (HADS) (Zigmond & Snaith 1983) is bi-dimensional, and the Depression Anxiety and Stress Scale (DASS) (Lovibond & Lovibond 1995) is multidimensional. Homogeneity is assessed using one of four methods: item to total correlations; split-half reliability; Kuder-Richardson (KR-20) coefficient; or Cronbach's alpha (α).

Item to total correlations

Item to total correlations measure the relationship between each of the items and the total scale, reflected as a correlation coefficient. When item to total correlations are calculated, a correlation for each item on the scale is generated. Usually in a research study, not all the item to total correlations are reported unless the study is a report of how the researcher developed the tool (a methodological study). Typically the lowest and highest correlations are reported, or a table may present analysis of all items tested.

One aim of this test when developing a new or short-form version of an instrument is to eliminate items which have too low a correlation (e.g. <0.30), and accept other items that measure the same concept without being redundant. If item to total correlations are found to be too high (e.g. >0.70), there is also redundancy, as a specific item is measuring the same dimension as the total instrument (see Table 13.2). That is, they overlap rather than complement each other. This is unlike the other measures of reliability in which a higher correlation is generally desirable.

In a study that measured Australian student nurses' 'readiness for self-directed learning', ten items with an item to total correlation of <0.30 were deleted from the initial scale, resulting in a final version with 40 items (Fisher et al. 2001). Similarly, following testing of an initial 38-item questionnaire with a sample of 520 participants, ten items were deleted from a new instrument measuring the attitudes of ICU nurses in Korea to brain death and organ donation. Item to total scores were recalculated on the remaining 28 items, increasing the internal consistency to α = 0.88 (Kim et al. 2006a).

Split-half reliability

The split-half test also provides a measure of consistency (homogeneity) of an instrument's content. This test involves dividing the items of a scale into two halves and making a comparison between them. Th e halves may be odd numbered and even numbered items, division of the first from the second half, or items may be randomly selected. If the correlation coefficients for the two halves are approximately equal, the instrument is considered reliable.

Kuder-Richardson coefficient

The Kuder-Richardson (KR-20) coefficient is the estimate of homogeneity used specifically for instruments that have a dichotomous ('yes/no' or 'true/false') response format. The resulting correlation is based on the consistency of all items in the instrument. A 36-item instrument was developed to test the expertise

TABLE 13.2 Hypothetical example of item–total correlations

Item	Item to total correlation	Comment
1	0.5096	Keep item
2	0.4455	Keep item
3	0.7479	Correlation >0.7 — delete item
4	0.4369	Keep item
5	0.2939	Correlation <0.3 — delete item
6	0.4016	Keep item

and insight of Dutch and Canadian nurses (n = 157) in relation to a palliative care course (Adriaansen & van Achterberg 2004). An internal consistency (KR-20) coefficient of 0.71 reflected acceptable homogeneity of the instrument.

Cronbach's alpha

The most commonly used test of internal consistency for an instrument which uses a Likert-scale response format is Cronbach's alpha (α), where each item in the scale is compared simultaneously with all other items. In an RCT testing the effectiveness of a brief midwife-led counselling intervention for 103 women who perceived that their childbirth experience was traumatic, the internal consistency for a postnatal depression and a depression anxiety and stress scale demonstrated coefficients >0.8 (Gamble et al. 2005). Women who received the counselling reported decreased trauma, depression and stress symptoms, and feelings of self-blame at 3 months, when compared to the control group.

Equivalence

Equivalence is the consistency or agreement among different observers using the same or alternate forms of a measuring instrument. The two methods to test equivalence are inter-rater reliability and alternate or parallel form. An instrument demonstrates equivalence when there is a high percentage of agreement of an observed behaviour. The procedures for assessing equivalence using parallel forms are the same as those for assessing stability (see previous section on 'Parallel form reliability').

Inter-rater reliability

Measurement instruments that use direct observations and systematic recording of variables from more than one observer need to be tested for inter-rater reliability. To accomplish inter-rater reliability, two or more individuals observe the same behaviour or event to ensure that there is consistency of observations between observers. Observers are trained to observe and record the behaviour in a standard, consistent manner. When establishing inter-rater reliability, it is the reliability of the observers rather than the reliability of the instrument that is being tested. Inter-rater reliability is expressed as a percentage of agreement between scorers,

kappa (κ; for categorical-level data) or as an intraclass correlation coefficient (for interval-level data) between scores assigned to the observed behaviours. The strength of agreement for kappa and intraclass coefficients have been interpreted as: >0.80 = very good agreement; 0.61 – 0.80 = good agreement; and 0.41 – 0.60 = moderate agreement (Altman 1999).

Research in brief

A six-category pressure ulcer and skin classification scale was tested using 378 paired assessments undertaken by 116 nurses in a British multi-centre study. Using kappa statistics, agreement between expert nurses and ward nurses varied by skin site and ranged from 94–100% ('very good agreement'). There were however instances of disagreement by two or more categories on 87 occasions (Nixon et al. 2005).

TT Tutorial trigger 1

A student in your class asks a nurse researcher why research assistants who participate in a clinical research study as data collectors need to be trained. What rationale would you offer to support the establishment of inter-rater reliability?

Validity

Validity examines the accuracy of a measuring instrument in reflecting all aspects of the construct of interest. The quality and rigour of any quantitative study is judged in part by the ability of the instruments used to measure what they were designed to measure. Importantly, instrument validity is not a dichotomous state (present or absent), but more of a continuum where there is continuing and stronger evidence developed for the validity of an instrument as more studies use and examine the instrument.

Point to ponder

▶ Measurement (instrument) validity is the extent to which an instrument measures what it was designed to measure; a valid instrument truly reflects the concept of interest.

A valid measure correctly measures the construct of interest. A measure can however be reliable but not valid. A valid instrument that is supposed to measure anxiety does so; it does not measure some other construct, such as stress. Consider an illogical hypothesis where a researcher wanted to measure anxiety in patients by measuring their body temperatures. The researcher could obtain highly accurate, consistent and precise temperature recordings, but such a measure could not be a valid indicator of anxiety. The high reliability of an instrument (in this case, a thermometer) is not necessarily congruent with evidence of validity. Conversely, for an instrument to be considered valid, it must also demonstrate acceptable reliability. An instrument cannot validly measure the attribute of interest if it is erratic, inconsistent and imprecise; that is, if it demonstrates poor reliability.

Evidence-based practice tip

Measurement validity should not be confused with study validity, which relates to the rigour of the study approach (internal validity) and the generalisability of the study findings to the wider population of interest (external validity).

The dominant contemporary view of measurement validity focuses on the central unitary concept of construct validity (Messick 1995), with varying levels of evidence to support the validity of a specific instrument (American Educational Research Association, American Psychological Association & National Council on Measurement in Education 1999). Establishment of construct validity is a complex process, involving numerous studies and different approaches over time.

Previous explanations of validity included the major sub-types: content validity; criterion-related validity; and construct validity. This artificial distinction was confusing, however, as the types were interrelated with an overlap of assessment approaches. Recent articles, various texts and other resources still use these old terms as well as others to describe the concept of validity. The CINAHL database still includes the terms content validity, criterion-related validity, and construct validity in their keywords (from 1991), with no update to a more contemporary view. In contrast, the PsycINFO database replaced the terms 'concurrent', 'construct', 'factorial' and 'predictive validity' with the encompassing term 'statistical validity' in 2000. There is, however, still continuing debate about the merits and limitations of these approaches for measuring validity (e.g. Borsboom et al. 2004; Kelly et al. 2005; Sechrest 2005).

Point to ponder

▶ 'Construct' validity is the central theme or over-arching concept under which differing assessment approaches operate.

A research consumer evaluates whether sufficient evidence of validity is present and whether the type of validity is appropriate to the design and instruments used in the study. Instrument (measurement) validity is examined according to:

- establishing evidence about the content of a measure
  - content (using experts)
  - structure (using factor analysis)
- establishing evidence of relationships between the measure and other variables
  - criterion-related (concurrent/predictive)
  - discriminant (convergent/divergent)
  - differences between groups — contrasted/known groups
  - hypothesis testing.

(American Educational Research Association, American Psychological Association & National Council on Measurement in Education 1999; Goodwin 1997.)

Research in brief

Development of a new instrument to examine responses of patients experiencing acute coronary syndrome included validity testing of items individually and collectively over a number of phases using exploratory interviews, expert review, factor analysis and a concurrent instrument. This multi-method testing resulted in a final 35-item instrument that measured the health domains of physical activity, insecurity, emotional reaction, dependency, diet, medication concerns and side effects (Thompson & Roebuck 2001).

Establishing evidence about the content of a measure

The ability of an instrument to represent the universe of content or the domain of a given construct reflects the 'content' of the measure. Approaches used to establish this include content experts and factor analysis.

Content experts approach

This approach includes the old term 'face validity', a rudimentary type of validity verified by intuitive judgment from people who are not necessarily experts that an instrument appears 'on face value' to measure the concept. This procedure is useful in the early phase of instrument development as the readability and clarity of content are examined. However, it is only a beginning component and not an alternative to other forms of evidence. The use of expert professionals enables more formal evaluation of the substance and content of an instrument in relation to reflecting the entirety of the concept of interest.

Factor analysis approach

This statistical analysis approach provides quantitative assessment about the extent to which a set of items measure the same underlying construct or dimension of a construct, and whether the items in the instrument reflect a single construct or several constructs. Factor analysis assesses the degree to which the individual items on a scale truly cluster together around one or more dimensions (Strickland 2003). Items designed to measure the same dimension should load on the same 'factor'; those designed to measure different dimensions should load on different factors. The process of factor analysis is also discussed in the following chapter on data analysis.

Factor analysis (principal component analysis) was conducted to establish the construct validity of a previously developed list of competency standards for specialist critical care nurses in Australia. The instrument consisted of 58 elements across 20 competency statements and 6 domains. Participants were 532 members of a specialty professional organisation. A 7-point Likert Scale compared how the competency elements reflected the participants' practice.

Factor analysis did not support the theoretical framework of 20 competency statements — a 10-factor model accounted for 64% of the variance in the instrument. All 58 elements loaded onto the first factor and were split randomly across the remaining nine factors (Fisher et al. 2005, p 34). Similarly, the 20 competency statements did not align with the theoretically derived six domains — a 4-factor model ('enabling', 'problem-solving', 'professional practice', 'leadership') accounted for 50% of the variance and improved the internal consistency of the instrument. The authors therefore recommended a re-specification of the model and cautioned against the use of the current instrument for measuring the clinical competence of critical care nurses (Fisher et al. 2005).

Establishing evidence of relationships between the measure and other variables

A range of approaches assesses the similarities or differences in performance between an instrument and other similar measures (related to the superseded term 'criterion-related validity') — concurrent, predictive, convergent/divergent, contrasted groups and hypothesis testing.

Concurrent approach

This approach examines the degree of correlation between two measures of the same concept administered at the same time. This process is used to assess the performance of a new instrument compared to an established instrument — the 'gold standard'. The gold standard label is given to an instrument or test that is the best available measurement of a concept, attitude, behaviour or physical state. Sometimes the established gold standard may be a long or complicated measurement process, and a researcher may decide to construct a shorter instrument with less respondent burden (i.e. the amount of effort and time required from the participants).

A randomised controlled trial (RCT) assessed the concurrent validity of three different psychometric measures for the concept of anxiety, in a sample of 56 patients admitted to a coronary care unit with ischaemic chest pain (Elliott 1993). The State-Trait Anxiety

Inventory (STAI) (Spielberger 1973) has 20 items (questions); the Hospital Anxiety and Depression (HAD) Scale (Zigmond & Snaith 1983) has seven items related to anxiety; and the Linear Analogue Anxiety Scale (LAAS) is a 10 cm line with anchor descriptors of 'no anxiety' and 'extreme anxiety'. The respondent burden was therefore different for each instrument.

Correlation of instruments was assessed using the product moment correlation coefficient (Pearson's r) which examines the strength of a straight line association between two variables; in this case, paired correlations of the three instruments — STAI, HAD, LAAS. The STAI had previously established validity and reliability, and therefore acted as the gold standard criterion (see Table 13.3).

TABLE 13.3 Correlation coefficients for three instruments measuring anxiety

	HAD		LAAS	
	Pre-test	Post test	Pre-test	Post test
STAI	0.64	0.48	0.70	0.67
HAD	–	–	0.48	0.28
LAAS	–	–	–	–

Modified from Elliott, D (1993). Comparison of three instruments for measuring patient anxiety in a coronary care unit. *Intensive Critical Care Nursing*, 9, 195–200; used by permission of the publisher Churchill Livingstone.

As noted in Table 13.3, the above study demonstrated high correlation between the 20-item STAI and the one-item LAAS, but less correlation between the STAI and the HAD Scale. The HAD and LAAS demonstrated a moderate to low relationship. The simple LAAS therefore was as effective as the longer instruments for measuring anxiety in this sample of patients with acute coronary syndrome, with less respondent burden.

● **Evidence-based practice tip**

Correlation coefficients greater than 0.50 indicate a strong inter-instrument relationship, coefficients of 0.30–0.50 reflect a moderate relationship, while 0.10–0.30 indicate a weak relationship.

Predictive validity

Predictive validity explores the degree of correlation between the measure of the construct of interest and some future measure or outcome of the same construct. With this passage of time, correlation coefficients are likely to be lower for predictive validity studies.

Research in brief

The ability of a 33-item self-report breastfeeding self-efficacy scale to predict actual breastfeeding practices was tested in a sample of 300 Australian women. Mothers with high antenatal scores were significantly more likely to be breastfeeding at one week and four months than were mothers with lower scores on the instrument (Creedy et al. 2003).

Convergent and divergent approaches

Convergent validity tests measures of a construct when no gold standard exists. Two or more instruments that theoretically measure the same construct are identified and administered to the same participants. A correlation analysis is performed to assess whether each participant's scores for both instruments change in the same way; that is, when one increases so does the other. If the measures are positively correlated, convergent validity is supported. See the earlier example of the study comparing instruments measuring anxiety in cardiac patients, where the STAI had a high positive correlation with the LAAS (0.67–0.70) and HAD (0.48–0.64) (Elliott 1993), reflecting convergent validity.

Divergent (discriminant) validity assesses the differentiation from one construct to another that may be potentially equivalent. A researcher may sometimes want to use instruments that measure the opposites of a construct. If the divergent measure is negatively related to other measures, validity for the measure is strengthened. Data from a factor analysis can also be used to determine divergent validity.

A specific method of assessing convergent and divergent validity is the multi-trait–multi-method approach. Similar to the approaches previously described, this method involves examining the relationship between indicators that should measure the same construct, and between those that should measure different constructs (Campbell & Fiske 1959). Anxiety, for example, can be measured by a variety of strategies, such as:

- a questionnaire — e.g. the State-Trait Anxiety Inventory (STAI)
- heart rate and blood pressure readings
- asking a participant directly about their anxious feelings
- observing a participant's behaviour
- measuring urinary or serum catecholamines.

The results of one of these measures can be correlated with results of each of the others in a multi-trait–multi-method matrix (Daly & Carnwell 2001; Waltz et al. 2004). The use of multiple measures such as self-report, observation, interview and collection of physiological data, will also decrease the effect of systematic error, improving instrument validity.

Contrasted-groups approach

This 'known-groups' approach identifies two groups of individuals who are expected to score extremely high and low in the characteristic being measured by the instrument. The instrument is administered to both the high-scoring and low-scoring groups and the differences in scores are examined using a t test or analysis of variance (ANOVA). If the instrument is sensitive to individual differences in the trait being measured, the two groups will differ significantly and evidence of construct validity is supported.

Hypothesis testing approach

This approach uses underlying theory of the instrument's design to develop and test hypotheses regarding the behaviour of individuals with varying scores on the measure. Empirical testing supports or rejects the relationships predicted among concepts and provides support for the construct validity of the instrument measuring those concepts. Data collected test the hypotheses and enable inferences about whether the rationale underlying the instrument's construction is adequate to explain the findings.

> **Point to ponder**
> ▶ Is it possible to have a valid instrument that is not reliable? Is the reverse possible?

Research in brief

Hypothesis testing was used to examine the validity of the 25-item Family Caregiving Factors Inventory for home health assessment in a Taiwanese population (Shyu 2000). Instrument domains (resources, expectations, task difficulty and knowledge) were examined in relation to the balance of caregivers' competing needs, and the quality of the relationship between caregiver and care receiver. The findings indicated a significant positive relationship between the domains and competing needs and the care-giving relationship. The instrument therefore appropriately measured the variables of interest within the hypothesised conceptual framework.

Responsiveness

Responsiveness is the ability of an instrument to detect small but clinically important changes in a patient's status (Guyatt et al. 1987; Guyatt et al. 2002). Responsive instruments demonstrate:

- maximum change when clinically important changes in status occur
- minimal change on repeated applications to stable patients.

Responsiveness is therefore the magnitude of change in a participant's score on an instrument that corresponds to a minimal important difference (MID) (Barrett et al. 2005; Guyatt et al. 2002). Responsiveness is measured by comparing instrument scores before and after a treatment of known efficacy. Effect size (change in scores due to treatment effect) can also be used to examine responsiveness, as it relates to changes in the mean score compared to the standard deviation of baseline scores or score changes among stable patients (Guyatt et al. 2002). The positioning of responsiveness as a separate psychometric property however remains debatable, with some opponents suggesting that it is an aspect of validity (e.g. Hays and Hadorn 1992) or internal consistency reliability (e.g. Lindeboom et al. 2005; recently disputed by Puhan et al. 2005).

The responsiveness or precision of an instrument is limited by 'floor and ceiling effects' (i.e. the range of responses possible) — the end-points (extremes) of the scale limit the responses that truly reflect a participant's status for that domain. This was illustrated earlier with Figure 13.3, where a probable ceiling effect was evident for the HRQOL instrument 15D. This instrument used only one item (question) per concept, and as a consequence participants' scores clustered primarily between 1 and 2 for most concepts. This was despite a data collection period of over 6 months that included measurements before and after cardiac surgery. Clearly, this instrument demonstrated a lack of precision in measuring any improvements in health status over time (Elliott et al. 2006).

Knowledge of previous responsiveness characteristics of instruments aid in instrument selection and allow for more accurate sample size and statistical power estimations. However, assessment and reporting of responsiveness has been minimal when compared to the evaluation of reliability and validity. It is therefore often difficult to select an instrument based on its comparative responsiveness against other measures. Responsiveness can be improved by:

- increasing the number of response categories
- disaggregation of scores within a multi-dimensional instrument
- the inclusion of transition questions
- the use of individualised questions.

Developing a measuring instrument

An enormous number of instruments exist for measuring a wide range of clinical, psychological and educational constructs that are relevant to nursing and midwifery researchers. As noted earlier, reliable, valid and responsive instruments require substantial development and testing, involving a suite of testing processes and related studies, often over a number of years. Despite a plethora of available instruments, a researcher cannot sometimes locate an instrument or method with acceptable reliability and validity that measures their variable of interest. This may be the case when examining an element of

a theory or when evaluating the effect of a clinical intervention. When deciding to develop a new instrument, a researcher needs to balance the disciplinary and academic need against the complex and time-consuming processes required. The development process includes:

- defining the construct of interest, a concept developed for a specific research purpose
- constructing items that reflect elements of the construct
- validation of the items
- pilot testing
- formal testing for reliability and validity of the entire instrument.

Defining the construct

A construct is an abstract entity used to describe or hypothesise about observations or relationships. Examples of constructs are suffering, comfort, or health-related quality of life. Defining a construct requires an extensive review of the theoretical literature as well as the existing knowledge base for all instruments developed to measure the concept. This background information enables the construct to be operationalised for measurement purposes. A well-constructed instrument consists of an objective, standardised measure of a clearly defined variable (e.g. a behaviour or characteristic).

> **Point to ponder**
> ▶ The measurement value of an instrument depends on the degree to which it reflects the broad construct or concept.

Item construction

Once the construct is defined, individual items (questions) can be developed. The collection of items should be comprehensive in covering all aspects of the construct. More items are initially developed than needed to address each aspect of the construct or sub-construct. In general, there should be a minimum of ten items for each independent aspect of the construct. Items need to:

- reflect the operational definition of the construct (the extent items appear to accomplish this reflects the validity of the instrument)

- be unambiguous, concise, exact statements with only one idea per item (negative stems or items with negatively phrased response possibilities that result in a double negative may cause ambiguity)
- use a limited numbers of formats (errors may occur if respondents are confused by shifting from one format to another)
- be neutral in style so as to not influence a respondent (unless carefully constructed, an item may indicate an expected response, or an expected response to a subsequent item)
- be not unnecessarily complex or require exact operations
- be appropriate to the educational level of participants.

Item validation

Newly constructed items are then evaluated by a panel of experts in the field to ensure that the items measure what they are intended to measure. During the process of item validation, the number of items will be decreased, as some items will not fit as intended and will be discarded. In this phase the researcher needs to ensure consistency among the items, as well as consistency in testing and scoring procedures.

Pilot test

The developing instrument is then commonly tested on a small, carefully chosen representative sample of participants that display the behaviour of interest. This process assesses the quality of the instrument as a whole (reliability and validity), as well as the ability of each individual item to discriminate between respondents (variance in item response). Instrument administration is standardised using a set of uniform items and response possibilities that are consistently administered and scored.

It is important that researchers who invest significant amounts of time in instrument development disseminate their findings. This type of research serves not only to introduce other researchers to the instrument but also to ultimately enhance the discipline, as our ability to conduct meaningful research is supported by our ability to measure important variables in a reliable and valid way.

Research in brief

A series of studies examined the knowledge and attitudes of Korean intensive care nurses to brain death and organ donation, including the construction and testing of a new instrument. The phases of the study included:

- a review of the literature to determine the construct and relevant factors influencing attitudes on brain death and organ donation (Kim et al. 2002)
- interviews with key informants to determine their views on professional (Kim et al. 2004a) and Korean socio-cultural factors influencing knowledge and attitudes (Kim et al. 2004b)
- constructing items from a review of the literature and the previous key informant interviews
- validating items with an expert panel and pilot test, item reduction, final revision of the instrument, into two sub-scales — knowledge and attitudes
- testing the instrument with a representative sample of Korean ICU nurses (n = 520), examining the reliability and validity of the attitudes (Kim et al. 2006a) and knowledge sub-scales (Kim et al. 2006b)
- confirmation of the reliability and validity of the scales, using a student nurse cohort (n = 292) (Kim et al. 2006c).

Assessing instruments

Reliability and validity are the crucial aspects when assessing a measuring instrument (see Box 13.1). An effective critique includes establishing the instrument's level of reliability and validity and comparing the setting to the context under investigation. In a research report the reliability and validity for each measure should be presented. If not, a reviewer must seriously question the merit and use of the tool and the study's results. If appropriate, responsiveness of the instrument should also be reported.

BOX 13.1 Criteria for evaluating psychometric properties of instruments

1. Was an appropriate method used to test the reliability of the instrument?
2. Is the reliability of the instrument adequate?
3. Was an appropriate method(s) used to test the validity of the instrument?
4. Is the validity of the instrument adequate?
5. If the sample from the developmental stage of the instrument was different from the current sample, were the reliability and validity recalculated to determine if the tool is still adequate?
6. Are strengths and weaknesses of instrument reliability and validity appropriately addressed in the Discussion, Limitations or Recommendations sections of the paper?
7. Is the precision or responsiveness of the instrument discussed in relation to clinically important differences?

Appropriate reliability tests should be reported in the original and subsequent reports of the instrument. If the initial testing sample and the current sample have different characteristics, a reader would expect that a:

• pilot study for the present sample was conducted to confirm that the reliability was maintained
• reliability estimate was calculated on the current sample.

Point to ponder

▶ The validity of an instrument is limited by its reliability; less confidence can be placed in scores from instruments with low reliability coefficients.

Satisfactory evidence of validity is probably the most difficult aspect for a reviewer to determine, but it is this that is most likely to not meet the required criteria. Validity studies are time-consuming, as well as complex, and researchers may only present minimal validity data in a published paper. A reader should therefore closely examine the item content of an instrument when evaluating its strengths and weaknesses and try to find evidence of its validity. Articles may however not include the instrument, or provide only a few sample items available for review. In this case, a reviewer will need to review other articles that examine the instrument more fully.

A reader would expect to see reliability and validity discussed in relation to other instruments devised to measure the same variable/construct. The relationship of the findings to strengths and weaknesses in instrument reliability and validity would be another important discussion point. Finally, recommendations for improving future studies in relation to instrument reliability, validity and responsiveness should be proposed.

T_T Tutorial trigger 2

The researchers in an article you are reading in a refereed journal state that the validity and reliability of the instruments used in their study were established at an acceptable level. You are unfamiliar with the instruments used. You believe that to critically review this section of the report it is necessary to find out how the validity and reliability of these instruments were determined and the criteria used to determine acceptability. How would you proceed? Include in your discussion how you could use technology to help you; support your position with examples.

Summary

The concepts of reliability, validity and responsiveness are complex, and often difficult for a beginning research consumer to assess with confidence. This chapter described the systematic assessment of the psychometric aspects of an instrument. Discussing these issues with colleagues is also a useful approach to assist research consumers in critically appraising the merits and shortcomings of existing, as well as newly developed, instruments that are reported in the nursing or midwifery literature. These exchanges promote understanding of the basic concepts of psychometrics as well as the exploration of alternative methods of observation and the use of reliable and valid tools in clinical practice.

ⓀEY POINTS

- Reliability examines varying attributes of a measuring instrument — stability, homogeneity and equivalence, using tests such as test–retest, parallel or alternate form, split-half, item to total correlation, Kuder-Richardson, Cronbach's alpha and inter-rater reliability.

- The selection of a method for establishing reliability depends on the purpose of the study, the characteristics of the instrument, and the testing method used for collecting data from the representative sample.

- Validity refers to whether an instrument measures what it is purported to measure and it is a crucial aspect of evaluating a tool.

- Testing of instrument responsiveness is an under-researched area, but is an important issue for determining appropriate sample size and power calculations.

Learning activities

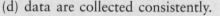

1. Which of the following statements are true? An instrument can be:
   i. valid but not reliable
   ii. reliable but not valid
   iii. neither reliable nor valid
   iv. both reliable and valid.
   (a) i, ii and iii
   (b) ii, iii and iv
   (c) i, iii and iv
   (d) i, ii, iii and iv.

2. A test score or measurement consists of:
   (a) random errors plus constant errors
   (b) random errors plus the true score
   (c) constant errors plus error variance
   (d) error variance plus the true score.

3. A researcher used an instrument to measure self-esteem in adolescent mothers. To measure the validity of this instrument, a second instrument known to measure self-esteem in adult women was also used. What type of validity was being tested?
   (a) predictive validity
   (b) face validity
   (c) concurrent validity
   (d) hypothesis-testing validity.

4. A Cronbach's alpha coefficient of 0.80 indicates that the:
   (a) frequency in each category is different from what would be expected by chance
   (b) instrument actually measures the concepts it was intended to measure
   (c) the instrument is consistent

   (d) data are collected consistently.

5. The degree of consistency in data collection between two researchers is called:
   (a) inter-rater reliability
   (b) reactivity
   (c) de-briefing
   (d) cross-rater validity.

6. Either random error (R) or systemic error (S) may occur in a research study. For each of the following examples, identify the type of measurement error and how the error might be corrected.
   (a) The scale used to obtain daily weights was inaccurate by 500 g less than actual weight.
   (b) Students chose the socially acceptable responses on an instrument to assess attitudes toward AIDS patients.
   (c) Confusion existed among the evaluators on how to score the wound healing.
   (d) Participants were nervous about taking the psychological tests.

7. Homogeneity is a measure of internal consistency. All items on an instrument should be complementary and measure the same characteristic or concepts. For each of the following examples, identify which of the following tests for homogeneity is described:
   • Item–total correlation
   • Split-half reliability

- Kuder-Richardson (KR-20) coefficient
- Cronbach's alpha.
  (a) The odd items of the test have a high correlation with the even numbers of the test.
  (b) Each item on the test using a 5 point Likert Scale had a moderate correlation with every other item on the test.
  (c) Each item on the test ranged in correlation from 0.62 to 0.89 with the total.
  (d) Each item on the true–false test had a moderate correlation with every other item on the test.

8. Tests that are used to estimate the stability of an instrument include:
   i. test–retest reliability
   ii. Kuder-Richardson (KR-20) coefficient
   iii. parallel reliability
   iv. Cronbach's alpha.
   (a) i and ii
   (b) i and iii
   (c) ii and iii
   (d) i and iv.

9. In reliability testing, what test is used for items with a dichotomous response format?
   (a) Cronbach's alpha
   (b) hypothesis-testing
   (c) alternate-form
   (d) Kuder-Richardson.

10. When a variety of measurement strategies is used to examine the relationships between instruments that purport to measure the same construct and between those that should measure different constructs, this approach is called a:
    (a) contrasted groups approach
    (b) convergent approach
    (c) multi-trait–multi-method approach
    (d) divergent approach.

Additional resources

Considine J, Botti M, Thomas S 2005 Design, format, validity and reliability of multiple choice questions for use in nursing research and education. *Collegian* 12:19–24

Health and Psychosocial Instruments (HaPI), Behavioral Measurement Database Services: a database distributed by Ovid; sourced by library subscription

Journal of Applied Measurement. Publishes scholarly work from all disciplines that relate to measurement theory and its application to constructing variables

Journal of Nursing Measurement. Publishes reports on instruments, approaches and procedures developed or utilised for measuring variables in nursing

Messick S 1995 Validity of psychological assessment: validation of inferences from persons' responses and performances as scientific inquiry into score meaning. *American Psychologist* 50:741–9

Munro B H 2005 *Statistical methods for health care research*, 5th edn. Lippincott, Philadelphia

Nunnally J C, Bernstein I 1994 *Psychometric Theory*, 3rd edn. McGraw Hill, New York

Patient-Reported Outcomes and Quality of Life Instruments Database (PROQOLID). Public and subscriber-level access; lists over 400 instruments, covering specific dimensions, therapy, conditions or illnesses (Emery 2005). Online. Available: http://www.proqolid.org

Sechrest L 2005 Validity of measures is no simple matter. *Health Services Research* 40:1584–604

Strickland O L, DiIorio C 2003 *Measurement of Nursing Outcomes Volume 2: Client Outcomes and Quality of Care*, 2nd edn. Springer, New York

US Veterans Affairs Health Service Research & Development Service. Measurement Excellence and Training Resource Information Center (METRIC). Online. Available: http://www.measurementexperts.org

Waltz C F, Strickland O L, Lenz E R 2004 *Measurement in Nursing and Health Research*. Springer, New York

References

Adriaansen M J M, van Achterberg T 2004 A test instrument for palliative care. *International Journal of Nursing Studies* 41:107–17

Altman D G 1999 *Practical statistics for medical research*, 2nd edn. London, Chapman & Hall

American Educational Research Association, American Psychological Association, National Council on Measurement in Education 1999 *Standards for educational and psychological testing* Washington, DC. American Educational Research Association

Barrett B, Brown D, Mundt M, et al. 2005 Sufficiently important difference: expanding the framework of clinical significance. *Medical Decision Making* 25:250–61

Borsboom D, Mellenbergh G J, van Heerden J 2004 The concept of validity. *Psychological Review* 111:1061–71

Campbell D, Fiske D 1959 Convergent and discriminant validation by the matrix. *Psychological Bulletin* 53:273–302

Creedy D K, Dennis C, Blyth R, et al. 2003 Psychometric characteristics of the Breastfeeding Self-Efficacy Scale: data from an Australian sample. *Research in Nursing & Health* 26:143–52

Daly W M, Carnwell R 2001 The case for a multi-method approach. *Nurse Researcher* 30–44

Elliott D 1993 Comparison of three instruments for measuring patient anxiety in a coronary care unit. *Intensive and Critical Care Nursing* 9:195–200

Elliott D, Lazarus R, Leeder S R 2006 Health outcomes of patients undergoing cardiac surgery: repeated measures using Short Form-36 and 15 Dimensions of Quality of Life questionnaire. *Heart & Lung* 35:245–51

Emery M-P, Perrier L-L, Acquadro C 2005 Patient-Reported Outcome and Quality of Life Instruments Database (PROQOLID): frequently asked questions. *Health and Quality of Life Outcomes* 3:12. Online. Available: http://www.hqlo.com/content/pdf/1477-7525-3-12.pdf [accessed 9 January 2007]

Fisher M J, Marshall A P, Kendrick T S 2005 Competency standards for critical care nurses: do they measure up? *Australian Journal of Advanced Nursing* 22(4):32–9

Fisher M, King J, Tague G 2001 Development of a self-directed learning readiness scale for nursing education. *Nursing Education Today* 21:516–25

Gamble J, Creedy D, Moyle W, et al. 2005 Effectiveness of a counselling intervention after a traumatic childbirth: a randomized controlled trial. *Birth* 32:11–19

Goodwin LD 1997 Changing conceptions of measurement validity. *Journal of Nurse Education* 36:102–7

Guyatt G H, Osoba D, Wu A W, et al. 2002 Methods to explain the clinical significance of health status measures. *Mayo Clinic Proceedings* 77:371–83

Guyatt G, Walter S, Norman G 1987 Measuring change over time: assessing the usefulness of evaluative instruments. *Journal of Chronic Disease* 40:171–8

Hays R D, Hadorn D 1992 Responsiveness to change: an aspect of validity, not a separate dimension. *Quality of Life Research* 1:73–5

Katsuki F, Goto M, Someya T 2005 A study of emotional attitude of psychiatric nurses: reliability and validity of the Nurse Attitude Scale. *International Journal of Mental Health Nursing* 14:265–70

Kelly P A, O'Malley K J, Kallen M A, et al. 2005 Integrating validity theory with use of measurement instruments in clinical settings. *Health Services Research* 40:1605–19

Kim J R, Elliott D, Hyde C 2002 Korean nurses' perspectives of organ donation and transplantation: a review. *Australian Transplant Nurses Journal* 11:20–4

—— 2004a Korean health professionals' attitudes and knowledge toward organ donation and transplantation. *International Journal of Nursing Studies* 41:299–307

—— 2004b The influence of socio-cultural factors on organ donation and transplantation in Korea: findings from key informant interviews. *Journal of Transcultural Nursing* 15:147–54

Kim J R, Fisher M, Elliott D 2006a Attitudes of Korean intensive care nurses towards brain death and organ transplantation: development and testing of an instrument. *Journal of Advanced Nursing* 53:571–82

—— 2006b Knowledge levels of Korean intensive care nurses towards brain death and organ transplantation. *Journal of Clinical Nursing* 15:574–80

—— 2006c Undergraduate nursing students' knowledge and attitudes towards organ donation in Korea. *Nurse Education Today* 26:465–74

Lindeboom R, Sprangers M A, Zwinderman A H 2005 Responsiveness: a reinvention of the wheel? *Health and Quality of Life Outcome* 3:8

Lovibond P, Lovibond S 1995 The structure of negative emotional states: comparison of the Depression Anxiety Stress Scale (DASS) with the Beck Depression and Anxiety Inventories. *Behavioral Research and Therapy* 33:335–43

Messick S 1995 Validity of psychological assessment: validation of inferences from persons' responses and performances as scientific inquiry into score meaning. *American Psychologist* 50:741–9

Nixon J, Thorpe H, Barrow H, et al. 2005 Reliability of pressure ulcer classification and diagnosis. *Journal of Advanced Nursing* 50:613–23

Puhan M A, Bryant D, Guyatt G H, et al. 2005 Internal consistency reliability is a poor predictor of responsiveness. *Health and Quality of Life Outcomes* 3:33

Sechrest L 2005 Validity of measures is no simple matter. *Health Services Research* 40:1584–604

Shyu Y L 2000 Development and testing of the Family Caregiving Factors Inventory (FCFI) for home health assessment in Taiwan. *Journal of Advanced Nursing* 32:226–34

Sintonen H 2001 The 15D instrument of health-related quality of life: properties and applications. *Annals of Medicine* 33:328–36

Spielberger C D 1973 *Manual for the state trait anxiety inventory*. Consulting Psychologists Press, Palo Alto, California

Strickland O L 2003 Using factor analysis for validity assessment: practical considerations. *Journal of Nursing Measurement* 11:203–5

Thompson D R, Roebuck A 2001 The measurement of health-related quality of life in patients with coronary heart disease. *Journal of Cardiovascular Nursing* 16:28–33

Waltz C F, Strickland O L, Lenz E R 2004 *Measurement in Nursing and Health Research*. Springer, New York

Zigmond A S, Snaith R P 1983 The hospital anxiety and depression scale. *Acta Psychiatrica Scandinavica* 67:361–70

Answers

TT Tutorial trigger 1

In quantitative studies, it is important that data collection and assessment of the outcome variables is consistent. If more than one assessor is used to measure an outcome variable, the researcher needs to be confident that each assessor will assess in the same and consistent way. The process of inter-rater reliability assesses how close each of the assessors measures the outcome. Each assessor independently measures the outcome variable with the same set of participants (possibly in a pilot test). The researcher then checks for the level of agreement.

TT Tutorial trigger 2

To check the reliability and validity (psychometric properties) of a previously developed instrument used in a subsequent study:

- check the reference list of the paper you are reading for the original or previous report/s of the instrument
- access the previous reference/s that describe the development and/or testing of this instrument
- in addition, you could search the internet for the instrument, using an online bibliographic database (e.g. CINAHL, Medline) or a generic search engine
- review the available information about the instrument
- note whether other researchers have also used the instrument and conducted psychometric testing
- check whether the numerous testing yielded similar or conflicting results
- check whether you can apply these findings to your population of interest
- question how this information influences your reading and critical review of the initial paper.

Examples of instruments will vary.

Learning activities
1. b   2. d   3. c
4. c   5. a
6. (a) S
   (b) S
   (c) R
   (d) R
7. (a) Split-half reliability
   (b) Cronbach's alpha
   (c) Item–total correlations
   (d) Kuder-Richardson (KR-20) coefficient
8. b   9. d   10. c

Analysing data in quantitative research

MURRAY FISHER AND ZEVIA SCHNEIDER

Learning outcomes

After reading this chapter, you should be able to:

- describe the differences between and state the purposes of descriptive and inferential statistics
- identify the statistical procedures appropriate for each level of measurement
- describe the differences between parametric and non-parametric tests
- explain the concept of probability as it applies to the analysis of sample data
- explain the relationship between sample size, effect size, and confidence levels as determinants of error
- determine whether the results are objectively reported and include generalisations and limitations.

Introduction

This chapter is designed to provide an understanding of statistical procedures commonly used in nursing and midwifery research: descriptive statistics and inferential statistics.

The research consumer does not need detailed knowledge of how to calculate these statistics but does need to understand what they mean, how they are used, how they are presented and their limitations.

An added impetus for nursing and midwifery research consumers to understand how to critically read and evaluate a research article came from the increasing pressure on health professionals, in general, to engage in evidenced-based practice. Notwithstanding factors which impede the enthusiasm of nurses and midwives, research utilisation in the interests of providing the best possible patient care necessitates becoming informed and knowledgeable as research consumers.

Descriptive statistics

Statistical procedures are used to give organisation and meaning to numerical data. Procedures that allow researchers to describe, organise and summarise raw data are known as descriptive statistics. Statistical methods that allow researchers to estimate how reliably they can make predictions and generalise their findings based on the data are known as inferential statistics.

There are many ways to describe data: the purpose of descriptive statistics is to order and summarise the data. As mentioned in Chapter 10, the design, data collection and data analysis strategies used depend on the research question. In the main, there are two important reasons for using descriptive statistics. The first refers to the graphical and numerical techniques for organising and interpreting the data; that is, the organisation of the data into various figures (e.g. pie charts, histograms, scatter plots, tables, line graphs).

Such graphical and numerical techniques enable trends and differences to be noted, and the calculation of simple statistics, such as frequency count, percentages and proportions of scores. The second use for descriptive statistics is to condense or reduce large quantities of numerical information into meaningful units. Data can be condensed and summarised using statistics like measures of central tendency (mode, median and mean), and measures of variability (range, semi-interquartile and standard deviation), and some correlational techniques, such as scatter plots). However, when undertaking research, investigators clearly need to understand the use of a particular set of techniques for data analysis. To evaluate the appropriateness of the statistical procedures used in a study, the research consumer should first develop an understanding of the levels of measurement that are appropriate for each statistical technique.

TABLE 14.1 Levels of measurement

Measurement	Description	Measures of central tendency	Measures of variability
Nominal	Classification	Mode	Modal percentage, range, frequency distribution
Ordinal	Relative rankings	Mode, median	Range, percentile, semi-quartile range, frequency distribution
Interval	Rank ordering with equal intervals	Mode, median, mean	Range, percentile, semi-quartile range, standard deviation
Ratio	Rank ordering with equal intervals and absolute zero	Mode, median, mean	All

Levels of measurement

Measurement is the assignment of numbers to objects or events according to certain rules. Measurement level is determined by the nature of the object or event being measured. Levels of measurement in ascending order are nominal, ordinal, interval and ratio (with the acronym NOIR). The higher the level of measurement, the greater the flexibility the researcher has in choosing statistical procedures. Every attempt should be made to use the highest level of measurement possible so that the maximum amount of information can be obtained from the data. Table 14.1 shows levels of measurement.

Nominal measurement

Nominal measurement is used to classify objects or events into discrete categories; but data are neither measured nor ordered. For example, male subjects may be assigned the number 1 and female subjects the number 2. The assignment of these numbers indicates that the categories of male and female are different and exclusive; and the object or event either has the characteristic or does not have it. The numbers assigned to each category are nothing more than labels (names), and therefore cannot be arithmetically manipulated; they do not give the reader any more information about the nature of the difference, they simply give a name to a category. Nominal measurement can be used to categorise a sample on such information as gender, hair colour, marital status, country of birth, occupation and religious affiliation. When measuring a phenomenon at the nominal level, the categories of response must be exclusive and exhaustive. A study (Pravikoff et al. 2005 p 44) of nurses' perceptions of their access to tools to obtain information about evidenced-based studies provides an example of nominal measurement to describe the work setting.

Hospital	60
Nursing home	6
Community or public health	6
School health	4
Non-hospital occupation health	1
Non-hospital ambulatory care	12
Other	11

The nominal level of measurement allows the least amount of mathematical manipulation, only frequencies and proportions. The most

FIGURE 14.1 Descriptive statistics decision path

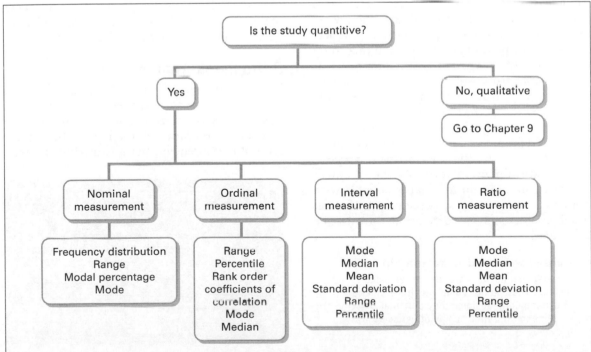

frequently used statistical procedure for nominal data is chi-square (X^2).

Ordinal measurement

Ordinal numbers convey more information than nominal measurement. Ordinal measurement is used to show the relative ranking of objects or events. The numbers assigned to each category can be compared and a member of a higher category can be said to have more of an attribute than one in a lower category. The intervals (space) between numbers on the scale are not necessarily equal, nor is there an absolute zero. For example, student nurses may be invited to place their clinical placement in order of preference on a Likert-type scale numbering 1 to 5, where number 1 is assigned to the least enjoyed placement and number 5 to the most enjoyed placement. Similarly, ordinal measurement is used to formulate class rankings where one student can be ranked higher or lower than another. However, the difference in actual score between students may differ widely. As for nominal level data, ordinal level categories are exclusive and exhaustive.

Fisher et al. (2005) used a 7-point Likert Scale to determine critical care nurses' clinical competence. Critical care nurses were asked to describe how closely each of the Australian College of Critical Care competency standards and the related elements reflected their view of their level of critical care nursing practice. The range of possible scores used in this study was from 1 to 7, where 1 referred to 'never or almost never true' and 7 referred to 'always or almost always true'. The limitation of ordinal measurement is that the intervals between the ranked categories cannot be treated as equal. Ordinal scales add 'greater than' and 'less than' to the measurement process. Mathematical manipulation of data is limited. However, in addition to what is possible with nominal data, medians, percentiles and rank order coefficients of correlation can also be calculated.

● **Evidence-based practice tip**

Correlational designs are non-experimental because they do not comply with the criteria of experimental designs; they permit an examination of relationships of variables in the study.

Interval measurement

In an interval scale, the differences between scores or measures can be treated as equal, as there is a specific numerical distance between each of the levels. However, the zero point remains arbitrary. For example, interval measurements are used in measuring temperatures on the Celsius scale. The distances between degrees are equal, but the zero point is arbitrary, reflecting the freezing point of water, which is not the same as having no heat. The Intelligence Quotient (IQ) is another variable that is treated as an interval scale.

In many areas of psychometric testing, including nursing and the social sciences, there is much controversy over the classification of the level of measurement of intelligence and aptitude and personality tests, with some regarding these measurements as ordinal and others as interval. The research consumer needs to be aware of this controversy and to look at each study individually in terms of how the data are analysed (Knapp 1990, 1993). Interval level data allow some manipulation such as addition and subtraction, but they do not necessarily allow multiplication and division. Examples of interval variables are test scores, age, and population size of a town or country. In these examples two values can be identified by comparison: Are they different and exclusive? (nominal); Is one value greater than another? (ordinal); Is there an equal numerical distance between intervals of the scale? (interval).

Ratio measurement

Ratio measurement shows ranking of events or objects on scales with equal intervals and absolute zeros; the zero point makes the ratio of scale values meaningful. This is the highest level of measurement, but it is usually achieved

> **Points to ponder**
>
> ▶ Nominal measurement is used to classify objects or events into discrete categories; data are not measured or ordered. The mode and frequency of scores are used to describe nominal measurement.
>
> ▶ Interval and ratio measurement show ranking of events or objects on scales with equal intervals.

only in the physical sciences and in describing characteristics of samples. Physical scales measuring height, weight, distance, pulse and blood pressure can usually be treated as ratio scales. Because there is a zero point in ratio scales, one can state that 'a baby weighing 4 kilograms is twice as heavy as one weighing 2 kilograms'.

Frequency distribution

A frequency distribution is the most basic way of organising data. In a frequency distribution the number of times each event occurs is counted or the data are grouped and the frequency of each group is reported. Although

not always reported, it is usually the first step researchers undertake when exploring and categorising their data. A lecturer reporting the results of an examination could report the number of students receiving each grade or could group the grades and report the number in each group. Table 14.2 illustrates the results of an examination given to a class of 51 students. The results of the examination are reported in several ways. The columns on the left give the raw data tally and the frequency for each grade, whereas the columns on the right give the grouped data tally and grouped frequencies.

When data are grouped, it is necessary to define the size of the group or the interval

TABLE 14.2 Frequency distribution

Individual			Group		
Score	Tally	Frequency	Score	Tally	Frequency
90	I	1	>89	I	1
88	I	1			
86	I	1	80–89	ﬂﬂﬂ ﬂﬂﬂ ﬂﬂﬂ	15
84	ﬂﬂﬂ I	6			
82	II	2	70–79	ﬂﬂﬂ ﬂﬂﬂ ﬂﬂﬂ ﬂﬂﬂ III	23
80	ﬂﬂﬂ	5			
78	ﬂﬂﬂ	5			
76	I	1	60–69	ﬂﬂﬂ ﬂﬂﬂ	10
74	ﬂﬂﬂ II	7			
72	ﬂﬂﬂ IIII	9	<59	II	2
70	I	1			
68	III	3			
66	II	2			
64	IIII	4			
62	I	1			
60		0			
58	I	1			
56		0			
54	I	1			
52		0			
50		0			
Total		51			51

Mean, 73.1, standard deviation, +12.1; median, 74; mode, 72; range, 36 (54–90).

width so that no score will appear twice in the same group. The grouping of the data in Table 14.2 prevents overlap; each score falls into only one group: that is, scores above 89; 80–89; 70–79; 60–69; and below 59. The interval widths should not be too large; very large interval widths lead to loss of data information and may obscure patterns in the data.

Research in brief

Fenwick et al. (2004) used an explorative descriptive design to describe the labour and birth expectations of a cohort of 202 Western Australian women in order to identify the factors that influenced their expectations. Data collected from telephone interviews were subjected to thematic analysis. Frequency counts and percentages were used to categorise their demographic data. Five major themes were identified, three of which revealed a positive outlook about birth. Major influences on expectations were public and private discourses of childbirth, the stories of mothers and sisters, professional discourses and women's own particular history. The findings challenge the anecdotal evidence that many women from Western society choose or expect birth to be a medicalised event.

Figure 14.2 shows an example of a histogram and a frequency polygon. The two examples are similar in that both plot scores against frequency. The greater the number of points plotted, the smoother the resulting graph. The shape of the resulting graph allows for observations that will further describe the data, particularly in terms of normal distribution.

Measures of central tendency

A measure of central tendency is a single central score that enables us to summarise the distribution of a data set. Measures of central tendency describe the centre of a distribution of scores. The three measures most commonly used to describe the central point of a distribution are the mode, the median and the mean. The mode refers to the numerical score that occurs with the greatest frequency in a distribution; the median is that point on a scale where half the scores fall above and half fall below; and the mean is the average score. These measures summarise members of a sample and are therefore also known as summary statistics and are sample specific. Because they are sample specific, they change with each sample.

The characteristics of a sample in a study are described in terms of summary statistics. The mean test score reported in Table 14.2 ($\overline{X}$ = 73.1) is an example of such a statistic. If a different group of students were given the same test, it is likely that the mean would be different. Following is a more in-depth discussion of the mode, the median and the mean.

Mode

The mode is the most frequently occurring score in a frequency distribution and is the only measure of central tendency when the data are nominal; however, it can be used

FIGURE 14.2 Frequency distributions — A, histogram; B, frequency polygon

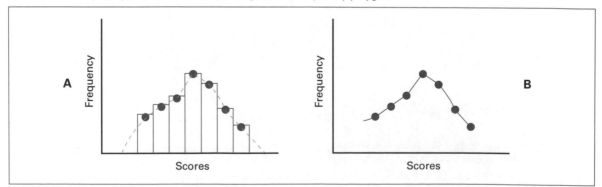

FIGURE 14.3 Symmetrical distributions

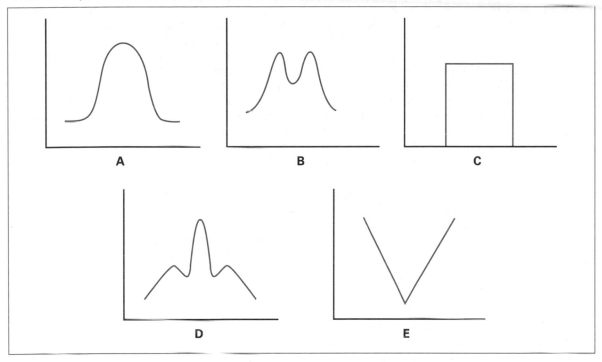

with all levels of measurement (see Table 14.1 above). A distribution can have more than one mode. The number of modes contained in a distribution is called the modality of the distribution. Figure 14.3, A and Figure 14.4 illustrate unimodal or one-peak distributions. Multimodal distributions having two or more peaks are shown in Figure 14.3, B and D.

TABLE 14.3 Measures of central tendency

Score	Frequency	Measure
35	‖‖‖	
36	‖‖‖ ‖‖‖	Mode
37	‖‖‖	Median, mean
38	‖‖‖	
39	‖‖‖	
40	‖‖‖ ‖	
35	‖‖‖	
36	‖‖‖ ‖‖‖	Mode
37	‖‖‖	Mean
38	‖‖‖‖	Median
39	‖‖‖ ‖‖‖	Mode
40	‖‖‖ ‖	

Table 14.3 illustrates how the change in a few scores can change the modality of a distribution from unimodal to bimodal. Since the mode takes account of only the most frequently occurring scores, it is not always a useful measure of central tendency.

𝑇𝑇 Tutorial trigger 1

1. The librarian wants to know how frequently the library is accessed by the 80 third-year nursing students during exam week. Your research group has been asked to provide the information. How could your group obtain these data?
2. You have recently covered measures of central tendency in your research course and your lecturer wants your research group to create a table showing the data collected for the librarian and to indicate which type of measure of central tendency you used.

Median

The median is the middle score or the score where 50% of the scores are above it and 50% of the scores are below it. In a set of an odd number of scores, the median is the middle score; in a set of an even number of scores, the median is the average of the two middle scores. For ordinal scale data, either the mode or the median can be used, however, the median retains more information about the distribution of scores by taking the rank order of the values into account. The median is not sensitive to extremes in high and low scores. In the series of scores in Table 14.2 the 26th score will always be the median regardless of the highest or lowest scores. It is best used when the data are skewed and the researcher is interested in the 'typical' score. For example, if age is a variable and there is a wide range of ages that may affect the mean, it would be appropriate to also report the median. The median is easy to find by either inspection or calculation and can be used with ordinal or higher level data, as shown in Table 14.1.

Mean

The mean is the arithmetical average of all the scores and is used with interval or ratio data (see Table 14.1), and is the only measure that reflects, and is affected by, all scores in the distribution. In a group of scores (e.g. age, income, height, test results), the mean (average) is calculated by adding all the scores and dividing the total by the number of scores in the group. The mean is the most widely used measure of central tendency and, of the three measures of central tendency, it is the most constant or least affected by chance. The larger the sample size, the less affected the mean will be by a single extreme score.

> ### Points to ponder
> ▶ The mode is the most frequently occurring score and can be used with all levels of measurement.
> ▶ The median is the middle score with an equal number of scores above and below.
> ▶ The mean is the only measure that reflects and is affected by all scores in the distribution.

Normal distribution

The concept of the normal distribution is a theoretical one, based on the observation that data from repeated measures of some interval or ratio level data group themselves about a midpoint in a distribution in a manner that closely approximates the normal curve (also

called Gaussian distribution), as illustrated in Figure 14.4. The vertical line or Y-axis represents the frequency of occurrences; that is, the values. The base line or X-axis shows values of the scores increasing in number from left to right. In addition, if the means of a large number of samples of the same interval or ratio data are calculated and plotted on a graph, that curve also approximates the normal curve. This tendency of the means to approximate the normal curve is termed the sampling distribution of the means. The mean of the population is derived from the means of the sampling distribution (see Chapter 11).

FIGURE 14.4 Normal distribution (mesokurtosis) with associated standard deviations

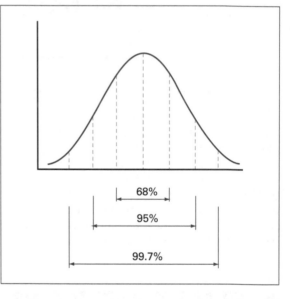

A normal distribution is bell-shaped, symmetrical about the mean and unimodal. The mean, median and mode are equal. Most of the values are clustered around the mean with smaller frequencies moving away from the mean or centre on either side. A characteristic of the normal curve is that a fixed percentage of the scores falls within a given distance of the mean. As shown in Figure 14.4, about 68% of the scores or means will fall within 1 standard deviation (SD) of the mean; 95% will fall within 2 SDs of the mean; and 99.7% will fall within 3 SDs of the mean. The mean and the standard deviation are known as the parameters of a normal distribution. The mean provides the central point of the distribution and the standard deviation determines the spread.

Skewness

Skewness refers to a measure of the asymmetry of a distribution of scores. Not all samples of data approximate the normal curve. Some samples are non-symmetrical and have the peak off-centre. If one tail is longer than the other, the distribution is described in terms of skew. In a positive skew, the bulk of the data are at the low end of the range and there is a longer tail pointing to the right or the positive end of the graph. Individual income has a positive skew, with most individuals in the low-to-medium range and very few in the upper range. The mean in a positive skew is to the right of the median. In a negative skew the bulk of the data are in the high range and there is a longer tail pointing to the left, or the negative end, of the graph. Age at death in Australia has a negative skew because most deaths occur at older ages. In a negative skew, the mean is to the left of the median. Figure 14.5 illustrates positive and negative skews. In each diagram the peak is off-centre and one tail is longer.

Most statistical packages are capable of measuring skewness. When skewness is reported to be between −1 and +1, the sample is said to be normally distributed. When the data are skewed, the mean and standard deviation do not describe the data very well, however, methods such as taking the logarithms of the data can be used to transform the data so that the transformed data approximate a near normal distribution.

> ### Research in brief
>
> In a study exploring medication knowledge and self-management by people with diabetes, Dunning and Manias (2005) analysed interval and categorical data using ANOVA and chi-square to detect significant relationships between the variables. Descriptive statistics — means, SDs and frequency counts were used for the demographic data. The Pearson correlation coefficient was used to reflect the degree of association between the interval level variables and content analysis was used to categorise the narrative data.

Symmetry

When the two halves of a distribution are mirror images of each other, the distribution is said to be symmetrical. The overall shape of the distribution does not affect symmetry. Although the shapes in Figure 14.3 are different, they are all symmetrical; however, only Figure 14.2, A approximates the normal curve. In addition, symmetry and modality are independent. Figure 14.3, A is unimodal and symmetrical, while the graphs in Figure 14.5 are skewed.

Kurtosis

Kurtosis is related to the peakness or flatness of a distribution. The peakness or flatness of a distribution is related to the spread of the data. The further the data are spread out on a scale, the flatter the peak. The distribution

FIGURE 14.5 Skewed distributions — A, positive skew; B, negative skew

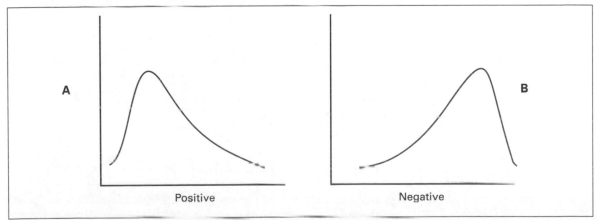

A   Positive

B   Negative

that peaks sharply is called leptokurtic, whereas a broad, flat distribution is called platykurtic. Figure 14.6 illustrates kurtosis. Neither the leptokurtic nor the platykurtic distributions approximate the normal curve or mesokurtic distribution.

> ### Points to ponder
> ▶ Non-symmetrical distributions (skewed data) have the peak off-centre and the mean and standard deviation no longer adequately describe the data.
> ▶ A mesokurtic distribution approximates the normal curve.

TT Tutorial trigger 2

You have collected data on the average hours students utilise the library in a given week. Below are the raw scores for 15 students who were surveyed. Calculate the mean, median and mode. What conclusions can be made of the distribution of scores?

Hours	Frequency of scores
2	1
3	2
4	5
5	3
6	2
7	1

Measures of variability or dispersion

Variability or dispersion is concerned with the spread of the data. Samples with the same mean could differ in both distribution (kurtosis) and skew. Variability measures answer the questions, 'Is a sample homogeneous or heterogeneous?' or 'Are the samples similar or different?'. If a researcher measures oral temperatures in two samples — one sample drawn from a healthy population and one sample from a population hospitalised with an infectious illness — it is possible that the two samples will have a similar mean temperature. However, it is likely that there will be a wider range of temperatures in the hospitalised sample than in the healthy sample. Measures of variation describe the extent to which individuals or scores in the sample vary. The most common measures used are the range, variance, standard deviation and semi-quartile range.

Range

The range is the simplest and most unstable measure of variability; it is simply the difference between the highest and lowest scores. The range in Table 14.2 is 36; that is, 90 − 54 = 36. The disadvantage of the range is that it depends upon the two extreme scores only, which may be 'outliers' (extreme cases), compared to the rest of the scores.

Variance

A strategy commonly used to permit mathematical manipulation of difference scores is to square them. Variance is a measure of variability that includes every score in the distribution rather than only two scores. Some of the scores will be greater than the mean and some smaller. When negative (smaller)

FIGURE 14.6 Kurtosis — A, leptokurtosis; B, platykurtosis

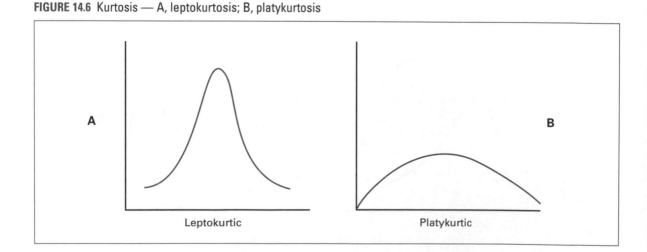

A — Leptokurtic

B — Platykurtic

scores are squared, they become positive. The squared scores are then summed. The variance then is the average or mean of the sum of squares. The following example illustrates variance.

Value	Mean	Actual deviation	Squared deviation
2	6	–4	+16
4	6	2	+4
7	6	+1	+1
9	6	+3	+9

Sum of squares = 30

Number of values: 4

$$\text{Variance} = \frac{\text{sum of squares}}{\text{number of values}} = \frac{30}{4} = 7.5$$

Because the deviations from the mean are squared, it will be noted that the variance is expressed in units different from the scores. In order to convert to the original set of data it is necessary to find the square root of the variance. The value thus obtained is the standard deviation.

$$\text{Standard deviation} = \text{square root of variance}$$
$$= \sqrt{7.5}$$
$$= 2.7$$

Standard deviation

The standard deviation (SD) is the most frequently used measure of variability and it is based on the concept of the normal curve (see Figure 14.4). It is a measure of average deviation or distance of each score from the group mean in a normal distribution and, as such, should always be reported with the mean. It takes all scores into account and can be used to interpret individual scores. Because the mean ($\bar{X}$) and standard deviation (SD) for the examination in Table 14.2 was 73.1 ± 12.1, a student should know that 68% of the grades were between 85.2 and 61. If the student received a grade of 88, he would know he did better than most of the class, whereas a grade of 58 would indicate he did not do as well as most of the class.

The SD allows the reader to get a feel for the variation the data contain. The SD is used in the calculation of many inferential statistics. One limitation of the SD is that it is expressed in terms of the units used in the measurement and cannot be used to compare means that

have different units. If researchers were interested in the relationship between height measured in centimetres and weight measured in kilograms, it would be necessary for them to convert the height and weight measurements to standard units or z scores.

z scores

The z score is used to compare measurements in standard units. z scores take account of the mean and SD of the distribution. Each of the scores is converted to a z score and then the z scores are used to examine the relative distance of the scores from the mean; this process is called *standardising the score*. The following formula will illustrate this concept:

$$z \text{ score} = \frac{\text{original value} - \text{mean}}{\text{standard deviation}}$$

Let us say the mean score on the drug calculation test was 70/100 and the standard deviation was 10. Mary's score on the test was 80. Using the above formula, from Mary's score (80) we subtract the mean (70), and divide it by the SD (10). We find then that Mary's score is 1 standard deviation above the mean. A z score of 1.5 means that the observation is +1.5 SD above the mean, whereas a score of –2 means that the observation is 2 SDs below the mean. By using z scores, a researcher can compare results from scales that use different units, such as height and weight.

Many measures of variability exist. The modal frequency is the easiest to calculate, but the SD is the most stable and useful. The SD and the semi-quartile range are unique for each sample. Most spreadsheets and all statistical software packages will calculate basic descriptive statistics including standard deviations and z scores. Examples of how to calculate the SD manually, can be found in Munro (2001), and the *Virtual Statistics Textbook* at: http://www.surfstat.newcastle.edu.au/surfstat/main/surfstat.html.

Semi-quartile range

The semi-quartile range (semi-interquartile range) indicates the range of the middle 50% of the scores. It is more stable than the range, because it is less likely to be changed by a single extreme score. It lies between the upper and lower quartiles; the upper quartile being the point below which 75% of the scores fall and the lower quartile being the point below which 25% of the scores fall. The middle 50% of the scores in Table 14.2 lie between 68 and 78 and the semi-quartile range is 10. This measure is used in conjunction with the median to describe the centre and dispersion of ordinal level data or interval/ratio level data that are skewed.

Percentile

A percentile represents the percentage of cases a given score exceeds. The median is the 50% percentile and in Table 14.2 it is a score of 74. A score in the 90th percentile is exceeded by only 10% of the scores. The zero percentile and the 100th percentile are usually dropped.

Inferential statistics

Descriptive statistics refer to various methods of summarising numerical data. Sometimes the researcher wants additional information: inferential statistics enable inferences and conclusions to be drawn from those data. Statistical inference is based on probability theory and permits the generalisation from a specific sample or samples, to the entire population. Statistical inference is generally used for two purposes: to estimate the probability that statistics found in a random sample accurately reflect the population parameter; and to test hypotheses about a population. In the first instance, a parameter is a characteristic of a population, whereas a statistic is a characteristic of a sample. Statistics are used to estimate population parameters.

An example will illustrate the difference between the two. Suppose we randomly sample 100 people with diabetes and use an interval scale to study their knowledge of the disease. If the mean (average) score for these subjects is 65/100, the mean represents the sample statistic. If we could contact every person with diabetes in Australia, we could also calculate a mean, and that score would be the parameter for the population. A researcher is rarely able to study an entire population, so inferential statistics allow statements about the larger population to be made from studying a random sample drawn from that population.

Statistical inference is inductive and indirect. We draw general conclusions (inductive) about populations on the basis of specific samples tested in our experiment; it is indirect because it begins by assuming the null hypothesis (H_0); that is, that any differences are due to chance. The null hypothesis is used because statistical tests are designed to reject, rather than accept, hypotheses. The null hypothesis (also referred to as a statistical hypothesis) is the hypothesis that is actually tested by statistical methods. The null hypothesis states that there is no actual relationship between the variables and that any observed relationship or difference is merely a function of chance fluctuations in sampling. The scientific hypothesis or research hypothesis is the researcher's expectation about the outcome of a study.

Hypothesis testing

The most common use of inferential statistics in experimental studies is hypothesis testing. Statistical hypothesis testing allows researchers to make objective decisions about the outcome of their study, and answers such questions as 'Is the difference between the two groups real?' or 'How strongly are these two variables associated with each other?'. Statistical hypothesis testing is a process of rejection or acceptance, not proof. It is impossible to prove that a scientific hypothesis is true, but it is possible to demonstrate that the null hypothesis has a high probability of being incorrect. However, making inferences about the population from a sample involves the possibility of sampling error because we cannot assume that the sample is an exact representation of the population. Remember that random assignment does not prevent differences occurring among subjects; however, it does result in a more equal distribution of any differences across the groups in the study. So, while sampling error cannot be excluded, its probable magnitude can be calculated by using inferential statistics (see Chapter 16).

Probability and the level of significance

The concept of probability derives from probability theory and is central to our understanding of inferential statistics. Probability is given the symbol p and is expressed as a proportion between 0 (the event will not occur) and 1 (the event will occur). The probability of an event is the event's long-run relative frequency in repeated trials under similar conditions. It is the notion of repeated trials that allows researchers to use probability to test hypotheses. In other words, the statistician does not think of the probability of obtaining a single result from a single study, but rather of the chances of obtaining the same result from an idealised study that can be carried out many times under identical conditions.

The probability that is chosen to indicate that an outcome is statistically significant is called the level of significance (alpha level α). Three levels of significance ca~~~~orted: namely, the 0.05 level of sig~~~~(α = 0.05); the 0.10 level (α = 0.10~~~~0.01 level (α = 0.0¹) The level of sign~~~~must be chosen pr~~~~e commenc~~~~the study, not af~~~~ical analys~~~~een completed.~~~~of signific~~~~the probability~~~~g a type~~~~the probability o~~~~a true null~~~~s). The minimur~~~~significance~~~~le for all scient~~~~lines, includ~~~~g and midwife~~~~5. If the rese~~~~ts the alpha (α)~~~~of significance at 0.05, the researche~~~~g to accept the fact that if the study~~~~peated 100 times, the decision to r~~~~null hypothesis would be wrong five times out of those 100 trials.

Statistical probability is based on the concept of sampling error, and inferential statistics are based on random sampling. However, even when samples are randomly selected, there is always the possibility of some errors in sampling. Therefore the characteristics of any given sample may be different from those of the entire population. Suppose a group of clinical nurses had access to a large number of patients with decubitus ulcers and wanted to find out the average length of time the ulcers would take to heal with the usual nursing care. If the nurses studied the entire population, they might obtain an average healing time of 50 days, with a standard deviation (SD) of 10 days; that is, between 40 and 60 days. Suppose too, that there were insufficient funds to study all the patients and instead the nurses conducted several consecutive studies on the group of patients. They would first sample a group of 25 patients, calculate the mean and SD, then return the sample to the main group before selecting the next sample. This

Research in brief

Jirojwong et al. (2005) conducted a cross-sectional study to assess health outcomes of home follow-up visits after postpartum discharge and the relationship between home visits and selected outcomes among women who birthed at two Queensland regional hospitals. The authors used descriptive data analysis, non-parametric tests and an alpha of 0.05 as a criterion for rejecting a null hypothesis. Power calculations were not mentioned in the their article.

process would be repeated many times and they might end up with a number of different means. If the nurses then placed the means in a frequency distribution, it might appear as in Figure 14.7 as the number of samples drawn increases, the curve will approximate the normal curve. This frequency distribution is called the sampling distribution of the means. It shows that the nurses might find that one sample's mean is 50.5 days, the next sample is 47.5 days, the next sample is 62.5 days, and so on. The tendency for statistics to fluctuate from one sample to another is called 'sampling error'.

In practice, researchers do not routinely draw on consecutive samples from the same population; usually they compute statistics and make inferences based on the one sample. However, the knowledge of the properties of the sampling distribution — if these

FIGURE 14.7 Sampling distribution of the means

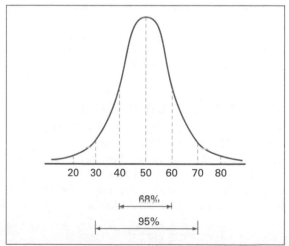

repeated samples are hypothetically obtained — permits the researcher to draw a conclusion based on one sample. This is possible because the sampling distribution of the means follows a normal curve and the mean of the sampling distribution will be the mean of the population. The fact that the sampling distribution of the means is normal tells us several important things. When scores are normally distributed we know that 68% of the cases will fall between +1 SD and –1 SD or that the probability is 68 out of 100 that any one randomly drawn sample mean will lie within the range of values between ±1 SD. The SD of a theoretical distribution of sample means is called the 'standard error of the mean'. The word 'error' is used because the various means that make up the distribution contain some error in their estimates of the population mean. The error is considered to be standard because it implies the magnitude of the average error, just as a standard deviation implies the average variation from one mean.

Although researchers rarely construct sampling distributions, standard error can be estimated because it bears a systematic relationship to the sample SD and the size of the sample. This tells us that increasing the size of the sample will increase the accuracy of our estimates of population parameters. The other reason that the sampling distribution is so important is that there are sampling distributions for all statistics. Researchers consult these distributions when making determinations about rejecting the null hypothesis.

> ● **Evidence-based practice tip**
>
> A standard deviation of a distribution indicates the average amount by which all the values deviate from the mean. Inspection of a polygon or histogram will show if the data are skewed.

95% confidence interval

A derivation of the SD is the 95% confidence interval (95% CI). This statistic is the range around the mean (point estimate) in a sample where it can be inferred that there is a 95% chance that the 'real' difference lies between the two points. The formula is:

$$95\% \text{ CI} = \frac{x \pm 1.96 \text{ SD}}{\sqrt{n}}$$

The following example (Figure 14.8) provides a graphical representation of the advantages of calculating the 95% CI. The physical role functioning scale of SF-36 (Ware 2000) ranges from 0–100: the higher the score, the better functioning. Figure 14.8 provides the mean score (small dark square) and the 95% interval (whisker plot) for each measurement point.

As illustrated, physical role functioning was lower at hospital discharge than prior to surgery, but at 6 months it was markedly improved. Note that there is overlap of the CIs between the first two scores — this means there is no statistically significant difference (i.e. the difference is >0.05). However, as there is no overlap between the CIs for measurement 3 and the other two measures, the functioning had significantly improved at 6 months ($p<0.05$).

FIGURE 14.8 95% CI of physical role functioning for a sample of cardiac surgery patients

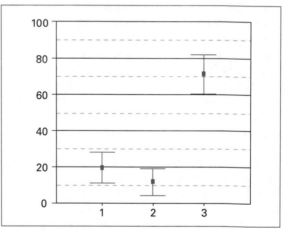

Odds ratio

Another way of presenting probabilities is the 'odds ratio'. The odds ratio (OR) is a statistic used to assess the risk of a particular outcome and is widely used in healthcare literature, particularly epidemiology, because it can be calculated for case-control studies, in studies using logistic regression, and as a way of presenting the results of a meta-analysis. The odds ratio is a measure of strength of association for case-control studies. This is the odds of exposure in the diseased, divided by the odds of exposure in the non-diseased. If the odds are greater than one, then the event is more likely than not to happen. In an observational study by McKinley et al. (2004), odds ratios were used to assess the variables studied for the risk of delay in arrival to the emergency department following symptom onset in women with acute myocardial infarction.

Errors in statistical inference: type I and type II errors

Suppose that a researcher decides to accept or reject the null hypothesis on the basis of how probable it is that the observed differences are the result of chance alone. Because data on the entire population are not available, the researcher cannot categorically assert that the null hypothesis is or is not true. It is possible, therefore, that statistical decision-making may result in incorrect decisions. There are two types of error in statistical inference: type I error and type II error. A type I error occurs when the null hypothesis is rejected when it is actually true. A type II error is the acceptance of a null hypothesis that is actually false (see Figure 14.9).

Figure 14.9 shows the relationship between the two types of error. In a practice discipline, type I errors are usually considered more serious because if the researcher says that there are differences where none are present, the potential exists for patient care to be adversely affected. As noted above, failure to reject a false null hypothesis is a type II error. Type II errors occur because of a stringent level of significance, a small sample size, or a small difference in measured effect.

Power analysis

Statistical power analysis refers to procedures and formulas that identify a number (of subjects/

> ### Research in brief
>
> A type II error is also possible in a study that compared patient satisfaction between two models of nursing care (team allocation and team nursing) (Wu et al. 2000). A medium effect was assumed *a priori* but little rationale was provided for this decision, and a sample size was determined ($n = 137$). The resulting finding was acceptance of the null hypothesis for each of the three hypotheses.

participants) that indicates the likelihood of achieving statistical significance. Power analysis and a related concept, sample size estimation (effect size), together are important in experimental designs, because the rejection or acceptance of the null hypothesis is dependent upon their correct computation. Broadly defined, *power* is the probability that a study will reject a false null hypothesis. Specifically, power is $1 - \beta$, and ranges from 0 to 1. The significance level is usually alpha = 0.5, and the minimal acceptable level for power to detect an effect is 0.80. An adequate level of power strengthens the meaning of a study's findings. For further discussion on low power (too few subjects, too little data) and high power (too much data) and related software programs see the websites http://cc.uoregon.edu/cnews/summer2000/statpower.html and http://www.statsoft.com/textbook/stpowan.html.

Power is influenced by the parameters (Cohen 1988; Rudy 1991):
- α level (usually set at 0.05)
- *n* (sample size)
- ES (effect size)

FIGURE 14.9 Outcome of statistical decision-making

	Reality	
Conclusion of test of significance	Null hypothesis is true	Null hypothesis is not true
Not statistically significant	Correct conclusion	Type II error
Statistically significant	Type I error	Correct conclusion

Effect size

Effect size equates to the magnitude of the effect of an intervention or treatment, compared to the control. Small effect sizes are common for nursing or psychological interventions such as muscle relaxation or music therapy. Unfortunately, most nursing and midwifery papers do not report effect sizes or the power of studies, thus making it difficult for researchers to establish appropriate sample sizes or the effect of nursing interventions. Effect sizes have been calculated for a variety of parametric tests (see Table 14.4). One method of calculating the effect size is by determining the difference between the sample mean and the population mean and dividing it by the sample standard deviation and is expressed in standard units, which is known as the Cohen's d.

TABLE 14.4 Parametric tests and effect size

Sample of parametric tests	Effect size values		
	Small	Medium	Large
t test	0.20	0.50	0.80
ANOVA	0.10	0.25	0.40
correlation	0.10	0.30	0.50
(Adapted from Cohen 1988 pp 40, 79, 85–7.)			

Research in brief

Chien et al. (2006) report on a Hong Kong study that used a quasi-experimental design to examine the effects of a needs-based education program on anxiety levels and satisfaction of psychosocial needs of families of individuals with a critical illness. Power analysis based on the results of two previous studies indicated that to achieve a power of 80% for detecting a large effect in the reduction of anxiety between the treatment and control groups at the 0.05 significance level, a sample size of 64 subjects (n = 32 in each group) was required. Based on their analysis of covariance results (p 47) a large effect size ($\eta^2 > 0.14$) was found for both a reduction in anxiety level ($\eta^2 = 0.18$) and an increase in satisfaction in family needs ($\eta^2 = 0.21$) in their treatment group.

Various power analysis resources are available, including 'Web resources on power analysis' at http://www.im.nbs.gov/powcase/powlinks.html and a Manchester Metropolitan University site at http://149.170.199.144/resdesign/power.htm.

Practical significance versus statistical significance

It is important to recognise the difference between statistical significance and practical or clinical significance. When a researcher tests an hypothesis and finds that it is statistically significant, it means that the finding is unlikely to have happened by chance. In other words, if the level of significance for a sample has been set at 0.05, the odds are 19 to 1 that the conclusion the researcher reaches is correct. The conclusion would be incorrect only 5 times in 100; that is, this result would be obtained by chance alone only 5 times in 100. If, as is sometimes done, the researcher wants to have a smaller risk of rejecting a true null hypothesis, the level of significance may be set at 0.01. In this case, the researcher is willing to be wrong only once in 100 trials. The decision on how strictly the alpha level should be set depends on how important it is to not make an error. For example, if the results of a study are to be used to determine whether a great deal of money should be spent in an area of nursing care, the researcher may decide that the accuracy of the results is so important that an alpha level of 0.01 is chosen. In most studies, however, alpha is set at 0.05.

Tests of statistical significance

Tests of significance may be either parametric or non-parametric. Parametric tests are used to analyse interval data or ratio scale data, and non-parametric (distribution free) tests are used for analysing nominal data and ordinal scale data. In both tests, researchers aim to discover the probability that the findings of their experiment occurred randomly by chance. There are many different statistical tests of significance that researchers use to test hypotheses. The procedure and the rationale for their use are similar from test to test. Once the researcher has chosen a significance level and collected the data, the data are used to compute the appropriate test statistic.

For each test there is a related theoretical distribution that shows the probable and improbable values for that statistic. On the basis of the statistical results and the values in the distribution, the researcher either accepts or rejects the null hypothesis and then reports both the statistical result and its probability.

> ### Points to ponder
> ▶ Effect size refers to the magnitude of the effect of an intervention compared to the control.
> ▶ Power is the probability that a study will reject a false null hypothesis and prevent a type II error.
> ▶ In both parametric and non-parametric tests researchers aim to discover the probability that the findings of their experiment occurred randomly by chance.

The format in which the statistical results are presented is commonly used in refereed journals, and once the student is familiar with this format it becomes easy to interpret reported findings from any statistical test. The abbreviations for some of the commonly used tests of difference are: t test (t), chi-square test (X²), ANOVA (F), Mann-Whitney U test (U) and Wilcoxon test (W). These are the most commonly used inferential statistics. The test that is used depends on the level of the measurement of the variables in question and the type of hypothesis being studied. Basically these statistics test two types of hypotheses — that there is a difference between groups or that there is a relationship between two or more variables:

- tests of difference
  - means
  - proportions
- tests of relationships
  - associations
  - predictive relationships.

Tests of difference

Suppose a researcher using an after-only (post-test) design wanted to find out if two randomly assigned groups are different after the introduction of the experimental treatment. If the measurements were at the interval level, the researcher would use the t test to analyse the data. If the t statistic was found to be high enough to be unlikely to have occurred by chance, the researcher would reject the null hypothesis and conclude that the two groups were indeed more different than would have been expected on the basis of chance alone. In other words, the researcher would conclude that the experimental treatment caused the difference (see Table 14.5).

Parametric tests

Parametric tests are commonly used to examine whether the mean scores of two groups (t test) or three or more groups (ANOVA) are different. To use these tests, the variables must have been measured at the interval or ratio level and the groups must be independent, that is, nothing in one group helps to determine who is in the other group(s). Parametric tests have the following three attributes:
1. they involve the estimation of at least one parameter
2. they require measurement on at least an interval scale

TABLE 14.5 Tests of differences between means

Level of measurement	One group	Related	Independent	More than two groups
		TWO GROUPS		
Non-parametric Nominal	Chi square	Chi-square Fisher exact probability	Chi-square	Chi-square
Ordinal	Kolmogorov–Smirnov	Sign test Wilcoxon matched pairs Signed rank	Chi-square Median test Mann-Whitney U	Chi-square
Parametric Interval or ratio	Correlated t ANOVA (repeated measures)	Correlated t	Independent t ANOVA	ANOVA ANCOVA MANOVA

3. they make certain assumptions about the variables being studied. This last attribute assumes that variances of scores (when two or more groups are being compared) are the same among the groups, that is, normally distributed in the population. This is called homogeneity of variance.

The advantages of using parametric tests are that the mathematical calculations are more sophisticated and robust than non-parametric tests. They permit analysis of interactions between two or more variables, and are usually more powerful in identifying significant differences. They are also most likely to reject the null hypothesis when it is false (less susceptible to type II errors). ANCOVA also measures differences among group means and uses a statistical technique to equate the groups on an important variable. Another expansion of the notion of analysis of variance is multiple analysis of variance (MANOVA), which is used to determine differences in group means when there is more than one dependent variable.

Non-parametric tests

The position taken by most researchers and statisticians is that non-parametric statistics are best used when the data cannot be assumed to be at the interval level of measurement, or when the sample is small and the normality of the underlying distribution cannot be inferred. Non-parametric tests are based on fewer assumptions than parametric tests and are also less powerful and, therefore, less likely to identify significant differences. Because they are 'distribution-free', they can be used to analyse data when the distribution of the population is unknown.

When data are at the nominal level and the researcher wants to determine whether groups are proportionally different, the chi-square (X^2) statistic is used. Chi-square is a non-parametric statistic that is used to determine whether the frequency in each category is different from what would be expected by chance. As with the t test and ANOVA, if the calculated chi-square value is high enough, the researcher would conclude that the frequencies found would not be expected on the basis of chance alone and the null hypothesis would be rejected. This test can be used in many different situations, but cannot be used to compare frequencies when sample size is small. In this instance, the Fisher's exact probability test is used. The chi-square test should not be used when 20% of the response categories have a frequency of less than five or if any category of response has a zero frequency. In these cases the researcher may collapse the data into fewer categories.

When the data are ranked at the ordinal level, researchers may use several other non-parametric tests, including the Kolmogorov–Smirnov test, the sign test, the Wilcoxon matched pairs test, the signed rank test for related groups, and the median test and the Mann-Whitney U test for independent groups. These tests use the ranks of raw scores and then the sum of ranks to determine difference. A general statistics book will provide more detailed information about these tests.

T_T Tutorial trigger 3

A study was designed to compare the frequency of medication errors between two methods of administering medication: medication trolley vs the bedside medication draw. Based on your knowledge of statistical power, how confident are you in the interpretation of the following results? What is required to improve the power of this study?

Method of medication storage		Medication error type cross-tabulation			
Count		Medication error type			
		Prescription error	Dispensing error	Administration error	Total
Method of medication storage	Medication trolley	12	16	37	65
	Bedside draw	10	21	25	56
Total		22	37	62	121

($X^2_{(2)} = 2.525$ p = 283)

The chi-square test resulted in the acceptance of the null hypothesis; that is, no statistical difference in medication errors was found between the two methods of medication storage. In small tutorial groups discuss these results.

Research in brief

Stahl and Hundley (2003) conducted a prospective, cross-sectional, non-experimental, case-control study in Germany, to investigate whether pregnant women's psychosocial state was affected by being labelled 'high risk'. A sample of 111 women (57 were classified as 'high risk' and 54 as 'no risk' according to the risks documented in their antenatal records) between 22 and 41 weeks gestation completed the *Abbreviated Scale for the Assessment of Psychosocial State In Pregnancy* questionnaire. Analysis of covariance (ANOVA) tested the effect of the risk label on psychosocial state. Findings indicated the effect of the risk label on psychosocial state, after adjusting for age, was statistically significant — p = 0.001. Also identified was the need to re-evaluate the risk catalogue in the German antenatal record.

Evidence-based practice tip

Recommendations in a research article provide consumers with an opportunity to assess the relevance of the study in terms of its usefulness for clinical practice.

Tests of bivariate relationships

Correlations are used to answer the question, 'To what extent are the variables related or connected to each other?'. When the relationship between two or more variables is explored, statistics are used to determine the correlation or the degree of association between the variables. Correlations are used most commonly with ordinal or higher level data. Tests of the relationships between variables are sometimes considered to be descriptive statistics. This is the case when they are used to describe the magnitude and direction of a relationship of two variables in a sample and the researcher does not wish to make statements about the larger population. Such statistics can also be inferential when they are used to test hypotheses about the correlations that exist in the target population (see Table 14.6).

Suppose a researcher is interested in the relationship between the age of patients and the length of time it takes them to recover from surgery. In this example, age and length

TABLE 14.6 Tests of association

Level of measurement	Two variables	More than two variables
Non-parametric		
Nominal	Phi coefficient Point-biserial	Contingency coefficient
Ordinal	Kendall's tau Spearman rho	Discriminant function analysis
Parametric		
Interval or ratio	Pearson *r*	Multiple regression Path analysis Canonical correlation

of time until recovery can be considered to be interval level measurements, and a test called the *Pearson correlation coefficient* (Pearson *r* or Pearson product moment correlation coefficient) would be used. Once the Pearson *r* is calculated, the distribution for this test is examined to determine whether the value obtained was likely to have occurred by chance. This is also calculated automatically in statistical analysis packages. Again, both the value of the correlation and its probability occurring by chance alone (the *p* value) would be reported.

Correlation coefficients can range in value from −1.0 to +1.0, including zero. A zero coefficient means that there is no relationship between the variables. A perfect positive correlation is indicated by a +1.0 coefficient and a perfect negative correlation is indicated by a −1.0 coefficient. Figure 14.10 provides graphical illustration, known as scatter plots, which shows the strength and direction of the relationship between two variables.

The example of age and length of time until recovery will illustrate the meaning of these coefficients. If there were no relationship between the age of the patient and the time he or she requires to recover from surgery, a correlation of zero would be found (with a wide scatter plot of data points). If, however, the correlation was close to +1.0, this would mean that the older the patient, the longer it would take him or her to recover. A negative correlation would suggest that the younger the patient, the longer it would take him or her to recover. Relationships are rarely perfect.

FIGURE 14.10 Scatter plots

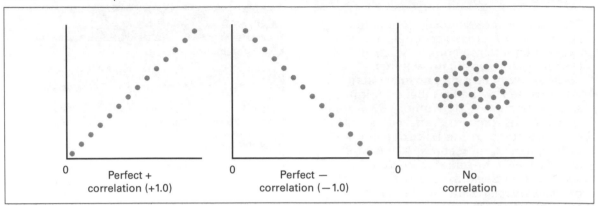

The magnitude of the relationship is indicated by how close the correlation comes to the absolute value of 1. Thus, a correlation of +0.76 is just as strong as a correlation of − 0.76, but the direction of the relationship is opposite (or inverse). As with other statistical tests of significance, the larger the sample, the greater the likelihood of finding a significant correlation. Therefore, the degrees of freedom associated with the test are also reported. An example of what is meant by degrees of freedom follows. Suppose that ten nurses need medical ward placements. When nine nurses have been placed, the tenth nurse must take the tenth place: there is no choice. So, although there are ten nurses (n), there are only nine (n–1) degrees of freedom.

Nominal and ordinal data can also be tested for relationships by non-parametric statistics. When two variables are being tested that have only two levels (e.g. male/female, yes/no), the phi coefficient can be used to express relationships. When the researcher is interested in the relationship between a nominal variable and an interval variable, the point–biserial correlation is used. Spearman rho is used to determine the degree of association between two variables at the ordinal level (sets of ranks), as is Kendall's tau. All of these correlation coefficients may range in value from −1.0 to +1.0 (see Figure 14.10).

Tests of multivariate relationships

Nursing problems are rarely so simple that they can be explained by bivariate relationships, the relationship between two variables. For studying complex multivariate relationships, relationships among more

than two variables, techniques other than those so far discussed are used. Examples of multivariate techniques include multiple regression, multiple discriminant analysis and logistic regression, principal component and exploratory factor analysis, and multivariate analysis of variance and covariance.

Structural equation modelling techniques

Structural equation modelling (SEM) is an umbrella term for various methods (e.g. path analysis, confirmatory factor analysis and structure models) used to test theory expressed in the form of a systematic set of relationships between multiple observed or non-observed (latent), dependent or independent variables. SEM requires specific software such as LISREL (linear structural relations) or AMOS. As many of the variables of interest to nursing are not easily defined and measured and because we are interested in causal models, software such as AMOS, LISREL and generalised linear modelling are becoming more commonly used in nursing studies. Many other statistical techniques are available to nurse and midwifery researchers, including the *Electronic Statistics Textbook*, available at http://www.statsoft.com/textbook/stathome.html.

Summary

Descriptive statistics are statistical procedures used to organise and give meaning to data and illustrated in a variety of visual ways (e.g. frequency distributions, skewed distributions and measures of variability). Inferential statistics allow researchers to estimate population parameters, test hypotheses and make objective decisions about the outcome of a study based on the acceptance or rejection of the null hypothesis. Statistical inference permits a conclusion about a population to be made based upon a sample of that population. Statistical hypothesis testing is subject to two types of error; the results of tests are reported to be significant or non-significant depending upon the level of significance set. Tests of statistical significance may be parametric (used

to determine the mean scores of two or more groups), or non-parametric (used when the data cannot be assumed to be at the interval level of measurement), which are used according to specific criteria. Levels of significance, power analysis, effect size, and sample size are briefly introduced. Techniques used to study complex multivariate relationships are briefly described together with more sophisticated statistics such as structural equation modelling (SEM), AMOS and LISREL.

KEY POINTS

- Inferential statistics allow researchers to estimate population parameters, test hypotheses, and make objective decisions about the outcome of a study based on sample data. Such decisions are based on the acceptance or rejection of the null hypothesis.

- Descriptive statistics refer to the measures used to describe raw data. Data can be presented in tables, histograms, bar charts, pie charts, polygons and scatter plots.

- Acceptance of the null hypothesis indicates that the findings are likely to have occurred by chance. If the null hypothesis is rejected, the researcher accepts the scientific hypothesis of a relationship being present between the variables and that this relationship is unlikely to have been found by chance.

- Statistical hypothesis testing is subject to two types of error — type I and type II. Type I error occurs when the researcher rejects the null hypothesis that is actually true. Type II error occurs when the researcher accepts a null hypothesis that is actually false. The risk of making a type I error is controlled by setting the alpha level or level of significance. Reducing the risk of a type I error by reducing the level of significance increases the risk of making a type II error.

- The results of statistical tests are reported to be significant or non-significant. Obtaining a probability value of less than 0.05 or 0.01 (depending on the level of significance set by the researcher)

indicates a statistically significant result.

- Commonly used parametric and non-parametric statistical tests include those that test for differences between means, such as the t test and ANOVA, and those that test for differences in proportions, such as the chi-square test.

- Tests that examine data for the presence of relationships (association) include the Pearson r, the sign test, the Wilcoxon matched pairs, signed ranks test, and regression.

- The most important aspects to consider when one critiques statistical analyses are the relationship of the statistics used to address the problem, and the design and method used in the study. Clues to the appropriate statistical test to use should stem from the researcher's hypotheses. The reader should also determine if all of the hypotheses have been presented in the paper.

- The frequency distribution presents data in tabular or graphic form and allows for the calculation of observations of characteristics of the distribution of the data, including skewness, symmetry, modality and kurtosis.

- The standard deviation is the most stable and useful measure of variability for interval and ratio level data. It is derived from the concept of the normal curve.

- The analysis of the findings is the final step of a research investigation. It is in this section that the consumer will find the results reported in a straightforward manner.

Learning activities

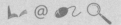

1. The distribution of sample means will approximate to the:
   (a) population mean
   (b) curve of the distribution
   (c) normal distribution
   (d) sample mean.

2. Variance is a measure of variability that includes:
   (a) every score in the distribution
   (b) the highest scores in the distribution
   (c) the lowest scores in the distribution
   (d) most of the scores in the distribution.

3. A non-parametric test can operate:
   (a) when measurements assume a normal curve
   (b) without the assumptions about the normality of the distributions
   (c) with any measurement of central tendency
   (d) only when means and SDs are calculated.

4. Parametric tests are not:
   (a) used with ordinal scale measurements
   (b) more robust than non-parametric tests
   (c) more likely to reject the null hypothesis
   (d) better at identifying significant differences.

5. If measurements were at the interval level what test of difference would be used to analyse the data?
   (a) the sign tests
   (b) chi-square test
   (c) *t* test
   (d) median test.

6. If the power of a study is low, what could the researcher manipulate to improve power?
   (a) increase the sample size
   (b) decrease the effect size
   (c) decrease the sample size
   (d) alter the significance level from 0.05 to 0.01.

7. Power is a measure of:
   (a) the probability of making a type I error
   (b) the probability of making a type II error
   (c) the probability of accepting the null hypothesis
   (d) the probability of rejecting the null hypothesis when the null hypothesis is true.

8. If measurements were at the ordinal level, what test of difference would be used to compare two independent groups?
   (a) chi-square
   (b) one-way analysis of variance
   (c) *t* test
   (d) Mann-Whitney *U* test.

9. Correlation is a measure of association, but does not determine:
   (a) the magnitude of the relationship
   (b) the direction of the relationship
   (c) cause and effect relationships
   (d) the significance of the relationship.

10. Multivariate analyses are used to establish relationships between several variables based on:
    (a) common variance shared amongst variables
    (b) error variance of each variable
    (c) unique variance of each variable
    (d) bivariate relationships.

Additional resources

Crichton N 2001 Information point: regression analysis. *Journal of Clinical Nursing* 10(4):462

Ratcliffe P 1998 Using the 'new' statistics in nursing research. *Journal of Advanced Nursing* 27:132–9

Virtual statistics textbook. Online. Available: http://www.surfstat.newcastle.edu.au/surfstat/main/surfstat.html

References

Chien W T, Chiu Y L, Lam L W, et al. 2006 Effects of a needs-based education programme for family carers with a relative in an intensive care unit: a quasi-experimental study. *International Journal of Nursing Studies* 43:39–50

Cohen J 1988 *Statistical power analysis for the behavioral sciences*, 2nd edn. Lawrence Erlbaum Associates, Hillsdale, New Jersey

Dunning T, Manias 2005 Medication knowledge and self-management by people with type 2 diabetes. *Australian Journal of Advanced Nursing* 23(1):7–13

Fenwick J, Hauck Y, Downie J, et al. 2004 The childbirth expectations of a self-selected cohort of Western Australian women. *Midwifery* 21:23–35

Fisher M J, Marshall A P, Kendrick T S 2005 Competency standards for critical care nurses: do they measure up? *Australian Journal of Advanced Nursing* 22(4):32–9

Jirojwong S, Rossi D, Walker S, et al. 2005 What were the outcomes of home follow-up visits after postpartum hospital discharge? *Australian Journal of Advanced Nursing* 23(1):22–9

Knapp T R 1990 Treating ordinal scales as interval scales: an attempt to resolve the controversy. *Nursing Research* 39(2):121–4

—— 1993 Treating ordinal scales as ordinal scales. *Nursing Research* 42(3):184–6

McKinley S, Dracup K, Moser DK, et al. 2004 International comparison of factors associated with delay in presentation for AMI treatment. *European Journal of Cardiovascular Nursing* 3:225–30

Munro B H 2001 *Statistical methods for health care research*, 4th edn. Lippincott, Philadelphia

Pravikoff D S, Tanner A B, Pierce S T 2005 Readiness of US Nurses for Evidence-Based Practice. *American Journal of Nursing* 105(9):40–51

Rudy E B 1991 Unravelling the mystique of power analysis. *Heart & Lung. The Journal of Acute & Critical Care* 20(5):517–22

Stahl K, Hundley V 2003 Risk and risk assessment in pregnancy — do we scare because we care? *Midwifery*. 19(4):298–309

Ware, J E Jr. 2000 SF-36 health survey update. *Spine* 25(24):3130–9

Wu M-LW, Courtney M, Berger G 2000 Models of nursing care: a comparative study of patient satisfaction on two orthopaedic wards in Brisbane. *Australian Journal of Advanced Nursing* 17(4):29–34

Answers

ᵀᵀ Tutorial trigger 1

Answer to part 1
Design a short questionnaire stating:
1. The librarian would like to know how frequently you visited the library during exam week on the following days:
   Monday (.....); Tuesday (.....); Wednesday ( ); Thursday (.....); Friday (.....) Total days: .....
2. Hours spent in the library on:
   Monday (.....); Tuesday (.....); Wednesday (.....); Thursday (.....); Friday (.....) Total hours: .....
3. At what times did you visit the library most often?
   (a) Morning (09.00–12.00)
   (b) Mid afternoon (12.00–15.00)
   (c) Late afternoon (15.00–18.00)
   (d) Evening (18.00 onwards)
   A frequency count will give you the total number of days the library was used by the nurses.
   Let's assume the following:
1. Monday 15; Tuesday 32; Wednesday 20; Thursday 13; Friday 10: Total:90
2. Hours spent in library:

Monday 20 hrs; Tuesday 35; Wednesday 40; Thursday 20; Friday 10: Total hours: 125
3. Times visited
   Morning (09.00–12.00) 21 nurses
   Mid afternoon (12.00–15.00) 50 nurses
   Late afternoon (15.00–18.00) 13 nurses
   Evening (18.00 onwards): 6 nurses

Answer to part 2

Days of the week	Number of students
Monday	15
Tuesday	32
Wednesday	20
Thursday	13
Friday	10

The mode is most likely to be used with categories; the mode is the most popular (frequent) value. In the above example, Tuesday would be the modal category when 32 nurses visit the library. The median would simply indicate the centre of the distribution, and the mean would give us the average number of nurses visiting the library each day, which isn't helpful in planning staff rosters and availability of facilities.

ᵀᵀ Tutorial trigger 2

Mean = 4.43   Mode = 4   Median = 4

When the mean, median and mode are equal, the solution of scores approximates a normal distribution. As the mean is to the right of the median and mode, this solution is positively skewed.

ᵀᵀ Tutorial trigger 3

On the face of it there appears to be a difference in the amount and type of medication errors between the two storage sites. Proportionately more dispensing errors occurred from the bedside draw and more administration errors occurred from the medication trolley. The chi-square test is less powerful than other statistics and requires larger sample sizes to ensure power. In this case the sample may be too small to detect the difference between the two storage sites and a type II error may have occurred. Further data collection is required to increase the sample size in order to detect the difference or alternatively the Fisher's exact probability test could be used.

Learning activities

1. c	**2.** a	**3.** b	**4.** a
5. c	**6.** a	**7.** b	**8.** d
9. c	**10.** a		

15

Mixed-methods research

DEAN WHITEHEAD AND DOUG ELLIOTT

KEY TERMS

action research
case study
Delphi technique
methodological
    triangulation/pluralism
mixed-methods research
Q methodology

Learning outcomes

After reading this chapter, you should be able to:

- understand the principles and issues underpinning mixed-methods research
- appreciate the value, benefits and dilemmas when using both qualitative and quantitative designs and methods in a single study
- explain the structures and processes that underpin action research
- explain the structures and processes that underpin Delphi technique research
- describe the purpose and processes of less common nursing-related mixed-method approaches, such as case studies and Q methodology.

Introduction

An exploration of past nursing and midwifery research literature has noted broad acceptance of one epistemological position to the exclusion of another and, consequently, the separating out of both quantitative and qualitative research. The consequence of this separation of paradigms and viewing each approach in isolation, where it occurs, means that nursing and midwifery research can not truly provide the evidence for understanding humans and their health-related needs, problems or required nursing support. This situation has led to the paradigm tension mentioned previously in this book (see Chapter 2) and a subsequent attempt by many researchers to reconcile this position. Method or methodological triangulation (mixing research methods and paradigms) has been suggested as the main means of reconciling this position of 'paradigmatic separatism' (Cowman 1993; Williamson 2005). When compared to other health professions, nursing and midwifery have concertedly begun to embrace mixed-methods research in a constructive and purposeful manner (Foss & Ellefsen 2002; Deery 2005; Annells 2007) — and hence the need for a detailed chapter like this in a nursing and midwifery research text.

Selecting methodology

There are immediate and immense benefits to be gained from not separating quantitative and qualitative research into distinct categories but, instead, acknowledging and understanding their inter-related nature and processes. The important thing is that researchers do not restrict themselves to a limited range of conventional research approaches or methods. Traditionally, a state of affairs has existed whereby nursing and midwifery research has predominantly steered towards qualitative research, whereas medicine has almost exclusively steered towards quantitative methodology. Health professional researchers, regardless of discipline, however, can and should choose from an increasingly wide and diverse range of research activities — from both paradigms, and within single studies, to address increasingly complex clinical issues (Whitehead 2005). Mixed-methods research offers a means for making research more meaningful, complete and purposeful than is the case when using either a singular qualitative or quantitative approach, and provides the nurse with other valuable tools to add to their research armoury. Annells (2007) and McKellar et al. (2006) have highlighted the notable increase in nursing and midwifery-related mixed-methods research.

TT Tutorial Trigger 1

What effects, for and against, might it have on nursing and midwifery research if medical research continues to predominate in the quantitative paradigm, while nursing and midwifery research predominates in the qualitative paradigm?

● Evidence-based practice tip

It is predicted here that nursing and midwifery will witness a steadily increasing amount of mixed-methods research. When reviewing your own nursing and midwifery-related literature, make a note of how often and when mixed methods are being employed.

Methodological triangulation/ pluralism

Historically, methodological triangulation (or pluralism), from its social science origins in the 1950s, was limited to just parts of a whole study. Denzin (1978) sought to expand the scope of mixed-methods research to the whole research design. His intention was to reduce the incidence of research error often associated with studies which used single methods, single researchers or single theories. In today's context, methodological triangulation/ pluralism are terms used to denote a single research study that uses a combination of research approaches, paradigms and/or methods. Essentially both terms refer to the same process although it is more common to see the term triangulation used, rather than pluralism. Risjord et al. (2002) refer to the process as a 'blending view' of methodological triangulation. This point is elaborated on by both Johnstone (2004) and Morse (2005).

Mixing approaches to achieve the best research outcome

As noted in Chapter 2, there is always going to be more than one way to investigate nursing issues in research and so the point of 'best fit' becomes the most important consideration. Each approach and method should also complement each other, and so are viewed as equally valuable in constructing research projects. However, with mixed-methods research, as with any research, it is never wise to re-construct and add/subtract approaches and methods as research progresses. A clear, well-planned and logical process, known from the beginning, is required in a research proposal (see Chapter 19). With many conventional mixed-method approaches, for example, Delphi (see later in this chapter), the structure and format is well established and known prior to study commencement.

TT Tutorial trigger 2

When considering the notion of 'best fit' for a mixed-methods research topic, what factors could be considered?

Different types, categories and combinations of triangulation research

As suggested earlier, there is always more than one way to approach a research issue — with the research question, statement or hypothesis guiding the approach (see Chapter 5). The same is true for mixed-methods/triangulation research. It is necessary to have a good understanding of different types, categories and combinations before commencing this type of research. Depending on what the main aims of any research study are, certain triangulation methods will work better than others.

There are a number of different 'types' of triangulation. Before commencing mixed-methods-based research then, the first step is in considering what type of triangulation will best suit the task at hand. Table 15.1 highlights the main types of triangulation to be considered. Each one is important in its own right and has the potential to produce different perspectives and outcomes than the next — hence the importance of choosing wisely. Triangulation research may attempt to use just one of the listed types or it can use a combination of some or all.

As well as different types of triangulation, there are also options for different paradigm combinations to consider. For instance,

TABLE 15.1 Types of triangulation

Type	Explanation
Data triangulation	The use of a variety of data sources in a study.
Investigator triangulation	The use of several different researchers or evaluators.
Theory triangulation	The use of multiple perspectives to interpret a single set of data.
Methodological triangulation	The use of multiple methods to study a single problem.
Multi-disciplinary triangulation	The use of multiple disciplines to inform the research process.

(Modified from Denzin 1978; Janesick 1994.)

simultaneous triangulation is the combination of qualitative and quantitative methods in one study at the same time, whereas sequential triangulation separates out the two paradigms, but combines them in the overall findings (see Table 15.2). Also, in sequential triangulation, only one approach is used in a study, but the researcher conducts multiple studies using different approaches in each.

Sometimes, it appears that two separate studies are conducted in triangulated research — such as a quantitative study followed by a qualitative study or vice versa. Where this is the case, the two studies are triangulated if they are both related to the same topic area, they are both planned prior to the research program commencing, one informs the other and, as a final outcome, they both equally expand the related field of inquiry. For instance, Symon et al. (2006) conducted an exploratory mixed-methods study of midwives' understandings and perceptions of clinical 'near misses' in maternity care settings. The first phase of this study was a survey-based questionnaire design, analysing quantitative data through simple descriptive statistic techniques. The second phase of the study followed up the questionnaire responses with follow-up group interviews (see Chapter 8), qualitatively analysed and transcribed. Another example sees Lukkarinen (2005) conducting a mixed-method longitudinal study on young people who had received treatment for coronary artery disease. She conducted two seemingly 'separate' studies, one quantitative and the

TABLE 15.2 Simultaneous and sequential combinations of quantitative and qualitative research methods

Combination	Rationale	Example
Simultaneous		
Qualitative + quantitative	There is a qualitative foundation and quantitative methods are used to provide complementary information.	The research is focused on the experiences of feeling depressed after miscarriage. Phenomenological methods could be used to address the question, and use of a depression scale would provide complementary information.
Quantitative + qualitative	There is a quantitative foundation and qualitative methods are used to provide complementary information.	The research is testing hypotheses about depression after miscarriage. The phenomenological method is used to uncover the experience for a select group who acknowledge feelings of depression.
Sequential		
Qualitative ⟶ quantitative	Findings from qualitative investigation lead to use of the quantitative approach.	The research has described the experience of feeling depressed after miscarriage. The themes emerging from the data are then used to create a depression scale, which is tested for reliability and validity.
Quantitative ⟶ qualitative	Findings from quantitative investigation lead to use of the qualitative approach.	The research has tested hypotheses linking miscarriage with depression and found no significant relationships. A qualitative study is undertaken to uncover the experience of living through miscarriage, in an effort to let the data lead to common thoughts and feelings.

(Modified from Morse 1991)

other qualitative, but then combined the findings of the two studies using the process of meta-analysis (see Chapter 4).

Tables 15.1 and 15.2 both offer a useful indication of the most common types and combinations of mixed-method triangulation. An Australasian study of note, for instance, investigated nursing workload-related issues using a simultaneous type data triangulation approach (Hegney et al. 2003). As is the case for much nursing and midwifery research, researchers attempt to push beyond conventional boundaries and extend the range of mixed-methods research options for future researchers. Maggs-Rapport (2000), for example, uses methodological triangulation as a means to combine two qualitative designs (ethnography and phenomenology) in a single study, rather than a more conventional combination of quantitative and qualitative approaches. Annells (2006) does the same with hermeneutical phenomenology and grounded theory, in her Australian-based study on how flatus affects people receiving nursing care. Henderson (2005) similarly combines a nested set of methodologies (ethnography, ethnomethodology and dramaturgy) to characterise the practices and interactions inherent in an Australian healthcare environment.

Research in brief

An Asian example of methodological triangulation, by Shih et al. (2005), explores the health needs of hospitalised Taiwanese older people with heart disease and, subsequently, develops an assessment instrument to measure these health needs and examine the relationships between the identified health needs. Three phases are involved in this 'between method' triangulation design. The first phase being an explorative qualitative method for exploring the contextual content of health needs, the second phase being the development and testing of their Health Needs Instrument (HNI), and the third phase tested the effects of implementation of the HNI tool. Table 15.3 helps to further break down the main components of the study in question.

TABLE 15.3 Use of triangulated approach in one study

Research process components	Qualitative approach First phase	Quantitative approach Second phase	Quantitative approach Third phase
Design	Descriptive, exploratory.	Correlational, Health Needs Instrument (HNI) tool development and testing.	Descriptive, correlational. Implementation of HNI tool.
Participants	Purposive sample of 34 elder patients.	Purposive sample of 32 elder patients.	Purposive sample of 54 elder patients.
Data collection	Semi-structured interviews.	Structured demographic data from HNI (35 nominal questions).	Structured interviews.
Analysis	Content/thematic analysis.	Internal consistency, content and concurrent validity.	Descriptive measures of variance and distribution.
Findings	Health needs included; help in managing tangible things, psychological support, health information, medical support and participation in decision-making.	A significant negative correlation with patients' tangible needs for help with activities of daily life (ADL) during hospitalisation transition. Strong correlation between educational level and the need for health-related information.	A significant correlation between psychological needs with the need for medical support, informational needs and maintaining ADLs during period of hospitalisation.

(Source: Shih et al. 2005)

The value of mixed-methods research

Perhaps the greatest value of mixed-methods research is the potential to offer wider scope for constructive, contained and appropriate research, with the potential to present as a more complete and comprehensive research opportunity. At the theoretical level, combining and triangulating methods produces research that 'provides completeness, abductive inspiration, and confirmation' (Risjord et al. 2002 p 269). It also assists in resolving the issue of methodological dominance and order, and enables a rich and comprehensive picture of the issue under investigation (Foss & Ellefsen 2002). Another argument for triangulation of methods assumes that weaknesses in one method can be counter-balanced by the strengths in another. This situation has challenged researchers to develop 'conceptual triangulation' as part of their planning. Here, each research approach that is incorporated into the overall research design is evaluated separately in accordance with its own methodological criteria. In this way, each component can stand alone while also being linked conceptually to other parts. This is of great value when researchers want to understand how parts of clinical issues that are investigated relate to the whole picture — again adding to the comprehensiveness of studies.

Nursing and midwifery practices and processes are viewed as complex and multifaceted. The humanistic and holistic nature of such practice, alongside its bio-scientific context, dictates that related clinical and academic issues are both eclectic and diverse. To reflect this, it is increasingly felt that contemporary nursing and midwifery research should be developed accordingly to reflect this multiplicity. Method triangulation is viewed as a very valuable tool in facilitating this transition (Foss & Ellefsen 2002).

Limitations associated with mixed-methods research

As with any area of research, accompanying the value and benefits of a research method, the researcher needs to also consider both the limitations and complexity of the task at hand. Undertaking mixed-methods research is usually far more complex than single design research. The limitations associated with mixed-methods research can be immediately obvious — such as being more time-consuming, involved, resource intensive and generating more complex data for collection and analysis.

Another limitation for mixed-method research lies not with the method, but the way that it is perceived by the wider research community and the fact that it still has to confirm its place within this community (Whitehead et al. 2003; Miller & Fredericks 2006). A perhaps cynical observation might be that 'purist' quantitative or qualitative researchers believe that mixing methods means that one paradigm taints or interferes with the other. Critical commentary subsequently may uphold the notion that rigour can be compromised in mixed-method studies (Williamson 2005; Miller & Fredericks 2006). This said, Jones and Bugge (2006) argue to the contrary. They state that triangulation leads to 'completeness', improved transparency and a more holistic understanding that, in turn, improves rigour through challenging findings. Added to this is the notion that some mixed-method research can be interpreted as more a style of research than a specific method — particularly with action research (Whitehead et al. 2003). A possible limitation for nursing and midwifery is that, while mixed-methods research is evolving at pace and increasing in frequency in all health professions, two particular designs currently predominate above all others — those of action research (AR) and the Delphi technique. The following sections in this chapter reflect this and, accordingly, focus on these two approaches. Other less common approaches, such as case study and Q methodology, are introduced later in the chapter.

While mixed-method approaches, such as action research and Delphi technique studies, are generally placed under the umbrella of qualitative research, it is argued here that this is often incorrect and misleading. Delphi studies tend to contain similar amounts of both quantitative and qualitative processes and outcomes, although some might argue that there are actually more quantitative than qualitative aspects. With action research and its participatory and empowering nature, it does tend to be derived more from an emancipatory qualitative approach — but not exclusively so, and again, studies may contain more quantitative than qualitative components. To illustrate this point, Miller and Fredericks

(2006 p 567) state the case for a particular mixed-methods design, called 'quantitative-dominant sequential analysis', as a means to conduct evaluation research.

Action research

Action research is fast becoming an important and well-established research approach for nursing practice. The term 'action research', underpinned by critical social theory (see Chapter 2), was coined in 1946 by the social psychologist Kurt Lewin — to describe the research program he developed in response to serious post–World War II social problems in America (Lewin 1946). Lewin's interest was in narrowing the gap between research recommendation and implementation, so that democratic inquiry could pave the way to group decisions and a commitment to organisational improvement (Lewin 1951). He wanted to develop a concrete procedure for translating evidence into action. Action research may be viewed as an umbrella term that can be, and often is, referred to using different terms.

Since its inception, many terms are now used to describe similar processes, and this has caused part of the confusion presented by action research. Research processes that cluster under the action research umbrella include *action science, action inquiry, action*

Research in brief

Deery (2005) uses an action research approach to explore the support needs of eight participant (co-researcher) community midwives, through interview, focus group and workshop sessions. Findings showed that recent organisational changes had placed increased managerial demands on the midwives that were detrimental to their working relationships and processes of clinical supervision. Subsequently, a clinical supervision support program was set up to address these issues. This article is a particularly useful example of how difficult it can be to translate and initiate organisational change and the dilemmas that participants (co-researchers) can face when conducting action research.

learning, participatory research, co-operative inquiry, transparent research, community development research and *organisational-change research* (Whitehead et al. 2003). From the last two stated terms, it should be noted that most action research is categorised into either a social/community development approach or an organisational-change process approach. Some of the different action research topics that nurses and midwives have recently investigated are found in Table 15.4. More recently, the emergence of 'practice development' and 'practice change', in clinical environments, has reinforced the use of action research processes as effective tools for engaging all health professionals to collaboratively solve practice-based issues (see Chapters 17 and 18).

Point to ponder

▶ Is it better to use a process like action research that 'forces' the researcher to apply change to the issue under investigation before final outcomes are known — or is it better, when using other research approaches, to be mindful of how change is actioned once the outcomes are known?

● **Evidence-based practice tip**

Action research is seen as one of the most effective research methods for clinical healthcare-related practice. Its processes demand that the researchers move away from the position where researchers often investigate issues but do not act upon the presented findings (instead merely reporting them), or conducting 'research for research's sake', towards the situation where research findings have to be evidenced, acted upon and notable strategies for change are implemented and evaluated. Action research requires action as part of the research process and is focused on the researcher's professional values rather than methodological considerations. Subsequently, action research is viewed as critical 'inside' research where researchers investigate and act upon their own professional actions.

The process of action research

While most forms of research are constructed in a series of linear steps from question/hypothesis through to recommendations for action, action research is depicted as a variation of a spiral/cycle design. It uses a cyclical research process that enables steps or actions to be carefully monitored, analysed and evaluated. This forms the basis for reflection on the success of the plan and the possibility of modifying it and starting another cycle of planning, action, data collection, analysis, evaluation and reflection. The spiral or cycle consists of a number of

TABLE 15.4 Nursing and midwifery examples of action research

Type	Authors	Focus
Organisational	Whitehead et al. 2004	Osteoporosis prevention in hospital.
	van Loon et al. 2004	Caring for female survivors of child sex abuse in EDs.
	Deery 2005	Supporting midwives' needs in clinical practice.
	Reed 2005	Discharge planning from hospital to home care.
	Waterman et al. 2005	Advancing ophthalmic nursing practice.
	McKellar et al. 2006	Improving parent postnatal education in a maternity hospital.
	Glasson et al. 2006	Establishing an evidence base for an evolving model of care for older hospitalised patients.
Socio-community	Walters & East 2001	Homelessness in young mothers.
	Choudhry et al. 2002	Accessing health services for South Asian immigrants.
	Parsons & Warner-Robbins 2002	Empowering the health of women recently released from prison.
	Garwick & Auger 2003	Culturally appropriate health care for Indian communities.
	Holkup et al. 2004	A collaborative model for working with native Americans.

stages, some of which are repeated until the situation under examination improves (see Figure 15.1). Figure 15.1 clearly delineates each continuing stage, starting with initial diagnosis of the clinical problem/s, through to data collection and analysis and resultant feedback to participants. Following on from this is the actioning of changes, leading to the processes of reflection and program evaluation, before planning further action and starting the cycle again. It is worth noting that, attached to the main spiral or cycle, many projects develop mini sub-projects with their own distinct spirals.

Research in brief

Schroyen & Finlayson's (2004) New Zealand-based action research study on implementing a practical change strategy, aimed at improving the teaching and learning relationships between nursing students and placement staff, identifies how they adapted and simplified Hyrkas' action research phase and cycle stages for their study. They are identified as; diagnosing the problem (reconnaissance), planning the action, carrying out the plan (implementation), evaluation of the results, and identification of central findings.

Action research involves the use of change experiments with real people and their real problems in their own social systems. The function of action research is to focus on 'real-world' events, as opposed to controlled environments (Kelly & Simpson 2001). Preliminary investigation demonstrates the extent of the problems in the situation under consideration and assists the research team to develop specific research question/s. In action research, the change/action cycles emerge from the creation of new knowledge constructed by the cyclical processes of consensus building. These processes are observing and reflecting on immediate experiences, forming abstract generalisations and concepts, and testing and applying these experiences in new situations.

TT Tutorial trigger 3

Why do you think that it is that some researchers might be reluctant to adopt a mixed-methods approach to their studies?

Action research stresses the importance of actively engaging its participants in the process of a democratic and reformatory social inquiry focusing on active partnerships and involvement. This is where the concepts of critical social theory and emancipatory research are demonstrated (see Chapter 2). The process is designed to be participatory and empowering for all its research participants — who are often referred to as 'co-researchers'. Action research, therefore, enjoys a collective ethos that actively encourages the shared learning of individuals and teams who are able to learn across the boundaries of any organisation, as and when new ideas and assumptions are presented to them (St Leger & Walsworth-Bell 1999). The key to participatory action research lies not with any given method but, rather, in the attitudes of researchers, which in turn affect how and for whom the research is constructed and conducted (Green et al. 2001). This connection between collecting evidence to understand a situation and collaborative action is the hallmark of an action research approach.

Action research is necessarily 'insider' research, in the sense that practitioners research their own professional actions. As action research aims to be democratic and inclusive of those the research outcomes are expected to affect, there are a number of strategies that are used to facilitate the widest possible involvement of representative stakeholders. Box 15.1 highlights how various stakeholder groups might interact with the action research process.

TT Tutorial trigger 4

Identify all the stakeholders who might be affected in a study on improving the sexual and reproductive health information for community-based teenagers — as part of preconceptual care.

With action research, as descriptive data are collected and analysed, the values, theories, attitudes and assumptions used in professional practice are exposed through a process of reflection. This capacity to generate 'theories-in-use' and build them into theories or conceptual models is a distinguishing trademark of action research — separating it from continuous quality improvement processes. The participant co-researchers usually share their reflective accounts and understandings with other group

FIGURE 15.1 An organisational-change action research cycle

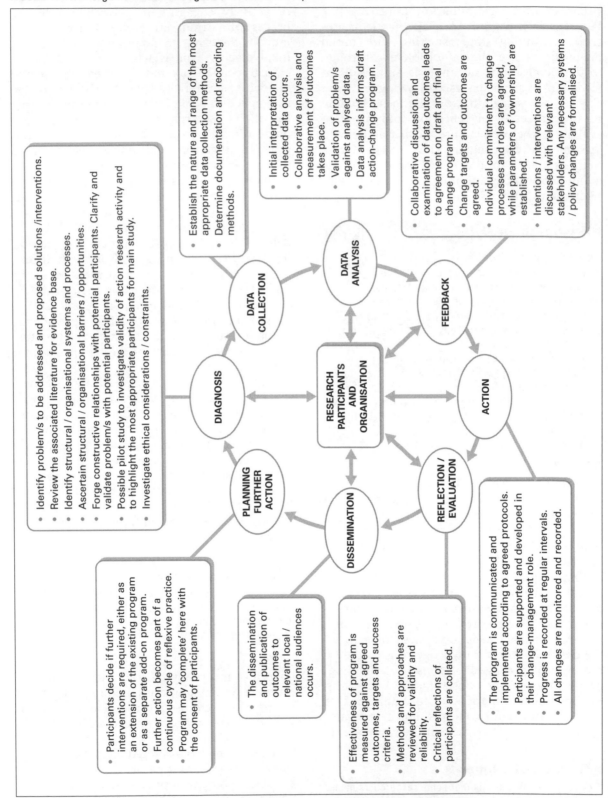

(Source: adapted from: Whitehead D et al. (2004) with kind permission from *Health Education Journal*)

BOX 15.1 Action research project structure

- Identify a health-related situation that needs improvement.
- Establish a collaborative research group concerned with addressing the situation.
- Establish a reference group composed of all key stakeholders.
- Conduct training action research workshops for participating researchers.
- Conduct a preliminary investigation to develop baseline data and understand the scope of the concern.
- Meet with the reference group to examine the data and assess the proposed plans.
- Implement the first action plan, collect and analyse data.
- Research group reflection and re-planning through the spiral or cycle.
- Meet with the reference group to discuss project results.
- Disseminate the findings in accessible formats to all stakeholders.

members. This sets up a retrospective group assessment of the progress that has been made in light of the wider research question and the values, theories and assumptions that inform the current and desired situation. This group reflection has an evaluative component, as the co-researchers judge progress in preparation for the next planning stage. It also has a responsive component. During reflection, researchers not only examine the analysed data, but also the research processes and the roles of all involved.

Reflecting on the main concerns at various cycles in the project can help to keep the team orientated. The interest is not only in what was discovered but how it was discovered, under what conditions, and how this relates to the wider concern. This 'lessons learnt so far' stage provides a rationale to underpin the next action plan. At this stage the group decides if the previous action plan needs to proceed with modifications or whether a new, but related plan, can be introduced to address the research question/s.

The value of action research

Perhaps the greatest value of action research is that it allows health professionals to learn about their local situation and facilitate the implementation and evaluation of research into this situation. Added to this, is the obvious benefit that this type of research approach lends to ongoing evidence-based practice change (see Chapters 17 and 18). Action research also offers the flexibility for research projects to evolve naturally. As the study evolves and changes, the co-researchers have the opportunity to further develop and refine the process and provide a much fuller and comprehensive picture of the problem at hand (Adami & Kiger 2005). Action research studies, therefore, have the potential to reach aims and outcomes that may not have been recognised or realised at project commencement. Many action research projects gain their own impetus and researchers want to keep working through more cycles to achieve better outcomes — usually until funding or support has ceased. As with some facets of action research though, this may be viewed as much as a limitation by some as it is of value to others. While action research works best when the intention is to effect wholesale community-wide or organisational change, it can be applied more manageably to a localised context, such as a single ward/unit (i.e. Deery 2005; Glasson et al. 2006).

Research in brief

Schroyen and Finlayson (2004) report on their New Zealand-based action research study. Using an education action research model, this study involved one lecturer, ten students and five supervising staff nurses and sought to identify, implement and evaluate a practice-change strategy aimed at improving teaching and learning relationships between students on clinical placement and their supervising staff nurses. In line with the abovementioned notions of reflection, one of the key aims of this study was to facilitate self-reflective teaching practice for the co-researchers. Findings demonstrated that contract learning improved the effectiveness of clinical learning and teaching relationships.

Limitations of action research

Action researchers will usually apply an action research-related study knowing the immense benefits that it can bring — especially in relation to measurable change in practice and structures. At the same time, action researchers are also acutely aware of the limitations that belie its nature. As one might already appreciate, action research is not easy to set up or instigate. Great effort, enthusiasm and widespread equal participation, over long periods, are necessary for effective action research (Karim 2001). The literature, however, can be critical of action research's ability to offer 'true' equality, empowerment and participation (Whitehead et al. 2003). The nature and intention of action research is often quite broad as it relates to the whole situation under investigation. This means that process and outcomes are often difficult to predict. Action researchers face situations where they may not know exactly what to investigate, when and where to start, or even when the research is likely to complete. Therefore, in action research, participants are often unaware of exactly where their research 'journey' will take them (Williamson & Prosser 2002). This aspect, therefore, has implications for gaining funding, organisational support and seeking ethical approval.

Action research can be viewed as an insensitive 'blunt tool' by the fact that it scrutinises and challenges organisations or communities. The inference, prior to the outset of action research, is that something is wrong and requires fixing/change — even though any criticism is intended to be constructive. In fact, action research is usually applied in situations where groups or communities are perceived to be powerless, vulnerable or oppressed by a dominant group, organisation or culture. Action research, therefore, with its intention of systematic inquiry made public, can appear threatening to the research participants and the viewed organisation/community. Imposed political or managerial agendas may work to oppose this type of scrutiny and hinder rather than assist research efforts. The need for many stakeholders to be involved at different levels can also provide organisational difficulties and may affect the willingness of some people to become involved.

The notion of methodological rigour has been challenged with action research. The dynamic and fluid aspect of action research and the involvement of stakeholders, as potentially novice and learning researchers, may mean that there are difficulties maintaining research rigour and validity. To offset this, many action researchers adopt several qualitative criteria including credibility, auditability and fittingness (see Chapter 9). The emphasis on finding concrete and practical solutions may, however, become the focus of the research to the detriment of systematic recording; that is, the researchers may be more focused on action than on research. The findings of action research are context-specific and therefore not generalisable from one setting to another. It is, however, certainly desirable to compare and contrast settings against each other while looking for commonalities as they may apply to all organisations/communities (Whitehead 2005).

> ● **Evidence-based practice tip**
>
> A useful exercise is to identify an issue that concerns you from your clinical experience and create an action research proposal. This exercise could include justification of your action research question, how you would conduct a preliminary investigation on this topic, what might an initial plan look like and what kind of data you would collect and analyse.

Delphi technique

The Delphi technique is named with reference to the Ancient Greek god Apollo, whose Delphi oracle was viewed as his most expert, truthful and trustworthy informant (Kennedy 2004). The Delphi technique is a research approach used to gain expert group consensus on a specific topic. It is an iterative, multi-stage, group facilitation process designed to transform opinion into group consensus (Hasson et al. 2000). The process involves a group of respondents providing expert opinion on a topic. This is achieved by extracting the viewpoints of all parties, enabling individual responses to the viewpoints and ultimately achieving a degree of consensus. The Delphi technique is a useful strategy for examining an area with a scant empirical research base and/or for where there are questions for which there may be no definitive answers. The technique, therefore, is particularly useful for determining best academic and practice standards and as a basis for policy-driven mechanisms.

Expert opinion, on a clinical practice issue, may be the only available evidence when no quality primary research findings are evident as stated above (NHMRC 2000). In Australasian terms, the Delphi technique is often used in nursing and midwifery studies for this very reason. For example, Williams and Clarke (2001) used a consensus method to determine staffing requirements for intensive care units in Australia. Sixteen critical care nurse experts were surveyed on four occasions to develop and refine a number of consensus statements on nursing workforce issues. Annells et al. (2005) also conducted a Delphi study to investigate the research priorities of 320 district nurses, throughout Australia, as a means of determining best research practice. Similarly, Rodger et al. (2004) performed a Delphi study with 115 emergency nurses, throughout Western Australia, to identify the most clinically relevant research questions for this professional group. Fenwick et al.'s (2006) midwifery-based Delphi study is detailed further in the following 'Research in brief' box.

Research in brief box

Fenwick et al. (2006) conducted a two-round Delphi study investigating the research priorities of over 100 midwives at five Perth-based public hospitals. Seventeen specific research topics, within four major categories, emerged from analysis of the first-round questionnaire. These topics were later ranked in round two in terms of importance to practising midwives. Research focusing on the evidence base for the postnatal experiences of women rated highest, while professional issues (such as preceptorship) scored lowest.

The Delphi process

A Delphi study involves a series (or rounds) of questionnaires, interspersed with controlled feedback from 'quasi-anonymous' participants — where names of the participants are known but their judgments remain anonymous (Löfmark & Thorell-Ekstrand 2004). Stages of the Delphi process include selection of the expert panel, formulation of the question(s), generation of statements, reduction and categorisation of statements, rating of statements, and analysis and iteration (Mead & Moseley 2001). A Delphi study is a mixed-method design in that both qualitative and quantitative techniques are used to collect and analyse the questionnaire data. It normally takes on the structure of a methodological triangulation/data triangulation with a sequential combination method (see Tables 15.1 and 15.2).

Typically with Delphi studies, the first round questionnaire collects qualitative data through unstructured questions seeking open responses. This type of data is needed initially to provide the necessary richness of data in order to formulate subsequent focused questions or statements. Qualitative content and thematic analysis processes of the collected first-round data are used as a basis to synthesise responses for each survey round (see Chapter 9). This analysis reveals a number of categories and themes which are, in turn, grouped and listed. Generally, the collated data from the first round are specific and structured, but then require quantification through descriptive quantitative survey design questionnaires. These are conventionally formulated as a list of Likert Scale questions, or sometimes visual analogue scale-related questions (see Chapter 12), and returned to the study participants for further feedback.

In many cases the initial first-round analysis reveals a large number of categories and therefore the second-round questionnaire may be very detailed. The aim of a Delphi study is to extract a fairly 'narrow' consensus on the investigated topic. Where this is the case, it usually requires a number of rounds of similarly structured Likert-style questionnaire rounds to help break the categories down into a manageable number. The lowest scoring questions are removed whereas the highest scores are kept for the following round/s. A predetermined consensus level or percentage is often set prior to analysing the data. Once the main points are manageable and/or cannot be broken down anymore, then this is when a degree of 'saturation' or consensus is deemed to have been met. In most cases it is by the second or third round that this situation occurs, but there is always the capacity to continue for a number of other rounds. The validity and rigour in Delphi is maintained during each round, as participants check and provide feedback that the interpreted data are consistent with their responses and overall position on the topic.

The value of the Delphi technique

The benefits of the Delphi technique include the ability to harness many opinions across geographical distance, the freedom of individuals to express their opinion without being influenced by other group members, allowing individuals to participate at a convenient time, and relatively small expense. Delphi can also be performed over relatively short periods of time — especially if conducted using electronic mail (Marsden et al. 2003). These benefits overcome the potential limitations of other consensus methods such as focus groups, nominal group technique or consensus conferences (Mead & Moseley 2001). It is a flexible technique and modifications can be made to suit the study at hand. Potentially small study groups can be used although the range can be anywhere from 4 to 3000 (Campbell & Cantrell 2001), although most commonly Delphi study participant numbers are usually anywhere from the range of 20 to 50. In McKenna et al.'s (2002) Delphi survey of midwives and midwifery students' identification of non-midwifery duties, they used a total of 275 participants.

Limitations of the Delphi technique

As well as a number of benefits, there are a number of methodological considerations to address with Delphi studies. These include inadequate descriptions of panellist characteristics (especially in terms of identifying who or what constitutes an expert), subjective researcher interpretation of definitions and measures of consensus, and high wastage of respondents due to response fatigue. It is also important to remember that the findings of a Delphi study represent expert opinion but not indisputable fact (Powell 2003).

Evidence-based practice tip

You might want to identify a clinically related issue that you think is not well defined, developed or researched in the literature, and that would benefit from the expert consensus that a Delphi study potentially offers.

Case study approach

The term case study has different meanings in research and clinical contexts. A case study research approach enables a detailed examination of a single 'case' or 'unit', within a real-life and contemporary context using multiple data sources (Bergen & While 2000; Hewitt-Taylor 2002). The case (phenomenon of interest) can be an individual/s (e.g. Hotham et al. 2005; Yoshioka-Maeda et al. 2006), a group or community, an organisation (e.g. Fullerton et al. 2003; Cooke 2006), a process (e.g. Gardner et al. 2003; Koch et al. 2005), or an event.

Point to ponder

▶ Do not confuse case study research with a 'case presentation' of a particular clinical case or a 'case-control' study of an epidemiological design (see Chapter 10).

Research in brief

Two midwifery-related studies utilise a case study approach. In one, Hotham et al. (2005), supplement their randomised controlled trial of nicotine replacement therapy with in-depth case studies of three pregnant smokers from the trial. The case studies were designed to demonstrate the unique difficulties and barriers that this group of women face when attempting to stop smoking. In another study, Fullerton et al. (2003) use an organisational case study design to investigate the effects of incorporating selected reproductive health services, on 24 family planning service delivery points, in Ghana. Service-related statistical data were supplemented with qualitative data by interviewing providers, managers and clients.

The case study approach is exploratory, observational and responsive to the context and therefore qualitative in terms of philosophical position (Fitzgerald 1999). Triangulation of methods, however, enables use of the full range of data collection strategies — such as interviews, field notes, participant observation, and contemporary documents (Bergen & While 2000). Data analysis can use a constant comparative approach (Hewitt-Taylor 2002; see Chapter 9) or be more structured (Yin 2003). Data can be examined in their own right, with no requirement for generalisability (Keyzer 2000), or the study procedure may include steps to ensure reliability, validity and generalisability (Yin 2003). The study examples mentioned already demonstrate the breadth of strategies available with this approach. Several of the mentioned studies are illustrated in the following 'Research in brief' boxes.

Research in brief

Yoshioka-Maeda et al. (2006) explored the tacit (implicit experiential) knowledge and skills of nine experienced public health nurses in Japan. Seven common approaches used by the cases were identified, and a model was constructed for identifying community needs and developing new services to meet those needs. The mixed-method profile of the study is reflected by both qualitative elements (i.e. theoretical sampling and confirmability of interview transcripts with a third interview) and quantitative elements (i.e. multiple case studies to improve reliability and validity and a protocol to standardise data collection). The case study approach enabled exploration of the sample nurses' informal undocumented knowledge of their work.

Q methodology

Q methodology uses a unique set of processes to reveal subjective attitudes and perspectives of participants about a particular topic (Brown 1996). A set of stimulus material (i.e. textual statements, pictures or recordings) amenable to appraisal are constructed — usually from prior interviews, to form the Q sample. Statements in the Q sample are representative, but not exhaustive, of the diversity of attitudes possible about the topic. Once the set of statements has been verified and finalised, each statement or material is placed on an individual card to enable the cards to be sorted into some order. Participants are instructed how to rank-order the set of Q sample statements or materials. This is referred to as the Q-sort technique. Ranking commonly follows a Likert Scale format (see Chapter 12); for example, from strongly agree to strongly disagree, using a quasi-normal distribution (Ryan & Zerwic 2004). That is, least cards are able to be assigned scores at the ends of the scale, while proportionally more can be located in the middle of the distribution.

Point to ponder

▶ Q methodology applies quantitative analysis to qualitatively derived data.

Figure 15.2 illustrates a hypothetical example for a 36-item Q sample, with an 11-point Likert Scale, from strongly disagree (−5) to strongly agree (+5). One card is placed per cell on the Q-sort diagram. In this example, only one card can be placed in the +5 location, while four statements can be located at −2,

FIGURE 15.2 Q-sort diagram

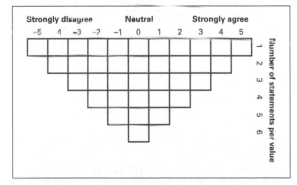

The resulting order of material is then analysed using quantitative techniques to produce correlational matrices and factor analysis solutions (see Chapter 13). The use of factor analysis enables the statements to be collated into factors for clearer interpretation (see the following 'Research in brief' box).

Research in brief

Ryan and Zerwic (2004) explored a cluster of symptoms that high-risk individuals and their significant others associate with an acute myocardial infarction (AMI). The Q sample statements were sourced from 141 transcripts of patients describing their actual AMI symptoms. A series of validation steps with patients and clinicians resulted in a set of 49 statements. Participants ($n = 63$) ranked the statements into 11 piles that ranged from 'most like a heart attack' to 'least like a heart attack'. A correlation matrix of the Q-sorts was constructed and a factor analysis applied. A four-factor solution accounted for 36% of the variance — where the factors were 'traditional symptoms', 'symptoms attributed to GI causes', 'non-specific symptoms', and 'variation on traditional symptoms.' A –5 to +5 Likert Scale (11 points), with a quasi-normal distribution, directed the participants in their Q-sort. The study demonstrated varied expectations regarding AMI symptoms, and the authors linked this finding to implications for practice, as the need for education to include differences in actual symptoms experienced by different demographic groups.

This approach has been used to examine a variety of clinical issues — although none could be found which incorporated specific midwifery elements. For example:

- decision-making of clinical nurses in caring for patients with an acute myocardial infarction (Bakalis et al. 2003)
- the attitudes of emergency department nurses to health promotion (Cross 2005)
- perceptions of caring behaviour by nurses from patients' and nurses' perspectives (Gardner et al. 2001)
- family care giving by women and the issue of non-support (Neufeld et al. 2004).

T_T Tutorial trigger 5

You or your study group is to present the steps involved in a Q methodology study, using a published paper to illustrate the concepts. Access two published Q methodology papers and identify the common steps undertaken. Provide a one-paragraph general description, with an accompanying example.

Summary

The value and contribution of mixed-methods research, to nursing and midwifery practice, is beyond question. Many researchers, with any understanding of mixed methods and triangulation techniques, will be able to appreciate the benefits of expanding research intentions and outcomes, to accommodate a range of paradigmatic approaches and methods. While researchers need to be aware that mixed-method research brings with it a unique series of challenges, it is argued that the benefits far outweigh the dilemmas. This is particularly in relation to higher likelihood of comprehensiveness, completeness and changes in practice. In bringing together the paradigms of both qualitative and quantitative research, this chapter 'completes the paradigmatic circle'.

Ⓚ EY POINTS

- Mixed-methods research is rapidly gaining recognition and approval in nursing and midwifery. Method triangulation/mixed-methods research combines methods, paradigms, and the approaches of qualitative and quantitative research — whereby triangulation of methods and data sources enable a broader and more comprehensive picture to emerge about the research topic.

- Action research is a useful method to use when researchers want to understand and improve a situation, as it is action-focused and context-specific, and therefore can address problems of practical concern. Action research uses a cyclical process in which the research, implementation, evaluation and theorising are linked to reduce the theory–practice gap.

- Delphi studies seek to gain expert consensus when there is little empirical evidence or understanding of a health-related issue, and typically combine qualitative and quantitative data from a series of questionnaire rounds.

- A case study approach enables a detailed examination of a single 'case' or 'unit' within a real-life setting. The 'case' can be an individual, social group, community, organisation, or event. Q methodology combines interview (qualitative) data to form statements about the topic of interest, which are then rank-ordered to produce quantitative data.

Learning activities

1. The main value of using mixed-methods research in nursing is it:
   (a) allows the researcher to understand a wider range of research methods
   (b) helps researchers champion particular research paradigms
   (c) offers a higher probability that the conducted research will be viewed as complete and comprehensive
   (d) assists in reducing research error.

2. Data triangulation involves:
   (a) prioritising data into discrete groups in a single study
   (b) using a variety of data sources in a single study
   (c) differentiating between data sources in a single study
   (d) using specific data sources in a single study.

3. A mixed-methods research study that sought to initially identify the lived health-related experiences of a group of patients and follow this up by using a tool to measure the extent of those health-related experiences, would be using which of the following combinations:

   (a) simultaneous — qualitative and quantitative
   (b) simultaneous — quantitative and qualitative
   (c) sequential — quantitative leading to qualitative
   (d) sequential — qualitative leading to quantitative.

4. Conventional Delphi studies have the following properties:
   (a) use experts, quantitative first-round, qualitative second-round, consensus
   (b) use clients, qualitative first-round, quantitative second-round, consensus
   (c) use experts, qualitative first-round, quantitative second-round, consensus
   (d) use clients, qualitative first-round, quantitative second-round, non-consensus.

5. With the Delphi technique, how many questionnaire rounds are most likely to occur:
   (a) 1
   (b) 2
   (c) 3
   (d) 4.

6. The main features of action research are:
   (a) mixed methods, participation, randomisation, change cycles
   (b) mixed methods, change cycles, participation, empowerment
   (c) participation, mixed methods, empowerment, organisational
   (d) change cycles, socio-community, mixed methods, empowerment.

7. An action research cycle or spiral would typically contain the stages:
   (a) diagnosis, data collection and analysis, feedback, actioning, reflection and evaluation, and further change cycles
   (b) diagnosis, evaluation, feedback, actioning, and further change cycles
   (c) diagnosis, data collection and analysis, feedback, actioning, reflection and evaluation
   (d) diagnosis, data collection and analysis, feedback, reflection and evaluation, and further change cycles.

8. Action research studies mainly focus on one of two broad areas. These being:
   (a) organisational development/ operational development
   (b) organisational development/ community development
   (c) procedural development/community development
   (d) organisational development/ procedural development.

9. With a case study, the phenomenon of interest can be:
   (a) an individual/s, a group or community, a conference, a process, an event
   (b) an individual/s, a nation, an organisation, a process, an event
   (c) an individual/s, a culture, an organisation, a process, an event
   (d) an individual/s, a group or community, an organisation, a process, an event.

10. With Q methodology, participants are instructed how to rank-order the set of Q sample statements or materials. This process is called the:
    (a) Q-filter technique
    (b) Q-sort technique
    (c) Q-sieve technique
    (d) Q-sift technique.

Additional resources

Badger T G 2000 Action research, change and methodological rigor. *Journal of Nursing Management* 8:201–7

Creswell J, Plano-Clark V 2006 *Designing and conducting mixed-methods research*. Sage Publications, Thousand Oaks, California

Crisp J, Pelletier D, Duffield C, et al. 1999 It's all in a name: when is a 'Delphi study' not a Delphi study? *Australian Journal of Advanced Nursing* 16:32–7

Keeney S, Hasson F, McKenna H 2006 Consulting the oracle: ten lessons from using the Delphi technique in nursing research. *Journal of Advanced Nursing* 53:205–12

Lax W, Galvin K 2002 Reflections on a community action research project: interprofessional issues and methodological problems. *Journal of Clinical Nursing* 11:376–86

Thurmond V A 2001 The point of triangulation. *Journal of Nursing Scholarship* 33:253–8

Williamson G R 2005 Illustrating triangulation in mixed-methods nursing research. *Nurse Researcher* 12:7–17

Yin R K 2003 *Case Study Research* (3rd edn). Sage Publications, Thousand Oaks, California

References

Adami MF, Kiger A 2005 The use of triangulation for completeness purposes. *Nurse Researcher* 12:19–29

Annells M 2007 What's common with qualitative research these days? (guest editorial). *Journal of Clinical Nursing* 16(2):223–4

—— 2006 Triangulation of qualitative approaches: hermeneutical phenomenology and grounded theory. *Journal of Advanced Nursing* 56:55–61

Annells M, DeRoche M, Koch T, et al. 2005 A Delphi study of district nursing research priorities in Australia. *Applied Nursing Research* 18:36–43

Bakalis N, Bowman G S, Porock D 2003 Decision making in Greek and English registered nurses in coronary care units. *International Journal of Nursing Studies* 40:749–60

Bergen A, While A 2000 A case for case studies: exploring the use of case study design in community nursing research. *Journal of Advanced Nursing* 31:926–34

Bowles N 1999 The Delphi technique. *Nursing Standard* 13:32–6

Brown S R 1996 Q methodology and qualitative research. *Qualitative Health Research* 6:561–7

Campbell S M, Cantrell J A 2001 Consensus methods in prescribing research. *Journal of Clinical Pharmacy and Therapeutics* 26:5–14

Choudhry UK, Jandu S, Mahal J, et al. 2002 Health promotion and participatory action research with South Asian women. *Journal of Nursing Scholarship* 34:75–81

Cooke H (in press) The surveillance of nursing standards: an organisational case study. *International Journal of Nursing Studies*

Cowman S 1993 Triangulation: a means of reconciliation in nursing research. *Journal of Advanced Nursing* 18:788–92

Cross R 2005 Accident and emergency nurses' attitudes towards health promotion. *Journal of Advanced Nursing* 51:474–83

Deery R 2005 An action research study exploring midwives' support needs and the affect of group clinical supervision. *Midwifery* 21:161–76

Denzin N K 1978 *The research act: a theoretical introduction to sociological methods*, 2nd edn. McGraw-Hill, New York

Fenwick J, Butt J, Downie J, Monterosso L, Wood J 2006 Priorities for midwifery research in Perth, Western Australia: a Delphi study. *International Journal of Nursing Practice* 12:78–93

Fitzgerald L 1999 Case studies as a research tool. *Quality in Health Care* 8:75

Foss C, Ellefsen B 2002 The value of combining qualitative and quantitative approaches in nursing research by means of method triangulation. *Journal of Advanced Nursing* 40:242–8

Fullerton J, Fort A, Johal K 2003 A case/comparison study in the Eastern Region of Ghana on the effects of incorporating selected reproductive health services on family planning services. *Midwifery* 19:17–26

Gardner A, Goodsell J, Duggan T, et al. 2001 'Don't call me sweetie!': patients differ from nurses in their perceptions of caring. *Collegian* 8:32–8

Gardner G, Carryer J, Gardner A, et al. 2006 Nurse practitioner competency standards: findings from collaborative Australian and New Zealand research. *International Journal of Nursing Studies* 43, 601–10

Gardner G, Gardner A, MacLellan L, et al. 2003 Reconceptualising the objectives of a pilot study for clinical research. *International Journal of Nursing Studies* 40:719–24

Garwick AW, Auger S 2003 Participatory action research: the Indian family stories project. *Nursing Outlook* 51:161–6

Glasson J, Chang E, Chenoweth L, et al. 2006 Evaluation of a model of nursing care for older patients using participatory action research in an acute medical ward. *Journal of Clinical Nursing* 15:588–98

Green L, Daniel M, Norvick L 2001 Partnerships and coalitions for community-based research. *Public Health Reports* 116:20–31

Hasson F, Keeney S, McKenna H 2000 Research guidelines for the Delphi survey technique. *Journal of Advanced Nursing* 32:1008–15

Hegney D, Plank A, Parker V 2003 Nursing workloads: the results of a study of Queensland nurses. *Journal of Nursing Management* 11:307–14

Henderson A 2005 The value of integrating interpretive research approaches in the exposition of healthcare context. *Journal of Advanced Nursing* 52:554–60

Hewitt-Taylor J 2002 Case study: an approach to qualitative enquiry. *Nursing Standard* 16:33–7

Holkup P A, Tripp-Reimer T, Salois E M, et al. 2004 Community-based participatory research: an approach to intervention research with a Native American community. *Advances in Nursing Science* 27:162–75

Hotham E D, Gilbert A L, Atkinson E R 2005 Case studies of three pregnant smokers and their use of nicotine replacement therapy. *Midwifery* 21:224–32

Janesick V J 1994 The dance of qualitative research design: metaphor, methodolatory, and meaning. In Denzin N K & Lincoln Y S (eds) *Handbook of qualitative research*. Sage Publications, Thousand Oaks, California

Johnstone P L 2004 Mixed-methods, mixed methodology health services research in practice. *Qualitative Health Research* 14:259–71

Jones A, Bugge C 2006 Improving understanding and rigour through triangulation: an exemplar on patient participation in interaction. *Journal of Advanced Nursing* 55:612–21

Karim K 2001 Assessing the strengths and weaknesses of action research. *Nursing Standard* 15:33–35

Keeney S, Hasson F, McKenna H 2006 Consulting the oracle: ten lessons from using the Delphi technique in nursing research. *Journal of Advanced Nursing* 53:205–12

Kelly D, Simpson S 2001 Action research in action: reflections on a project to introduce clinical practice facilitators to an acute hospital setting. *Journal of Advanced Nursing* 33:652–9

Kennedy H P 2004 Enhancing Delphi research: methods and results. *Journal of Advanced Nursing* 45:504–11

Keyzer D M 2000 Nursing research in practice: the case study revisited. *Australian Journal of Rural Health* 8:266–80

Koch T, Rolfe G, Kralik D 2005 Core elements of programmatic research in nursing: a case study. *Collegian* 12:7–12

Lewin K 1946 Action research and minority problems. *Journal of Social Issues* 2(4):34–46

—— 1951 *Field theory in social science*. Harper, New York

Löfman P, Pelkonen M, Pietila A-M 2004 Ethical issues in participatory action research. *Scandinavian Journal of Caring Sciences* 18:333–40

Löfmark A, Thorell-Ekstrand I 2004 An assessment form for clinical nursing education: a Delphi study. *Journal of Advanced Nursing* 48:291–8

Lukkarinen H 2005 Methodological triangulation showed the poorest quality of life in the youngest people following treatment of coronary artery disease: a longitudinal study. *International Journal of Nursing Studies* 42:619–27

Maggs-Rapport F 2000 Combining methodological approaches in research: ethnography and interpretive phenomenology. *Journal of Advanced Nursing* 31:219–25

Marsden J, Dolan B, Holt L 2003 Nurse practitioner practice and deployment: electronic mail Delphi study. *Journal of Advanced Nursing* 43:595–605

McKellar L V, Pincombe J I, Henderson A M 2006 Insights from Australian parents into educational experiences in the early postnatal period. *Midwifery* 22:356–64

McKenna H, Hasson F, Smith M 2002 A Delphi survey of midwives and midwifery students to identify non-midwifery duties. *Midwifery* 18:314–22

Mead D, Moseley L 2001 The use of Delphi as a research approach. *Nurse Researcher* 8(4):4–23

Miller S I, Fredericks M 2006 Mixed-methods and evaluation research: trends and issues. *Qualitative Health Research* 16:567–79

Morse J M 1991 Approaches to qualitative–quantitative methodological triangulation. *Nurse Researcher* 40:120–3

—— 2005 Evolving trends in qualitative research: advances in mixed-method design [editorial]. *Qualitative Health Research* 15:583–5

National Health and Medical Research Council (NHMRC) 2000 How to use the evidence: assessment and application of scientific evidence. NHMRC, Canberra

Neufeld A, Harrison M J, Rempel G R, et al. 2004 Practical issues in using a card sort in a study of nonsupport and family caregiving. *Qualitative Health Research* 14:1418–28

Nojima Y, Tomikawa T, Makabe S, et al. 2003 Defining characteristics of expertise in Japanese clinical nursing using the Delphi technique. *Nursing and Health Sciences* 5:3–11

Parsons M L, Warner-Robbins C 2002 Formerly incarcerated women create healthy lives through participatory action research. *Holistic Nursing Practice* 16:40–9

Powell C 2003 The Delphi technique: myths and realities. *Journal of Advanced Nursing* 41:376–82

Reed J 2005 Using action research in nursing practice with older people: democratizing knowledge. *Journal of Clinical Nursing* 14:594–600

Risjord M W, Dunbar S B, Moloney M F 2002 A new foundation for methodological triangulation. *Journal of Nursing Scholarship* 34(3):269–75

Rodger M, Hills J, Kristjanson L 2004 A Delphi study on research priorities for emergency nurses in Western Australia. *Journal of Emergency Nursing* 30:117–25

Ryan C J, Zerwic J J 2004 Knowledge of symptom clusters among adults at risk for acute myocardial infarction. *Nursing Research* 53:363–9

Schofield I, Knussen C, Tolson D 2006 A mixed-method study to compare use and experience of hospital and a nurse-led acute respiratory assessment service offering home care to people with an acute exacerbation of chronic obstructive pulmonary disease. *International Journal of Nursing Studies* 43:465–76

Schroyen B, Finlayson M 2004 Clinical teaching and learning: an action research study. *Nursing Praxis in New Zealand* 20:36–45

Shih S-N, Gau M-L, Kao C-H, et al. 2005 Health needs instrument for hospitalized single-living Taiwanese elders with heart disease: triangulation research design. *Journal of Clinical Nursing* 14:1210–22

St Leger A S, Walsworth-Bell J P 1999 *Change-Promoting Research for Health Services*. Open University Press, Buckingham, UK

Symon A G, McStea B, Murphy-Black T 2006 An exploratory mixed-methods study of Scottish midwives' understandings and perceptions of clinical near misses in maternity care. *Midwifery* 22:125–36

van Loon A M, Koch T, Kralik D 2004 Care for female survivors of child sexual abuse in emergency departments. *Accident and Emergency Nursing* 12:208–14

Walters S, East L 2001 The cycle of homelessness in the lives of young mothers: the diagnostic phase of an action research project. *Journal of Clinical Nursing* 10:171–9

Waterman H, Harker R, MacDonald H, et al. 2005 Advancing ophthalmic nursing practice through action research. *Journal of Advanced Nursing* 52:281–90

Whitehead D 2005 Project management and action research: two sides of the same coin? *Journal of Health Organization and Management* 19:519–31

Whitehead D, Keast J, Montgomery V, et al. 2004 A preventative health education programme for osteoporosis. *Journal of Advanced Nursing* 47:15–24

Whitehead D, Taket A, Smith P 2003 Action research in health promotion. *Health Education Journal* 62:5–22

Williams G, Clarke T 2001 A consensus driven method to measure the required number of intensive care nurses in Australia. *Australian Critical Care* 14:106–15

Williamson G R, Prosser S 2002 Action research: politics, ethics and participation. *Journal of Advanced Nursing* 40:587–93

Williamson G R 2005 Illustrating triangulation in mixed-methods nursing research. *Nurse Researcher* 12:7–17

Yin R K 2003 *Case Study Research* (3rd edn). Sage Publications, Thousand Oaks, California

Yoshioka-Maeda K, Murashima S, Asahara K 2006 Tacit knowledge of public health nurses in identifying community health problems and need for new services: a case study. *International Journal of Nursing Studies* 43:819–26

Answers

TT Tutorial trigger 1

Effects for nursing and midwifery	Effects for medicine
Building up an expertise in qualitative research.	Continued research dominance.
More able to align qualitative principles and philosophies with caring i.e. patients feelings, experiences, perceptions etc.	Quantitative methods support curative, reactive and biomedical principles.
	Dominant share of research funding.
	Greater claim to valid research credibility, testing and measurement.

Effects against nursing and midwifery	Effects against medicine
Continuing division between medicine and nursing/midwifery — lack of research collaboration.	Continuing division between nursing/midwifery and medicine — lack of research collaboration.
Accusations of residing within the 'weaker' paradigm — issues of research rigour, credibility, validity and efficacy.	
Less likely to secure large-scale funding for qualitative research.	

TT Tutorial trigger 2

1. What research has previously been conducted in the topic area — and how much of it is qualitative, how much quantitative?
2. Has mixed-methods research been used previously in the topic area? If so what type and combination?
3. What does the research need to do? What types of outcomes are required?
4. With mixed-methods approaches, would it be best if quantitative outcomes firstly informed followed by expanding qualitative investigation, or vice versa?
5. With mixed methods, what differing tools are required for collecting and analysing the data?

TT Tutorial trigger 3

1. Professional/methodological protectionism.
2. Traditional schooling, experience or expertise in just one or a few research approaches/methods.
3. The need to become conversant with a wider range of research theories and approaches.
4. Reluctance to move away from the security of the major opinion or current trend in research methodology.
5. Increased complexity that accompanies mixed-methods research.
6. More limited chance of securing large-scale funding.

TT Tutorial trigger 4

1. The teenagers themselves.
2. Their sexual partners.
3. The teenagers' families and relatives.
4. Various local and/or national youth organisations.
5. Sexual health organisations and health services (acute and community-based; nursing and midwifery).
6. Local/national sexual health policy-makers.
7. Media promoting positive sexual health.
8. The wider community.

Learning activities

1. c	**2.** b	**3.** d	**4.** c
5. b	**6.** b	**7.** a	**8.** b
9. d	**10.** b		

Critical evaluation
of research

ZEVIA SCHNEIDER

Learning outcomes

After reading this chapter, you should be able to:

- identify the reasons why it is necessary to critically analyse studies
- list the criteria used to review qualitative studies
- list the criteria used to review quantitative studies
- identify the strengths and weaknesses of a research report
- discuss the implications of the findings of a research report for nursing and midwifery practice.

Introduction

This chapter is designed to introduce you to the critical review guidelines for qualitative and quantitative studies and the stages of *understanding* relating to critical reading. The critique or critical review is the process of objectively, critically analysing a research report's content for scientific merit and application to practice or theory. It requires some knowledge of the subject matter, knowledge of how to read critically, and how to interpret appropriate criteria. It is above all a lucid and stringent cognitive process requiring a basic understanding of the research process and relevant terminology. The critical review guidelines provide a structured approach with specific information to facilitate reading research articles.

Two research articles, namely, a qualitative approach by Arthur et al. (2005), and a quantitative design by Middleton et al. (2005), presented in full in this chapter, will be analysed using the critical review criteria for each approach. Criteria necessary to adequately review an article are any measures, standards, evaluation guides or questions used to judge (critique) a product or behaviour. The reader, in analysing a research report, must evaluate each step of the research process and ask questions about whether the explanation of each step of the process meets or does not meet these criteria. For instance, one of the objectives of a literature review is to determine gaps, consistencies and inconsistencies in the literature about a subject, concept or problem. One question to guide the reviewer is, 'What gaps or conflicts in knowledge about the problem are identified and how does this study intend to fill those gaps?' Search strategies for accessing the relevant articles are explained in Chapter 3. Once articles have been selected and acquired, the process of review begins.

Critical reading

Reading contributes to the growth of consciousness. Through reading, recognition and understanding of previous unfamiliar concepts and steps of the research process gradually become increasingly clearer and more accurate and facilitate the next stage, which is to read critically. Critical reading has been described as 'an active, intellectually engaging process in which the reader participates in an inner dialogue with the writer' (Paul & Elder 2001). A critical reader therefore actively looks for assumptions, key concepts and ideas, reasons and justifications, supporting examples, parallel experiences, implications and consequences in the written text (Paul & Elder 2003). Critical reading involves making a judgment about the content of an article; that is, how the evidence provided is used and interpreted.

A critical reading of research articles requires the reader to assess how the author's purpose is developed and argued. Critical reading is difficult for the beginning research consumer and may be somewhat frustrating at first. To accomplish the purpose of critically reading a research study, the reader must have skilled reading, writing and reasoning abilities. These skills are experiential and cumulative — the

more practice and experience, the higher the skill level. It is quite common for a research article to require several readings. A minimum of three or four readings, with a research textbook by your side, facilitate an effective review and are necessary to do the following (Paul & Elder 2003):

- identify concepts
- clarify unfamiliar concepts or terms
- question assumptions and rationale
- determine supporting evidence.

No matter how difficult it may seem, read the entire article and reflect on it. Critically read for the *levels of understanding* described below. Most importantly, draw on previous knowledge, common sense and the critical thinking skills you already possess.

- Preliminary understanding is gained through a light reading.
- Comprehensive understanding relates to a recognition of relationships between different parts.
- Analysis understanding involves breaking the content into parts to facilitate processing the information.
- Synthesis understanding requires joining the parts to make a comprehensive whole.

Preliminary understanding

Preliminary understanding is gained by quickly or lightly reading an article to familiarise yourself with its content and to get a general sense of the material: the title and abstract are read carefully but the content is skimmed. Skimming includes reading the introduction, major headings, one or two sentences under the heading and the summary or conclusion.

Research in brief

When reading the article by Dunning and Manias (2004), it is important to know that structured in-depth interviews and observations of respondents performing medication self-management/help practices (including being able to open medicine packages, breaking tablets in half, administering insulin, and monitoring blood glucose levels), were used as a means of eliciting, first hand, medication knowledge and self-management practices of people with type 2 diabetes.

Some strategies for reading and evaluating a research report appear in Box 16.1.

Comprehensive understanding: content in relation to context

The purpose of comprehensive understanding is to understand the article — to see the terms in relation to the context or the parts of the study in relation to the whole article; the reader should be able to identify core concepts and themes. Reading for comprehension requires an understanding of the terminology and being able to state the main idea in your own words.

Analysis understanding: breaking into parts

The purpose of reading for analysis is to break the content into parts in order to understand each aspect of the study, and ultimately, a deeper understanding of the content. Some of the questions to ask during analysis of the research article include:

- Can the main idea or theme of this article be captured in one or two sentences?

BOX 16.1 Highlights of critical thinking and reading strategies

1. Read primary research articles from refereed journals.
2. Read secondary research (critique/response/commentary) articles from refereed journals.
3. Obtain primary and secondary articles (photocopy or print copies) and make notations directly on the copy.
4. While reading articles:
   - keep a research text and a dictionary by your side
   - list key variables at the top of the article
   - highlight or underline new terms, unfamiliar vocabulary and significant sentences
   - look up the definitions of new terms and write them on the article copy
   - review old and new terms before subsequent readings
   - highlight or underline identified steps of the research process
   - identify the main idea or theme of the article — state it in your own words in one or two sentences
   - continue to clarify terms that may be unclear on subsequent readings
   - make sure you understand the main points of each reported step of the research process you identified before you critique the article.
5. Determine how well the study meets the criteria:
   - ask fellow students to analyse the same study using the same criteria and compare results
   - consult faculty members about your evaluation of the study.
6. Type a one-page summary and critical review of each study:
   - cite bibliographical information of the reference at the top of the summary according to relevant reference style (e.g. APA, Harvard, Vancouver)
   - briefly summarise each reported research step in your own words
   - briefly describe strengths and weaknesses in your own words (bibliographical databases allow you to write a narrative for each paper reviewed).

- How are the major parts of this article organised in relation to the research process?
- What is the purpose of this article?
- How was this study carried out? Can it be explained step by step?
- What are the main conclusions of the author(s)?
- Is each section understood and can it be summarised or paraphrased into your own words?

In a sense you are determining how the steps of the research process are presented or organised in the article and what the content related to each step is all about. You are beginning the process of critically analysing the merit of the study. It may require some knowledge of the subject matter, but knowledge of how to critically read is the most important consideration.

Synthesis understanding

Synthesis involves combining parts into a complex whole. The purpose of reading for synthesis is to make sense of the whole. It is during this final step that you decide how well the study meets the criteria, its contribution to nursing and/or midwifery and how useful it is in practice.

Reading for synthesis is facilitated by the following strategies.

- reviewing your notes on the article on how each step of the research process measures up against the established criteria
- briefly summarising the study in your own words: the components of the study and the overall strengths and weaknesses
- limit your summary to one page, including the citation at the top of the page in the specified reference style, and staple the summary to the photocopied article.

Points to ponder

▶ Read whole sentences to gain an overall understanding of the idea/content before concentrating on single words.

▶ Practise expressing ideas/concepts in the text in your own words.

▶ Your ability to summarise text content indicates understanding of the concepts.

Consumer perspective

Nurses, midwives and other health professionals have long recognised the importance of utilising research on which to base their practice. Evidence-informed practice is a key factor in contributing to accountability and benchmarking by providing answers and evidence to questions about current and traditional practices and processes. Furthermore, evidence-based practice should be viewed as a quality improvement process (Pravikoff et al. 2005). Not all nurses and midwives are committed to conducting research and some may think that they therefore do not have to read and analyse the literature. Being able to critically read and understand research articles is different from conducting research and remains crucial to the improvement of patient care, management and administration.

DiCenso et al. (2004) define evidence-based nursing as 'the process by which nurses make clinical decisions using the best available research evidence, their clinical expertise and patient preferences and values, in the context of available resources'. The same concepts and contexts apply to midwifery-orientated evidence-based practice (evidence-based midwifery). In fact, Webster et al. (1999), in their Royal Women's Hospital Brisbane study, invited both midwives and gynaecology

Research in brief

Campbell and Torrance (2005) conducted a descriptive survey to explore self-reported changes in coronary risk factors in a group of self-selected patients 3 to 9 months following coronary artery angioplasty. The data collection tool was a questionnaire designed to elicit the perceptions, knowledge and experiences of patients undergoing percutaneous transluminal coronary angioplasty (PTCA). Of a total of 560 questionnaires, 41.7% were returned representing a fair response rate. Although generalisation is limited because of the sample being self-selected, important issues about lifestyle and life-promoting behaviours were identified for clinical practice.

nurses to participate in their Evidence-Based Practice Project. Their intention here was to evaluate and improve the overall quality of services, through translating research findings to develop practice guidelines (see Chapter 18). Clearly, the concept of evidence-based practice is concerned with patient inclusivity in decision-making, accountability, using the best available information for improving patient care, and benchmarking through a critical evaluation of the evidence (see Chapter 17). The requirement that all health professionals engage in critical reading, to enhance their understanding of the research process and the format of research articles, becomes clear.

TT Tutorial trigger 1

Describe the levels or stages of *understandings* involved in reading critically.

Critical review of qualitative research studies

A careful reading of the qualitative approaches in Chapters 7, 8 and 9 will highlight issues of data collection, analysis, interpretation and rigour in these approaches. In general, a critique of qualitative research studies includes:

1. identifying the phenomenon
2. structuring the study
3. gathering the data
4. analysing the data
5. describing the findings.

Notwithstanding the difference in terminology, qualitative studies require a different kind of critical analysis from quantitative designs. Suggestions for critique appear in Box 16.2.

Points to ponder

▶ While qualitative research findings may be specific to particular patients, the information contributes to understanding the phenomenon and to nursing's and midwifery's knowledge base.

▶ Qualitative research findings can be used to generate nursing and midwifery interventions; interventions can then be tested in practice.

Evidence-based practice tip

In-depth interviewing is a qualitative data-gathering technique that permits exploration of a person's feelings, ideas and thoughts. The interview or conversation is a strategy for creating knowledge.

Research in brief

Fenwick et al. (2004) explored the labour and birth expectations of a cohort of Western Australian women in order to identify the factors that influence these expectations; 202 women who were pregnant or birthed within the last 12 months self-selected to participate in the study. A qualitative, exploratory descriptive design was used to collect data through telephone interviews. Selection effects are a problem and introduce bias in studies in which individuals themselves decide whether to participate. Some advantages of a telephone interview are that the researcher knows who is giving the answers and this helps to ensure data are reliable. If interpretation of data match what has been recorded in the interview, validity becomes a question of credibility. While not generalisable, the findings that some women are anxious and frightened of the childbirth experience are strongly supported by the literature.

Introduction to critical reviews

The article 'A primary healthcare curriculum in action: The lived experience of primary healthcare nurses in a school of nursing in the Philippines: A phenomenological study' (Arthur et al. 2005) is critically reviewed for its design and contribution to healthcare and nursing knowledge. The critical review guidelines appear in Box 16.2.

Title and abstract

The title identifies the participants, their domicile and the nature of their work; that is, primary healthcare (PHC) nurses, and the research approach. The abstract provides the motivation for the study; that is, primary healthcare is practised widely in the Philippines yet little has been published by the practitioners

BOX 16.2 Critical review guidelines for qualitative studies

Title and abstract
1. Is the title of the research paper congruent with the text?
2. Were the aims and/or objectives stated? What are they?
3. Did the abstract contain sufficient information about the stages of the research process (e.g. aims, research approach, participants, data collection, data analysis, findings)?

Identifying the phenomenon
1. Is the phenomenon focused on human experience within a natural setting?
2. Is the phenomenon relevant to nursing, midwifery and/or health?

Structuring the study
1. Is it clear that the selected participants are living the phenomenon of interest?
2. How is published literature used in the study?
3. Does the question identify the context (participant/group/place) of the method to be followed?
4. Is the theoretical framework clearly stated?
5. Does the theoretical framework fit the research question?
6. Is the method of data collection and analysis clearly specified?
7. Does the qualitative method of data collection chosen fit the research question (e.g. grounded theory, ethnography)?
8. Are the limitations of the study stated?

Research question and design
1. Was the research question determined by the need for the study? How was this determination made?
2. Are the data collection strategies appropriate for the research question?
3. Do the data collection strategies reflect the purpose and theoretical framework of the study (e.g. in-depth interviewing, focus groups)?

4. Can the data analysis strategy be identified and logically followed?

Participants
1. How were the participants and setting selected (e.g. sampling strategies)?
2. How was confidentiality of the participants assured?
3. How was the anonymity of participants assured?
4. What ethical issues were identified in the study?
5. How were the ethical issues addressed?

Data analyses
1. How were the data analysed?
2. Is the analysis technique congruent with the research question?
3. Is there evidence that the researcher's interpretation captured the participants' meaning?
4. Did the researcher say how the criteria for judging the scientific rigour of the study were maintained in terms of credibility, auditability, fittingness and confirmability?

Describing the findings
1. Does the researcher demonstrate to the reader the method (e.g. audit trial) by which the data were analysed?
2. Does the researcher indicate how the findings are related to theory?
3. Is there a link between the findings to existing theory or literature, or is a new theory generated?

Researcher's perspective
1. Are the biases of the researcher reported (e.g. researcher/participant expectations, researcher bias (objectivity/subjectivity) and power imbalance)?
2. Are the limitations of the study acknowledged?
3. Are recommendations suggested for further research?
4. Are implications for healthcare mentioned?

themselves or about the work they do. A PHC curriculum and the experiences of nurses working as faculty and also providing service to the local community are described. Specified are type of sample and methods of data collection and data analysis. Findings are stated with recommendations for future research.

Identifying the phenomenon/ phenomena of interest

Three phenomena within the context of the lived experience of PHC nurses are examined: (1) the experiences of faculty in two universities in the Philippines, engaged in PHC nursing;

(2) a description of a PHC curriculum that they implemented; and (3) the environment in which the program operates.

The nurses were practising PHC in a natural setting; that is, their community and homeland. Primary healthcare has the potential to empower patients through understanding and knowledge of their own health and that of their families and communities. For this reason it is important and highly relevant to healthcare practitioners.

Structuring the study

The motivation for the study is the perceived lack of published information about PHC nurses and their practices. Research previously undertaken (Chalmers et al. 1997; Simpson et al. 2002; Twinn 2001) was region specific and therefore not generalisable to other communities. The present study fills a gap in the literature regarding PHC practices in the Philippines. Limitations are indicated by reference to similar studies which the authors consider unique with findings appropriate only to the particular people and locality in which the studies were conducted.

The research question and design

Motivation for the study was made explicit; that is, the paucity of studies on PHC practice.

The research approach best suited to examine the lived experience of PHC nurses in this study is through in-depth interviewing and the phenomenological approach (see Chapter 7).

The participants

Purposeful sampling was used to recruit five registered nurse participants from the College of Nursing at Silliman University, experienced in the provision of PHC nursing in a region of the Philippines. No information is provided about a plain language statement, consent forms or how confidentiality was assured, or that the participants could withdraw from the study without prejudice. There is no indication that the study was submitted to a human research ethics committee (HREC). It is simply reported that faculty, local village leaders, and members of a management committee met to 'identify problems, plan strategies and implement action' (p 108).

Data collection

In-depth interviews were used to collect information about the nurses' personal and professional experiences. Participants were asked to respond to the question: 'Tell me about the PHC activities in the school?' Prompts were used to encourage conversation and judgment was suspended; that is, the interviewer keeps an open mind to new unexpected phenomena, rather than having preconceived concepts and interpretations (Kvale 1996). Notes were taken during the interview, transcribed and returned to the participants for verification.

Data analysis

Data were analysed using Huserrlian (descriptive) phenomenology and Colaizzi's method of data analysis. One hundred and two meanings were organised first into themes then into four theme clusters: *teaching PHC*; *external influences*; *the working reality*; and *practising PHC*. Little information is provided about how the statements were 'formulated'. An important omission is the lack of evidence for judging the scientific rigour of the study (e.g. credibility, fittingness).

Describing the findings

The four theme clusters are described with exemplars from the interviews. *Teaching PHC* included education issues experienced by both faculty and students; *External influences* referred to government policies and services with which PHC interacts; *Working reality* related to working with people in the community and the constraints experienced, and *Practising PHC* referred to the experiences of faculty and students working in the field.

Discussion

The discussion draws on previous literature from Canada and Hong Kong about PHC practice and highlights commonalities in the Philippines situation. Recommendations are: testing some of the interventions explained in the four themes, for example, the effectiveness of herbal remedies; replicating the Chalmers et al. (1997) PHC Questionnaire to contrast student profiles with those of a Canadian sample; and a further in-depth qualitative examination of the Philippines communities to gain a deeper understanding of PHC in this region.

Available online at www.sciencedirect.com

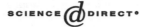

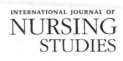

INTERNATIONAL JOURNAL OF
NURSING
STUDIES

International Journal of Nursing Studies 43 (2006) 107–112

www.elsevier.com/locate/ijnurstu

A primary health care curriculum in action: The lived experience of primary health care nurses in a school of nursing in the Philippines: A phenomenological study

David Arthur[a],*, John Drury[b], Maria Teresita Sy-Sinda[c], Ramonita Nakao[c], Arsenia Lopez[c], Grace Gloria[c], Rowena Turtal[c], Evelyn Luna[c]

[a]*The School of Nursing, The Hong Kong Polytechnic University, Hung Hom, Kowloon, Hong Kong*
[b]*The School of Nursing Edith Cowan University, Perth, Western Australia*
[c]*The College of Nursing, Silliman University, Dumagete City, The Philippines*

Received 2 March 2004; received in revised form 16 March 2005; accepted 22 March 2005

Abstract

Primary health care (PHC) nursing is widely practiced in the Philippines yet little is published about the nurses working in this field nor by these nurses. This paper describes a PHC nursing curriculum conducted in an island in the south of the Philippines and examines the experience of nurses working as faculty and simultaneously providing service to the local community. Data were collected from a convenience sample of faculty by interview and analysed using Husserlian (descriptive) phenomenology and Colaizzi's method of data analysis. From 102 formulated meanings emerged four theme clusters: *teaching PHC*; *external influences*; *the working reality* and *practicing PHC*, and these are presented with exemplars from the interviews. The data gives a clear impression of the experience of implementing PHC and working with small communities and highlights the educational and clinical issues inherent in this unique model. The insights gained from the analysis of the interviews are contrasted with current literature and recommendations for future research are made.

Keywords: Phenomenology; Philippine experiences; Primary health care curriculum

1. What the paper adds to the literature

- Contributes to limited literature on primary health care (PHC) nursing in the Philippines.
- Examines the experiences of nurses working within the faculty and simultaneously providing service to the community.

*Corresponding author. Tel.: +852 2766 6390;
fax: +852 2364 9663.
E-mail address: hsarthur@inet.polyu.edu.hk (D. Arthur).

2. Introduction

The literature on PHC in nursing reveals several papers theorising on aspects of the practice, written by the articulate privileged of the profession who profess knowledge of PHC but fail to translate this into practice, or evidence-based research (Kendall, 1997; Vilakazi et al., 2000; Perkins et al., 2001). Conversely, in the practice arena there are numerous nurses practicing PHC who do not have the privilege, the motivation, nor the opportunity to publish. PHC nursing is widely practiced in the Philippines yet little research has been

0020-7489/$ - see front matter © 2005 Elsevier Ltd. All rights reserved.
doi:10.1016/j.ijnurstu.2005.03.007

conducted to examine the lived experiences of the nurses who are providing the PHC (Sy Sinda, 1997).

Over the last 5 years, the authors of this paper have been privileged to witness PHC nursing practiced by two rural universities in the Philippines. Both the schools operate in private universities of different religious persuasions, but both have a curriculum which is based on PHC where students and faculty work together with local communities to deliver the service. This paper will present a view of the environment in which these schools of nursing operate, then the experiences of the academic staff at one of the universities will be presented using in-depth interviews.

The authors were moved to present the material in this way as it seemed a way of presenting this valuable work to the profession. Unfortunately many nurses in the Philippines are less likely, than their western colleagues to publish their work due to the priorities facing them and their communities. For, when working with a community in a remote region of the Philippines, what does a publication in a refereed journal mean compared to helping a community plan the building of a tiny health centre, a school or church, or a fresh water supply to a village (which by the way costs the equivalent of a western academic's monthly salary)? The authors were so moved by the impressive work of their colleagues in The Philippines and set out to describe and present it as follows.

3. Background

Before explaining the way the faculty conducts their empowerment model of PHC, some background of the country and region may help set the scene. The beautiful rural setting is dominated by rice paddies, corn fields, caribou pulled ploughs and simple farming techniques and scattered villages while in the towns, the smoke from numerous buses and motorbike taxis blend with the dust of poor roads and weak infrastructure to provide the colour, texture and smells found in many lesser developed Asian countries. These people live in a world touched but not privileged by the rampant global commercial capitalism evident in the developed world. These friendly, warm people are a blend of their Spanish ancestry and Asian roots and are hard working, optimistic and fanatical about the religion which plays a central part in community activities. Ironically, this has probably been the force which has kept them tightly knit and supportive while allowing the ravages of political exploitation, neglect and corruption to leave them apart from the developments enjoyed by many people in South-East Asia. The communities in this region of the Philippines have struggled with basic necessities such as fresh water, basic health care, schooling and have managed a subsistence lifestyle: a

reflection of the country's poverty, politics and land mismanagement. In one of the communities, (Baranguay) with a population of approximately 1100 in 1998, a government survey, as part of the Social Reform Agenda of the Minimum Basic Needs, revealed only 26% of children over the age 12 were attending school, and in 1992 they didn't have a fresh drinking water supply (without a long walk to a mountain spring), no electricity, no school, no health centre, an impossible walk to the town for emergency health care, little work and virtually no money. This was a community where many people are born and die without ever accessing the health care system. Currently, this community boasts of a proud management committee, a piped fresh water supply, a humble but efficient health centre with a full-time midwife, a school, a nearly completed church and a basic income coming from the acquisition of a rice thrasher. How? Through the empowerment model initiated in 1992 by the school of nursing and left to the community in 1998. Nurses from the local school of nursing practice PHC which in this sense are activities carried out in the home or community involving roles of health visitor/public health and clinic-based health centre work (Goodman et al., 2003). The faculty set up meetings with the local village leaders and worked together with members of a management committee to identify problems, plan strategies, and implement action. The definition of PHC nursing differs from country to country and is certainly unique in the Philippines. Relevant literature on these issues is reviewed in the next section.

4. Literature review

Much has been written about PHC, the theory, and principles to follow in order to achieve to the goals (WHO, 1978; Mahler, 1977) and implementation of projects (Degremont, 1987). Common models for implementing PHC have relied on lay community members to provide a bridge between formal health care programs and the local community (Bender and Pitkin, 1987). A frequent strategy has been to identify individuals from local communities to serve as lay or community health workers and varying forms of health education programs have been designed to prepared community health workers for such roles (McElmurry and Keeney, 1999). Community member models assume that: (a) basic health information can be learnt by individuals from within the community; (b) lay helpers can understand local culture, values and practices; (c) lay workers can communicate basic health information to their communities and (d) communities are more likely to accept new information from people they know and trust (WHO, 1978; Bender and Pitkin, 1987; Berman, 1984; Eng and Young, 1992; Giblin, 1989;

D. Arthur et al. / International Journal of Nursing Studies 43 (2006) 107–112   109

Swider and McElmurry, 1990; Werner and Bower, 1982).

While pursuing PHC, practitioners in different countries tend to use different terms such as empowerment, or partnership working, community development or community health nursing. Goodman et al. (2003), for example describing the situation in the UK suggested that community nursing and primary care nursing are umbrella terms that are often loosely applied to describe all aspects of nursing in primary care carried out by the district nurse. Hildebrandt et al. (2003) describe a US model of academic community nursing centres where nurses practice PHC and work in partnership with communities. The key to understanding PHC practice by nurses, irrespective of terminology or country is that it is holistic care consistent with the WHO (1978) definition of PHC which emphasises partnership with communities to provide access to services that promote, restore and maintain health.

The above are the foundations of practice and provide the guiding direction. The recent refereed English nursing literature tends to focus on descriptive educational issues such as the experience of students (Simpson et al., 2002); what is meant by PHC and evidence-based care (Goodman et al., 2003; Kendall, 1997; Mackenzie and Ross, 1997); integrating PHC into curricula and expanded nurses' roles (Tenn, 1995; Hannigan, 1997; Sy Sinda, 1997; Leonard, 1998; Vilakazi et al., 2000).

Evidence-based clinical nursing research on the experiences of nurses in implementing PHC is rare. Chalmers et al. (1997) developed the PHC Questionnaire to measure knowledge, attitudes and qualitative data on practices of PHC among 457 students and faculty in a western Canadian university. Simpson et al. (2002) outlined the process and outcomes of the experiences of eight nursing students in Hong Kong who developed and implemented a PHC project with older adults. Twinn (2001) aimed to better describe the developments in nursing practice in PHC in Hong Kong using three community-based research projects to identify the opportunities and challenges created for nurses working in these settings. Twinn's work was descriptive, however, there is evidence in her writing of active involvement in PHC in Hong Kong. Only one research project, which focused on the experiences of nurses conducting PHC, was found in the refereed literature.

Vukic and Keddy (2002) utilised 'institutional ethnography', in an attempt to investigate the nature of nursing work in northern indigenous communities in Canada to highlight the uniqueness of nursing experiences in different cultures around the world. They attempted to explore the social relations and the nature of northern nursing, using interviews and field notes. The findings of Vukic and Keddy (2002) are of course unique to that area and do not generalise, but do provide a fascinating picture of work in that region.

They highlight the themes which emerge in northern nursing literature and which certainly apply to PHC nursing in other areas. They include: the expanded role for nurses related to lack of back-up and the independent nature of the role; the cultural context and knowledge of the local culture; the context of the regional health care including the inequalities and social concerns which are a result of history and paternalistic and colonial ways; the changing role of nurses from health care provider to facilitator; and the quality of work life where there is high turn over and the main issues are lack of adequate preparation and professional isolation. One study (Hildebrandt et al., 2003) carried out on 11 years of practice of an academic community nursing centre in the US provided useful insights into faculty and student practice in this unique PHC model and the authors explained the expanded role of nurses in terms of a nursing framework.

Unfortunately, little has been written about the experience of implementing PHC by nurses and no literature has been produced for the English refereed literature describing what it is that nurses do in the Philippines when working with their communities and implementing PHC.

5. Method

5.1. Sample

The setting for the study was a School of Nursing, in a rural setting offering a 3-year Bachelor of Nursing degree. The students have a variety of theory and clinical practice typical of any international nursing school: however, in addition they undergo training and clinical placement in PHC settings in local communities. Each semester, two batches of students have a 9-week rotation with families in their assigned community. The faculty of the school work with the communities for approximately 3 years to provide the necessary continuity, and several of the faculty have worked in PHC settings in other parts of the Philippines and overseas in countries such as Africa. Purposeful sampling was used to recruit five registered nurse participants experienced in the provision of PHC nursing from the College of Nursing at Silliman University in the Dumaguette region of the island of Negros Oriental.

In-depth interviews generated data about the nurses' personal and professional experiences. Participants were asked to respond to the single question: 'Tell me about the PHC activities in the school?' Prompts were used to keep the interview flowing, judgement was suspended and notes were taken during the interview, then transcribed and given back to the participants for their verification. Once agreement was reached on the actual content of the interview, data was analysed as follows.

Interview data analysis incorporated the qualitative methods of Huserrlian (descriptive) phenomenology and Colaizzi's method of data analysis. One hundred and two meanings were formulated from statements significant to the participants' lived experiences of providing PHC. These formulated meanings were organised into themes which evolved into four theme clusters. At this point the authors decided that no further collapsing of the data was appropriate, as in doing so would lose richness that is contained in the data. The theme clusters were then described and enriched with exemplars from the interviews.

6. Results

The theme clusters from the interview data are: teaching PHC; external influences; the working reality and practicing PHC.

6.1. Teaching primary health care

Theme cluster one *teaching PHC* represents the educational issues which both the faculty and students experience. Respondents talked about the factual material which is taught at different points in the curriculum, the practical rotation of students, including the how and where of placements. This involves the structure of the curriculum, and the practical mechanics of clinical placement. For example *'the implementation is at the Purok level (a small community) and two students are assigned per Purok'*…*'we work with approximately five families for three years'*…*'we teach shiatsu and accupressure'*.

Apart from the mechanics of teaching PHC, two of the respondents remarked about the challenges and the maturity required by the students to work in PHC, saying: *'Students have difficulty grasping the concepts as it is too premature to expose them to the community…'* another commented *'it's a big challenge helping students understand concepts and application to real life circumstances'*.

6.2. External influences

The second theme cluster, *external influences* emerged from comments made about government policy and agendas with which PHC interacts. The policies and services provided by the government are influenced in a two-way process. For example one respondent remarked: *'…we follow the slogan 'health in the hands of the people'…'* another said: *'In some places there are no toilets so we encourage government involvement in this'*. Other comments included: *'At the livelihood level it is common to involve intersectoral linkages such as the Department of Agriculture or the Department of Social*

Welfare which might involve skills training for women for extra income or capitol money with training to open a store'… *'We need to have committed front line health care workers of all levels to lobby, advocate changes in health care policies'*.

Two of the respondents had valuable experiences working in other regions or countries in PHC. One participant found working in this way frustrating *' because of my experience, I was working with NGOs doing PHC in (another region) with indigenous people-….I lived with the people'*. This respondent also felt that the experience could be further developed but was constrained: *'One reason we haven't developed further is because our administration hasn't fully grasped the value…'*

6.3. Working reality

The third theme cluster, *working reality,* relates to the reality of working with the people in the community, the constraints, and the facts that dictate what can and can't be done. Several comments related to the actual produce of the communities: *'the communities are agricultural and most of their products are used for consumption leaving little left over to sell'*. Incomes are low in the families and it is the tradition for families to live within the family compound where there can be up to 40 families: *'There are approximately 6–8 children per family…sadly some families only have corn to eat with some salt'*. One summarised the frustration of watching and not being ale to help families: *'To see this lack of food and surrounding land which could be tilled is frustrating but the men are away working and women cannot till the soil as they are busy with child rearing'*

There were comments about the importance of gaining cooperation with the community: *'One of the difficulties with implementing PHC is the indifference in individuals, so we need to have the approval of the formal leaders…'*.…*'There are approximately 6 Puroks (40–50 households) in each Baranguay and each Purok has a leader who will inform the college representative what is the priority. This formal entry into the community is important and a meeting is held with the important people who are the contact points'*.…*'some have no or weak leadership structure and the activities have helped develop a leadership structure. It is also important to identify the informal leaders'*.

One respondent concluded that: *'Really, PHC should be an ongoing project with a community being adopted where we can have a staff member in an ongoing project so students can come and go and see PHC phases taking place. In this way the participant can see change and development of the working relationship with the people of the community'*.

D. Arthur et al. / International Journal of Nursing Studies 43 (2006) 107–112   111

6.4. Practicing primary health care

The *practicing PHC* theme cluster reveals the actual techniques and experiences that occurred while the students and faculty were working with the communities. At the community level one revealed that: *'a health plan is developed and the formal leaders are asked to identify three main concerns'.*

One respondent reflected on the links made between the PHC service and other professionals: *'We used to have a medical and dental clinic held in the Community but we found this was encouraging dependence rather than independence so we now make referrals and encourage Community members to visit the Doctor or Government clinic in the city'.* Some interventions were at the information level such as: *'We target special groups such as the elderly (60+) as we found that many were not aware or didn't have ID cards nor knowledge about the benefits available for elderly such as services/discounts'.* At the health level, one respondent explained how the use of medicinal, commonly occurring plants are woven into the practice: *'we introduce the appropriate technology, mainly to the women, such as the 10 or 12 medicinal plants and teach them recipes for coughs and colds and joint problems'.*

The following are respondents' explanations of what it is they do when practicing PHC: *'We have devised health clinics which are held annually where we examine BP, do physical assessment, test urine for glucose or albumin',* ...*'When we leave a Community there is a degree of self reliance with managing minor illnesses and increased awareness of services e.g. government agencies'.*

Interventions used include use of indigenous plants for coughs and colds and complementary treatments such as: *'performing health education (where each student conducts a session e.g. prevention of denghi), how to make herbal medicine, managing coughs and colds in children using a manual for respiratory problems and referral...'*... *'acupressure and 'ventussa' treatment which involves using a glass bowl, a wick of cotton and a slice of ginger which local people believe relieves wind or 'panohot'.*

One respondent concluded with what she saw as the value of this work: *'Now after 13 years people are proud of what they have done. They commented on failures in the past, aid projects which failed, church projects which failed, but this project gave them a boost to morale'.* And another reflected that: *'water is not a problem now'* and the challenge for the future was *'we don't want the community to feel they are our guinea pigs'.*

7. Discussion

Vukic and Keddy (2002) highlight the problems of nurses not being part of the community saying that nurses make decisions based on their past work/life experiences and they bring their ideals to the 'north' and the idea of the nurse as the 'other' on the community is a challenge. In this study the nurses were part of the community, of the same culture and therefore better able to become part and build trust. In the light of the five themes described by Vukic and Keddy (2002) in their Canadian study, these respondents projected a comfort and confidence with the skills necessary in the *expanded role*, the *cultural context*, the *context of the health care* and the *changing role* while *quality of work life* was somewhat cushioned by being employed by the university, although some of the respondents did feel the university could take a stronger position by having a full-time clinician working in the communities.

A comparison of the four themes which emerged here with the five themes in the Canadian study show some commonalities and some obvious differences. This study was with a sample of nurses who were also teachers, unlike those in the Canadian study, so the theme *teaching PHC* involved issues related to curriculum design, knowledge and placement. *External influences* were experienced in common and explained as the cultural context and the context of health care in the Canadian study. *Working reality* and *practicing PHC* and *external influences* were defined by Vukic and Keddy (2002) in the themes cultural context, and quality of work life, the context of (northern) health care and shared similar concepts while obviously being culture bound.

It is clear from the literature review and a critique of research by nurses in the area, that the body of knowledge is in its infancy. This may be due to the difficulty of generalising PHC practice from one culture to the next. While several authors have expounded the principles and skills needed in implementing PHC (McElmurry and Keeney, 1999; WHO, 1978; Bender and Pitkin, 1987; Berman, 1984; Eng and Young, 1992; Giblin, 1989; Swider and McElmurry, 1990; Werner and Bower, 1982) and clearly these were adhered to in our Philippine sample, different communities in different countries will have different needs related to their culture and unique environmental influences making replicable research difficult. Twinn (2001), for example explains some of the current PHC issues facing nurses and health needs of individuals in Hong Kong under the headings of cancer education, HIV/AIDS, and chronic health problems, issues which were not raised by our Philippine respondents.

8. Conclusion

This study emerged from an impression gained by outsiders observing valuable PHC being implemented by nurses in the Philippines which hitherto has been unreported. Nurses are obviously practicing PHC but the literature lacks evidence of what it is that nurses actually do and research into the effectiveness of these PHC interventions. Through interviewing a small sample of nurse academics working with their students in a rural area of the Philippines, some valuable insights into the 'what and how' of PHC has been revealed and explained in the four themes which emerged. Future studies could be implemented to test some of the interventions explained, such as the effectiveness of the herbal remedies, and a replication of Chalmers et al, (1997) PHC Questionnaire would help contrast the students profiles with that of a Canadian sample, while a further in-depth qualitative examination of the communities would help further deepen the understanding of PHC in this region.

References

Bender, D., Pitkin, K., 1987. Bridging the gap: the village health worker as the cornerstone of the primary health care model. Social Science and Medicine 24, 515–528.

Berman, P., 1984. Village health workers in Java, Indonesia: coverage and equity. Social Science and Medicine 19, 411–422.

Chalmers, K., Bramadat, I., Sloan, J., 1997. Development and testing of the Primary Health Care Questionnaire (PHCQ): results with students and faculty in diploma and degree nursing programs. Canadian Journal of Nursing Research 29, 79–96.

Degremont, A., 1987. Primary health care in the tropics. Tropical Medicine and Parasitology 38, 222–225.

Eng, E., Young, R., 1992. Lay health advisors as community change agents. Family and Community Health 15 (1), 24–40.

Giblin, P., 1989. Effective utilization and evaluation of indigenous health care workers. Public Health Reports 104, 361–368.

Goodman, C., Ross, F., Mackenzie, A., Vernon, S., 2003. A portrait of district nursing: its contribution to primary health care. Journal of Interprofessional Care 17 (1), 97–108.

Hannigan, B., 1997. A challenge for community psychiatric nursing: is there a future in primary health care? Journal of Advanced Nursing 26, 751–757.

Hildebrandt, E., Baisch, M., Lundeen, S., Bell-Calvin, J., Kelber, S., 2003. Eleven years of primary health care delivery in an academic nursing centre. Journal of Professional Nursing 19 (5), 279–288.

Kendall, S., 1997. What do we mean by evidence? Implications for primary health care nursing. Journal of Interprofessional Care 11, 23–34.

Leonard, L., 1998. Primary health care and partnerships: collaboration of a community agency, health department, and university nursing program. Journal of Nursing Education 37, 144–148.

Mackenzie, A., Ross, F., 1997. Shifting the balance: nursing in primary health care. British Journal of Community Health Nursing 2, 139–142.

McElmurry, B., Keeney, G., 1999. Primary health care. Annual Review of Nursing Research 17, 241–268.

Mahler, H., 1977. Primary health care. The New Zealand Nursing Journal (October, 3–6).

Perkins, I., Vale, D., Graham, M., 2001. Partnerships in primary health care: a process for re-visioning nursing education. Nursing and Health Care Perspectives 22, 20–25.

Simpson, P., Chan, M., Cheung, L., Hui, T., Li, K., Tang, H., Tong, N., Wong, S., Wong, P., 2002. Primary health care theory to practice: experience of first-year nursing students in Hong Kong. Journal of Nursing Education 41 (7), 302–309.

Swider, S., McElmurry, B., 1990. A woman's health perspective in primary health care: a nursing and community health worker demonstration project in urban America. Journal of Family and Community Health 13, 1–17.

Sy Sinda, M., 1997. Effective nursing in primary health care, women and health in the Philippines—from the nursing point of view. Philippine Journal of Nursing 68, 42–47.

Tenn, L., 1995. Primary health care nursing education in Canadian university schools of nursing. Journal of Nursing Education 34, 350–358.

Twinn, S., 2001. Developments in nursing practice in primary health care in Hong Kong: opportunities and challenges. Journal of Clinical Nursing 10, 345–351.

Vilakazi, S., Chabeli, M., Roos, S., 2000. Integration of the primary health care approach into a community nursing science curriculum. Curationis 23, 39–53.

Vukic, A., Keddy, B., 2002. Northern nursing practice in a primary health care setting. Journal of Advanced Nursing 40, 542–548.

Werner, D., Bower, B., 1982. Helping Health Workers Learn. Hesperian Foundation, Palo Alto, CA.

WHO/UNICEF, 1978. Primary Health Care (Alma-Ata, 1978). WHO/UNICEF, Geneva.

Research in brief

Simpson et al. (2001) undertook a double-blind, randomised, placebo-controlled trial to identify the effect and safety of raspberry leaf tablets, taken by nulliparous women from 32 weeks gestation until labour, on labour and birth outcomes. Approval from an ethics committee was obtained. The authors do not report power analysis and sample size calculation, however, they estimated their sample size on three assumptions: the average length of nulliparous labour is 12 hours; the SD of the length of labour is 5 hours, and the treatment reduction in length of labour will be about 2 hours. A convenience sample of women was randomly allocated to either the treatment (n = 96) or placebo (n = 96) group. The major dependent variable was length of labour. Raspberry leaf and placebo tablets were contained in bottles identical in appearance. Descriptive and inferential statistics were used. Findings revealed little difference in maternal blood loss at birth between groups. Analyses suggested that women taking raspberry leaf were more likely to experience spontaneous rupture of membranes, give birth vaginally and unassisted, and less likely to have a forceps delivery compared with the control group. While not statistically significant, this result was considered to be clinically significant. A limitation was reliance on the accuracy of self-reports. A recommendation was for further research to determine an optimal safe dosage of raspberry leaf.

Critical review of quantitative research studies

The following review process for quantitative studies (Box 16.3) is not exhaustive. As you read research papers or chapters in this book, additional pertinent questions may occur to you. Consider the size of the sample and remember that samples have to be large enough to permit the assumption of normality. If the sample is quite small, say, five to ten subjects, the assumptions necessary for inferential statistics may have been violated. The important question is whether the researcher has provided enough justification to use the statistics presented. As you read the 'Methods' section consider the level of measurement and statistical tests used to measure important variables.

Evidence-based practice tip

If the level of measurement was interval or ratio, the statistics most likely to be used will be parametric; however, if the variables are measured at the nominal or ordinal level, the statistics used should be non-parametric (see Chapter 14).

Finally, consider the results as they are presented. The first place to begin to critique the statistical analysis of a research paper is with the hypothesis. The hypothesis should indicate to you what statistics were used. If the hypothesis predicts that a relationship between the variables will be found, you should expect to find indices of correlation. If the study is experimental or quasi-experimental, the hypothesis would indicate that the author is looking for differences between the groups studied and you would expect to find statistical tests of difference between means or proportions. There would be serious implications for the study if the stated aims and hypotheses are written in a vague way. There should be enough data presented for each hypothesis studied to determine whether the researcher actually examined each hypothesis (see Chapter 5). The tables, procedures, analysis and text should be congruent. For example, the text should not indicate that a test reached statistical significance while the tables indicate that the probability value of the test was below 0.05.

Tutorial trigger 2

Beverley is in her postgraduate year of nursing. She works as a full-time theatre nurse and would like to conduct research in her clinical area. She has discussed a topic with the theatre manager and received approval to present a short paper outlining her plan. How should she proceed?

There are two other aspects of the data analysis section that the reader should review. The paper should not read as if it were a statistical textbook. The results in the text of the paper should be clear enough to the average reader so that determinations can be made about what was done and what the results were. In addition, the author should attempt to make a distinction between practical and statistical significance. Some results may be statistically significant, but their practical importance may be doubtful. If this is so, the author should note it. Alternatively, you may find yourself reading a research report that is elegantly presented, but you come away with a 'so what?' feeling. Such a feeling may indicate that the practical significance of the study and its findings have not been adequately explained.

Note that the critical analysis of a research paper's statistical analysis is not done in a vacuum. The adequacy of the analysis must be judged in relation to the other important aspects of the paper: the problem, the hypothesis, the design, the sample, and data collection methods. For example, a researcher may sometimes use a non-parametric statistic when it appears that a parametric statistic is appropriate. Because parametric statistics are more powerful than non-parametric statistics, the result of the parametric analysis may not have been what the researcher expected. However, the non-parametric result might be in the expected direction, so the researcher reports only that result, but this would be misleading (see Chapters 11 and 12).

● **Evidence-based practice tip**

Use whatever opportunities you can to examine and evaluate your clinical practice. Then, generate questions about your practice and share them with colleagues.

TT **Tutorial trigger 3**

Explain to your nursing or midwifery colleagues why, as research consumers, they need to know how to critically read research articles.

The next article 'Nursing intervention after carotid endarterectomy: a randomised trial of Co-ordinated Care Post-Discharge (CCPD)' (Middleton et al. 2005) is critically reviewed for its design and contribution to healthcare and nursing knowledge. Critical review guidelines appear in Box 16.3.

Title and abstract

The title specifies the design, a randomised trial, nursing intervention following the surgical procedure of endarterectomy, and time of the intervention. The aim of the study was to evaluate the short-term impact on patients of nursing-led care after discharge following carotid endarterectomy. The intervention was a telephone liaison with the patient by a registered nurse (RN) at 2, 6 and 12 weeks post operation, combined with an educational program. The control group did not receive a telephone contact from the RN, however their general practitioners received postoperative liaison.

There was a statistically significant positive effect on the intervention group regarding knowledge of stroke warning signs, self-reported changes to improve lifestyle and dietary modifications. Other outcomes showed statistically significant improvements in both groups. Further research in this area is recommended.

Structuring the study

Motivation for the study was the paucity of rigorous evaluation of nursing care models. Of the four CCPD models cited (within the last 12 years), all showed statistically significant patient improvements. Limitations of the four study trials conducted in American hospitals are discussed. No hypothesis was stated.

The sample/participants

Fifty-six vascular surgeons in NSW were invited to recruit participants for the study during their pre-operative visits. Patients were informed of the randomisation process — intervention group (n = 66) and control group (n = 67). No information is provided as to how sample numbers were determined or if number size was appropriate for the statistical tests used. Randomisation was managed by CONSORT principles to allocate patients to the two groups. Figure 1 CONSORT shows the flow diagram of the progress through the phases of the CCDP trial. Surgeons, patients and researchers were blinded to group allocation.

Patients who agreed to participate were given an information statement and asked to sign a consent form and complete a baseline (pre-operative) questionnaire. Ethics approval was obtained from an HREC.

Data collection

All patients received and completed a pre-operative questionnaire including questions about demographic information, health status, smoking status, physical activity, blood pressure and cholesterol level; and a follow-up questionnaire by mail 3 months post discharge. This questionnaire was identical to the baseline questionnaire with additional questions relating to changes made to lifestyle.

The intervention group had telephone contact from an RN at 2-, 6- and 12-week intervals following their operation and during these calls stroke risk factors were discussed.

Between the calls, extensive literature about stroke risk factors and its management were mailed e.g. National Stroke Foundation brochures, Personal Vascular Log Book to record their clinical information.

The control group had no telephone contact from the RN. However, the GPs of these patients were telephoned at 2 weeks postoperatively with details of the patients' immediate postoperative recovery.

BOX 16.3 Critical review guidelines for quantitative studies

The title and abstract
1. Is the title of the research paper congruent with the text?
2. Were the aims and/or objectives stated? What are they?
3. Did the abstract contain sufficient information about the stages of the research process (e.g. aims, hypothesis, research approach, sample, instruments, and findings)?

Structuring the study
1. Is the motivation for the study demonstrated through the literature review?
2. Is the literature review adequate? Are the references recent?
3. Are the stated limitations and gaps in the reviewed literature appropriate and convincing?
4. How was the investigation carried out?
5. Is the hypothesis stated?
6. Which hypothesis is stated: the scientific hypothesis or the null hypothesis?
7. Does the hypothesis indicate that the researcher is interested in testing for differences between groups or in testing for relationships?

The sample
1. Is the sample size large enough to prevent an extreme score from affecting the summary statistics used?
2. How was the sample size determined?
3. Was the sample size appropriate for the analyses used?

Data collection
1. How were the data collected (questionnaires or other data collection tools)?
2. Who collected the data?
3. What is the origin of the measurement instruments?
4. Are the instruments adequately described?

5. How were the data collection instruments validated?
6. How was the reliability of the measurement instruments assessed?
7. Were ethical issues discussed?

Data analysis
1. Are descriptive or inferential statistics reported?
2. What tests were used to analyse the data: parametric or non-parametric?
3. Were the descriptive statistics/inferential statistics appropriate to the level of measurement for each variable?
4. Were the appropriate tests used to analyse the data?
5. What is the level of measurement chosen for the independent and dependent variables?
6. Were the statistics appropriate for the research question and design?
7. Are there appropriate summary statistics for each major variable?
8. Were the statistics primarily descriptive, correlational or inferential?
9. Identify the outcome of each statistical analysis.
10. Explain the meaning of each outcome.

Findings
1. Were the findings expected? Which findings were not expected?
2. Is there enough information present to judge the results?
3. Are the results clearly and completely stated?
4. Describe the researcher's report of the findings.
5. Identify any limitations or gaps in the study.
6. Were suggestions for further research made?
7. Did the researcher mention the implications of the study for healthcare?
8. Was there sufficient information in the report to permit replication of the study?

ISSUES AND INNOVATIONS IN NURSING PRACTICE

Nursing intervention after carotid endarterectomy: a randomized trial of Co-ordinated Care Post-Discharge (CCPD)

Sandy Middleton BAppSc MN PhD RN
Professor of Nursing, Australian Catholic University, North Sydney, Australia

Neil Donnelly BSc MPH
Consultant Statistician, Division of Population Health, South Western Sydney Area Health Service, Sydney, Australia

John Harris MBBS MS FRACS FRCS FACS DDU
Professor of Vascular Surgery, Department of Surgery, University of Sydney, Sydney, Australia

Jeanette Ward MBBS MHPEd PhD FAFPHM
Director, Institute of Population Health, University of Ottawa, Ottawa, Canada

Accepted for publication 15 December 2004

Correspondence:
Sandy Middleton,
Australian Catholic University,
PO Box 968,
North Sydney,
New South Wales 2059,
Australia.
E-mail: s.middleton@mackillop.acu.edu.au

MIDDLETON S., DONNELLY N., HARRIS J. & WARD J. (2005) *Journal of Advanced Nursing* 52(3), 250–261
Nursing intervention after carotid endarterectomy: a randomized trial of Co-ordinated Care Post-Discharge (CCPD)

Aim. This paper reports a study evaluating the short-term impact of nursing-led, co-ordinated care after discharge following carotid endarterectomy.

Background. Patient education about stroke risk factors, combined systematically with carotid endarterectomy, holds unrealized potential to improve patient outcomes. Nurses are well-placed in the healthcare system to co-ordinate this type of education.

Methods. A randomized controlled trial was conducted between October 2001 and October 2002. Patients having carotid endarterectomy ($n = 133$) were randomized to either the intervention ($n = 66$) or control group ($n = 67$). The intervention consisted of telephone liaison with the patient by a Registered Nurse at 2, 6 and 12 weeks following carotid endarterectomy, combined with education about stroke risk factor management and structured liaison with the patient's surgeon and referring general practitioner. While patients allocated to the control group did not receive any postoperative telephone contact directly from the Registered Nurse during the study, their general practitioners received structured postoperative liaison.

Results. The co-ordinated care postdischarge intervention had a statistically significant positive effect on patient knowledge of stroke warning signs ($P = 0.002$), patient self-reported changes to improve lifestyle ($P = 0.006$) and diet modification ($P < 0.001$). Statistically significant improvements from baseline to follow-up were detected in both groups for other outcomes.

Conclusions. While nursing-led, co-ordinated care after discharge achieves important improvements for short-term outcomes, carotid endarterectomy itself may have been a catalyst for improved patient outcomes. Further research of nursing-led co-ordinated care initiatives for vascular surgery patients is needed.

Keywords: carotid endarterectomy, nursing, nursing-led, randomized trial, vascular surgery

Background

Stroke prevention and management are global health priorities (Murray & Lopez 1997, National Stroke Foundation 1997). While medical strategies reduce stroke risk factors (National Health and Medical Research Council (NHMRC) 1997a), surgical management by carotid endarterectomy (CEA) has demonstrated effectiveness in reducing rates of stroke for both symptomatic (Cina *et al.* 1999) and asymptomatic patients (Chambers *et al.* 2000). Patient education about stroke risk factors, combined systematically with CEA, holds unrealised potential to improve patient outcomes (Middleton *et al.* 2003).

Co-ordinated care models (Zwarenstein *et al.* 2002), also known as 'case management', show promise as an approach to improve patient outcomes through enhanced communication and interprofessional collaboration (Griffiths *et al.* 2002). Nurses are particularly well placed to co-ordinate care (Naylor *et al.* 1999) and assist patients achieve a smooth transition from hospital to home (Phillips 1993). Little rigorous evaluation of such models has been undertaken, however. Of four randomized trials of nursing-led, co-ordinated care postdischarge (CCPD) interventions published since 1992, all demonstrate statistically significant improvements for patients allocated to postdischarge care (DeBusk *et al.* 1994, Naylor *et al.* 1999, Escobar *et al.* 2001, Riegel *et al.* 2002). Only two trials recruited patients with vascular disease (acute myocardial infarction and cardiac failure) (DeBusk *et al.* 1994, Riegel *et al.* 2002), but did not focus on vascular surgery. Two trials (DeBusk *et al.* 1994, Riegel *et al.* 2002) failed to adjust for the clustered nature of their data (Campbell *et al.* 2000). All four trials were conducted in American hospitals, further limiting generalizability (DeBusk *et al.* 1994, Naylor *et al.* 1999, Escobar *et al.* 2001, Riegel *et al.* 2002). Only one study examined the effect of co-ordinated care after surgery (Naylor *et al.* 1999).

The study

Aim

The aim of the study was to evaluate the short-term impact of nursing-led, co-ordinated care for patients after discharge following CEA. Short-term outcomes at 3 months are reported here.

Design

A randomized controlled trial was carried out in 2001–2002.

Participants

Vascular surgeons in New South Wales, Australia (NSW) ($n = 54$) previously participating in a state-wide audit (Middleton & Donnelly 2002) were invited to recruit patients for this trial. Two vascular surgeons who had subsequently commenced specialist practice were also approached. Consenting surgeons recruited consecutive patients during their preoperative visits prior to CEA. Patients were informed that participation involved randomization to one of two groups, both of which would receive 'usual care' and one of two types of additional postdischarge care. Patients were ineligible for recruitment if they could not give informed consent or complete a self-administered questionnaire due to an insufficient level of English. Those having emergency operations were excluded.

Patients who agreed to participate were asked to sign a consent form and complete the baseline (preoperative) questionnaire before their CEA. They also were asked for permission to contact their general practitioner (GP). Evidence based follow-up strategies were employed for questionnaire non-responders, who were telephoned by a research assistant blind to group allocation 10 days after distribution of the baseline questionnaire (Edwards *et al.* 2002).

Surgeons provided clinical details and anticipated dates of surgery for consenting patients. One week after the proposed date of surgery, researchers ascertained the immediate outcome of the CEA from surgeons.

Randomization

We used CONSORT principles to allocate patients to the study groups (Moher *et al.* 2001) (Table 1). Using a random number table, a schedule of group allocation was prepared for each surgeon. All possible combinations of group allocation in permuted blocks of six patients were determined, using an allocation ratio of 1:1. SM generated the allocation sequence and assigned participants to groups and was, by necessity, the only person aware of group allocation. Surgeons, patients and research assistants were blinded to group allocation. Postoperative data entry was blinded, as was data analysis.

Co-ordinated care postdischarge intervention

Patient liaison and education
Patients allocated to the CCPD group received telephone contact by a Registered Nurse (RN) (SM) at 2, 6 and 12 weeks following the date of their CEA, and during this

S. Middleton et al.

Table 1 Components of CCPD intervention

Patient components	Clinician components
Two weeks postoperatively	*Two weeks postoperatively*
Patient telephone call:	GP telephone call:
Patients were asked about general post-op recovery, intention to make changes to lifestyle to decrease stroke risk & which risk factors. Patients' were prompted as follows:	GPs were informed that patients had undergone a CEA and that they had experienced an eventful or uneventful post-operative recovery according to information provided by surgeons.
• change diet	GP fax:
• increase physical activity level	Following patient telephone call at two weeks post-operatively, GPs were faxed individual summaries outlining the stroke risk factors each patient was particularly interested in attempting to modify. Any relevant health concerns expressed by the patient at this time also were fed back to the GP.
• take medications	
• visit GP to discuss risk factor management	
• stop smoking	
• decrease smoking	
• stop drinking alcohol	Surgeon fax:
• decrease alcohol intake	Following patient telephone call at two weeks post-operatively, surgeons were faxed individual summaries outlining the stroke risk factors each patient was particularly interested in attempting to modify. Any relevant health concerns expressed by the patient at this time also were fed back to the surgeon.
• get cholesterol level checked	

Written materials sent to CCPD patients following two week phone call:
National Stroke Foundation (NSF) brochures
(http://www.strokefoundation.com.au):
• 'Introducing the NSF and the National Stroke Research Institute
• 'Answers to the top ten questions about stroke'
• 'Stroke: Know the warning signs'
• 'What is Transient Ischaemic Attack (TIA)'
• 'High blood pressure medically known as hypertension and stroke'
• 'Atrial fibrillation increases your risk of stroke'
• 'Stroke treatment in an emergency'
Heart Foundation brochures (http://www.heartfoundation.com.au):
• 'Be active everyday'
• 'Weight loss checklist'
• 'Healthy eating for the heart'
• 'The low down on high blood cholesterol'
• 'Get the good eating habit'
• 'The Heart Foundation Cookbook'
• 'Kick the habit'
• 'High blood pressure – the facts'
• 'Women and heart disease'
• 'Stroke'
• 'How to have a healthy heart'
Personal Vascular Log Book for patients to record their own clinical data.
Six weeks postoperatively
Patient telephone call (identical content to the 2-week call)
Written materials sent to CCPD patients following six week phone call:
NHMRC 'Prevention of Stroke, A Consumer's Guide' (NHMRC 1997b)
National Heart Foundation Cook Book (James 2001)
List of eight internet addresses with a description of each site:
• National Stroke Foundation
• Heart Foundation
• Australian Consumer Association
• NSW Health
• Australian Institute of Health and Welfare
• Australian Council on Smoking and Health
• American Heart Association
• Cochrane Collaboration Consumer Network
Twelve weeks postoperatively
Patient telephone call (identical content to the 2 and 6 weeks call)

CCPD, co-ordinated care postdischarge; CEA, carotid endarterectomy; GP, general practitioner; NHMRC, National Health and Medical Research Council; NSF, National Stroke Foundation; NSW, New South Wales (Australia); TIA, transient ischaemic attack.

call stroke risk factors were reviewed (Table 1). Between telephone contacts, patients were mailed comprehensive information about stroke risk factors and their management (Table 1).

Clinician liaison

To co-ordinate care between the patient, surgeon and GPs, the RN telephoned each GP to inform them of their patient's immediate postoperative recovery. Both surgeon and GP were then faxed individual summaries for each patient outlining stroke risk factors s/he was particularly interested in changing. Any relevant health concerns expressed by the patient at this time were also communicated.

Control group

Patients allocated to the control group did not receive any postoperative telephone contact directly from the RN during the study. GPs of these patients received telephone contact from the RN only at 2 weeks postoperatively. They were informed only that the patient had undergone a CEA and given details of their immediate postoperative recovery.

Data collection

Baseline patient questionnaire

Our 26-page baseline (preoperative) questionnaire for patients began with questions about sociodemographics (six questions) and general health status (two questions). Next questions were asked about smoking status (one question), physical activity (six questions) (Armstrong *et al.* 2000), blood pressure (two questions) and cholesterol level (one question). Patients also were asked 33 questions to assess their knowledge of stroke.

Follow-up patient questionnaire

Our 23-page follow-up (postoperative) questionnaire and covering letter were mailed 3 months after discharge. This questionnaire was identical to the baseline questionnaire, with the addition of six questions: changes made to patient's lifestyle since their operation to further reduce their risk of stroke (two questions); written information patients had received following their CEA (three questions). Patients also were asked to recall verbal information received about stroke and stroke risk factor management since their operation (one question). Copies of questionnaires are available on written request. As at baseline, non-responders were telephoned by a research assistant blind to group allocation 10, 20 and 30 days after distribution of the follow-up questionnaire (Edwards *et al.* 2002).

Ethical considerations

Ethics approval was obtained from the Central Sydney Area Health Service Ethics Review Committee. Patients who were eligible for recruitment to the study were given an information statement. Those who agreed to participate signed a consent form prior to completion of the baseline questionnaire.

Data analysis

Data were analysed using SPSS (Norusis 1999), applying an intention-to-treat approach. Frequencies for stroke risk factors were analysed. 'Sufficient' time spent undertaking physical activity was defined as the accrual of ≥ 150 minutes of walking and/or moderate-intensity physical activity and/or vigorous-intensity physical activity per week (where vigorous-intensity physical activity was weighted by a factor of two to reflect its greater intensity) (Armstrong *et al.* 2000). 'Sufficient' number of sessions was defined as physical activity occurring over five or more separate sessions per week (Armstrong *et al.* 2000).

Patients' knowledge of physical symptoms as 'warning' signs of stroke was also measured (NHMRC 1997a, National Stroke Foundation 2000). Patients received one point for each correct response (minimum score, zero; maximum score, 18). Similarly, they were asked whether each of 10 conditions made it 'more likely' for somebody to have a stroke (NHMRC 1997a, National Stroke Foundation 2000). Patients received one point for each correct response (minimum score, zero; maximum score, 10). For the question 'What would you do if you thought you or someone you were with looked as though they were having a stroke?', responses were classified as 'correct' (either 'take the person to Emergency at the nearest hospital' or 'call 000 for an ambulance') or 'incorrect' (any of the five other response options).

For binary outcome variables, McNemar's test for paired proportions was calculated within each group to assess whether there had been a change in the proportion reporting the attribute of interest (Armitage & Berry 1994). In order to determine whether there was a difference between groups in the percentage reporting change in the attribute of interest, a repeated measures analysis for marginal proportions was conducted using the PROC CATMOD procedure in SAS Version 8.0 (SAS Institute Inc. 1999).

For interval scaled variables, within-group changes in the mean value over time were assessed using the matched paired *t*-test (Armitage & Berry 1994). In order to determine whether the intervention and control groups differed in their mean postscores, adjusting for baseline level, linear regres-

S. Middleton et al.

sion analyses were conducted regressing follow-up score on the GROUP variable and baseline score (Vickers & Altman 2001).

Results

Of 30 surgeons who agreed to participate, 10 did not perform any CEAs during the recruitment period. Of the remaining 20, all recruited patients (100% surgeon compliance).

Of the 151 patients seen during the study period (Figure 1), four were considered ineligible due to inability to complete a self-administered questionnaire in English ($n = 3$) or inability to give informed consent due to confusion ($n = 1$). Surgery was cancelled for another three patients, precluding entry to the trial. Of the 144 eligible patients, 11 declined to participate (92% response rate). There were no statistically significant differences between eligible patients who agreed to participate and those who did not in terms of sex ($\chi^2 = 1\cdot0$, d.f. = 1, $P = 0\cdot3$), age ($\chi^2 = 2\cdot3$, d.f. = 1, $P = 0\cdot13$) or symptom status ($\chi^2 = 0\cdot3$, d.f. = 1, $P = 0\cdot6$).

Of the participating 133 patients, 66 were randomized to the CCPD group and 67 to the control group. Completed baseline questionnaires were received for all 133 patients (100%) (Figure 1).

Baseline questionnaire

Table 2 displays characteristics of participating patients by group. The mean age was 70·4 years. The majority of patients undergoing CEA were men (61·1%) and symptomatic (62·4%) (Table 2). There were no statistically significant differences between the CCPD group and the control group in terms of patient age ($\chi^2 = 1\cdot7$, d.f. = 1, $P = 0\cdot19$), sex ($\chi^2 = 0\cdot2$, d.f. = 1, $P = 0\cdot67$) and level of education ($\chi^2 = 1\cdot5$, d.f. = 2, $P = 0\cdot47$) (Table 2). There were statistically significantly more symptomatic patients in the control group (70·1%) than in the CCPD group (54·5%) ($\chi^2 = 4\cdot1$, d.f. = 1, $P = 0\cdot04$). In addition, five patients (3·8%) were undergoing a second CEA on the same side (a 're-do' operation), all of whom were from the CCPD group (Fisher's Exact Test $P = 0\cdot03$).

In the first postoperative week, surgeons reported nine (6·8%) unexpected events as follows: return to operating theatre for removal of neck haematoma [$n = 4$, 3·0% (CCPD $n = 2$; Control $n = 2$)], postoperative stroke [$n = 2$, 1·5% (CCPD $n = 1$; Control $n = 1$)], acute myocardial infarction ($n = 1$, 0·8% CCPD $n = 1$), vocal cord paralysis [$n = 1$, 0·8% (CCPD $n = 1$)] and one case of dehydration ($n = 1$, 0·8% Control $n = 1$). Five of these events occurred in patients allocated to the CCPD group

and four in patients from the control group (Fisher's Exact Test $P = 0\cdot74$).

Follow-up questionnaire

Of the 133 patients participating in the trial, one patient died before our scheduled follow-up at 3 months and one withdrew due to a diagnosis of terminal cancer. Of the 131 follow-up questionnaires sent to patients, 129 were returned (overall response fraction 98%) (63 from the CCPD group and 66 from the control group).

Health status
The CCPD group showed a statistically significant increase from baseline to follow-up in the proportion of patients who rated their health 3 months after surgery to be either 'good', 'very good' or 'excellent' (56·7–75·0%) (McNemar's $\chi^2 = 9\cdot1$, d.f. = 1, $P = 0\cdot003$). While the control group also demonstrated an increase (50·0–64·1%) from baseline to follow-up, this was not statistically significant (McNemar's $\chi^2 = 3\cdot4$, d.f. = 1, $P = 0\cdot07$). The rate of increase in the CCPD group was not statistically significantly greater than that determined for the control group pre- to post-CEA ($\chi^2 = 0\cdot3$, d.f. = 1, $P = 0\cdot61$).

Patients were also asked to rate their health in general compared with 1 year ago. Both groups showed statistically significant increases in the proportion of patients who rated their health to be either 'somewhat' or 'much' better than a year ago. The CCPD group showed a statistically significant increase from 16·4% to 50·8% (McNemar's $\chi^2 = 17\cdot4$, d.f. = 1, $P < 0\cdot0001$). The control group showed a statistically significant increase from 11·1% to 49·2% (McNemar's $\chi^2 = 17\cdot6$, d.f. = 1, $P < 0\cdot0001$). Repeated measures analysis found no difference between groups in the magnitude of this increase at follow-up ($\chi^2 = 0\cdot1$, d.f. = 1, $P = 0\cdot71$).

Physical activity
The CCPD group showed a statistically significant increase from 33·9% at baseline to 54·2% at follow-up in the percentage of patients who exercised in excess of 150 minutes per week (McNemar's $\chi^2 = 6\cdot1$, d.f. = 1, $P = 0\cdot01$). The control group also showed a statistically significant increase from 37·3% at baseline to 52·5% at follow-up in the percentage of patients engaging in a sufficient number of minutes of exercise per week (McNemar's $\chi^2 = 3\cdot8$, d.f. = 1, $P = 0\cdot05$). There was no statistically significant difference between the groups at follow-up ($\chi^2 = 0\cdot3$, d.f. = 1, $P = 0\cdot60$) (Table 3).

At follow-up, the CCPD group also showed a statistically significant increase from baseline to follow-up in the number of patients engaging in both sufficient *time* and

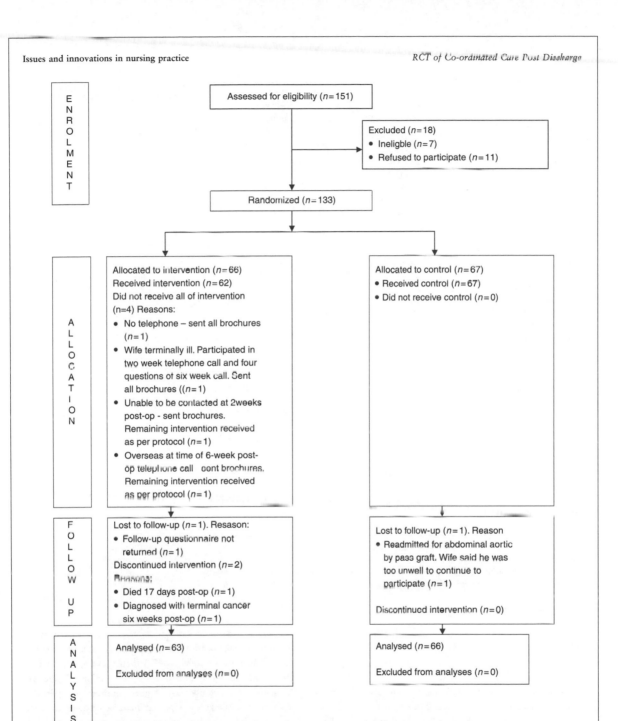

Figure 1 CONSORT Flow diagram of the progress through the phases of the co-ordinated care postdischarge trial (Moher *et al.* 2001).

sessions of physical activity (30·5–49·2%) (McNemar's $\chi^2 = 5\cdot3$, d.f. = 1, $P = 0\cdot02$). The control group increase was more modest (33·9–44·1%) and not statistically significant (McNemar's $\chi^2 = 1\cdot3$, d.f. = 1, $P = 0\cdot26$). There was no statistically significant difference between the two groups in terms of the magnitude of improvement in this

S. Middleton et al.

Table 2 Patient characteristics reported at baseline by group (*n* = 133)*

	CCPD group (*n* = 66), *n* (%)	Control group (*n* = 67), *n* (%)	Differences between groups
Age (years)			
<60	8 (12·3)	6 (9·0)	$\chi^2_3 = 1\cdot8$, $P = 0\cdot61$
60–69	23 (34·8)	18 (26·9)	
70–79	28 (42·4)	33 (49·3)	
≥80	7 (10·6)	10 (14·9)	
Sex			
Male	39 (59·1)	42 (62·7)	$\chi^2_1 = 0\cdot2$, $P = 0\cdot67$
Female	27 (40·9)	25 (37·3)	
Level of education			
Did not complete primary	0	3 (4·5)	$\chi^2_2 = 1\cdot5$, $P = 0\cdot47^\S$
Primary only	6 (9·1)	9 (13·4)	
No intermediate or school certificate	22 (33·3)	24 (35·8)	
Intermediate or school certificate	22 (33·3)	18 (26·9)	
Leaving or higher school certificate	6 (9·1)	7 (10 4)	
University, TAFE or college	8 (12·1)	5 (7·5)	
Symptom status			
Symptomatic	36 (54·5)	47 (70·1)	$\chi^2_1 = 4\cdot1$, $P = 0\cdot04$
Asymptomatic	30 (45·5)	20 (29·9)	
Type of symptoms[†]			
TIA	20 (30·3)	21 (31·3)	$\chi^2_1 = 0\cdot0$, $P = 0\cdot90$
Amaurosis fugax	12 (18·2)	19 (28·4)	$\chi^2_1 = 1\cdot9$, $P = 0\cdot17$
Previous stroke	7 (10·6)	9 (13·4)	$\chi^2_1 = 0\cdot3$, $P = 0\cdot62$
Non-specific symptoms	8 (12·1)	16 (23·9)	$\chi^2_1 = 3\cdot1$, $P = 0\cdot08$
Stenosis of operated artery			
50–69%	7 (10·6)	4 (5·9)	$\chi^2_1 = 1\cdot1$, $P = 0\cdot30$
70–99%	55 (83·3)	62 (91·2)	
Surgeon report of patient past history[†]			
Diabetes	11 (16·9)	19 (27·9)	$\chi^2_1 = 2\cdot6$, $P = 0\cdot11$
Hypertension	40 (61·5)	51 (75·0)	$\chi^2_1 = 2\cdot4$, $P = 0\cdot12$
Stroke or TIA	16 (24·6)	33 (48·5)	$\chi^2_1 = 6\cdot9$, $P = 0\cdot009$
CCF within last 100 days	0	0	N/A
AMI	13 (20·0)	15 (22·1)	$\chi^2_1 = 0\cdot0$, $P = 0\cdot96$

*Where totals do not add to 100%, data were missing.
[†]More than one option possible per patient.
[§]Did not complete primary, primary only, no intermediate or school certificate versus intermediate or school certificate versus leaving or higher school certificate, university, and TAFE or College.
CCPD, co-ordinated care post-discharge.

measure of physical activity at follow-up ($\chi^2 = 0\cdot7$, d.f. = 1, $P = 0\cdot41$) (Table 3).

Other stroke risk factors
Results for other stroke risk factors are also shown in Table 3. There were no statistical differences between groups in changes over time for level of last blood pressure reading, level of last cholesterol reading or change in smoking prevalence over time (Table 3).

Lifestyle changes
Fifty-six (43·4%) patients reported making changes to their lifestyle since their operation to further decrease their risk

of having a stroke. Patients in the CCPD group were statistically significantly more likely to report making changes to their lifestyle (57·4%) than those in the control group (32·8%) ($\chi^2 = 7\cdot6$, d.f. = 1, $P = 0\cdot006$) (Table 4). A statistically significantly higher number of patients from the CCPD group reported making changes to their diet at follow-up when compared with patients from the control group ($\chi^2 = 14\cdot6$, d.f. = 1, $P < 0\cdot001$) (Table 4). Point prevalence of smoking did not change within groups over time. There was no statistically significant difference between the two groups in the change in smoking prevalence at follow-up ($\chi^2 = 0\cdot1$, d.f. = 1, $P = 0\cdot81$).

Issues and innovations in nursing practice   *RCT of Co-ordinated Care Post-Discharge*

Table 3 Stroke risk factor data at baseline and follow-up by group

Group	Valid (n)	Baseline (%)	Follow-up (%)	McNemar's χ^2 (within group)	Group × time interaction (between groups)
Blood pressure last measured by your GP					
CCPD 'within last year'	63	96·8	93·7	$\chi_1^2 = 0·2, P = 0·68*$	$\chi_1^2 = 0·0, P = 0·98$
Control 'within last year'	66	97·0	93·9	$\chi_1^2 = 0·2, P = 0·68*$	
Level of last BP reading					
CCPD 'about right'	63	79·4	88·9	$\chi_1^2 = 1·8, P = 0·18^\dagger$	$\chi_1^2 = 0·0, P = 0·97$
Control 'about right'	65	70·8	80·0	$\chi_1^2 = 1·6, P = 0·21^\dagger$	
Level of last cholesterol reading					
CCPD 'about right'	63	47·6	58·7	$\chi_1^2 = 1·6, P = 0·21^\ddagger$	$\chi_1^2 = 2·7, P = 0·12$
Control 'about right'	66	54·5	50·0	$\chi_1^2 = 0·2, P = 0·65^\ddagger$	
Smoking status					
CCPD current smokers	59	22·0	18·6	$\chi_1^2 = 0·3, P = 0·62$	$\chi_1^2 = 0·1, P = 0·81$
Control current smokers	64	25·0	20·3	$\chi_1^2 = 0·6, P = 0·45$	
Sufficient time per week spent in physical activity (150 + mins)					
CCPD sufficient time	59	33·9	54·2	$\chi_1^2 = 6·1, P = 0·01$	$\chi_1^2 = 0·3, P = 0·60$
Control sufficient time	59	37·3	52·5	$\chi_1^2 = 3·8, P = 0·05$	
Sufficient time and sessions per week spent in physical activity (150 + minutes and 5 or more sessions)					
CCPD sufficient time and sessions	59	30·5	49·2	$\chi_1^2 = 5·3, P = 0·02$	$\chi_1^2 = 0·7, P = 0·41$
Control sufficient time and sessions	59	33·9	44·1	$\chi_1^2 = 1·3, P = 0·26$	
Proportion of sedentary patients					
CCPD sedentary	61	14·8	11·5	$\chi_1^2 = 0·1, P = 0·72$	$\chi_1^2 = 2·6, P = 0·11$
Control sedentary	62	33·9	17·7	$\chi_1^2 = 4·5, P = 0·03$	

*'Within last year' vs. 'over a year ago'
†'About right for my age' vs. 'too high', 'too low', 'can't remember'
‡'About right for my age' vs. 'too high', 'too low', 'can't remember', 'have never had level checked'.
CCPD, co-ordinated care post-discharge; GP, general practitioner.

Table 4 Lifestyle changes since CEA reported at follow-up by group (n = 129)*

	CCPD group (n = 63), n (%)	Control group (n = 66), n (%)	Differences between groups
Have you made any changes to your lifestyle since your CEA to further reduce your stroke risk?			
Yes	35 (55·6)	21 (31·8)	P = 0·006
No	19 (30·2)	34 (50·0)	
Unsure	7 (11·1)	10 (15·2)	
Please list changes made†			
'Changes to diet'	35 (55·5)	15 (22·7)	P < 0·001
'Increased exercise'	15 (23·8)	9 (13·6)	P = 0·14
'Decreased' or 'ceased smoking'	6 (9·5)	6 (9·1)	
'Resigned positions held in organizations'/ 'retired'/'decreased stress'/'relaxing more'	2 (3·2)	2 (3·0)	
Following my doctors advice	0	1 (1·5)	

*Where totals do not add to 100%, data were missing.
†More than one option possible per patient.
CEA, carotid endarterectomy.
CCPD, co-ordinated care post-discharge.

Knowledge of stroke warning signs

There were no differences in baseline mean knowledge scores according to symptom status (symptomatic or asymptomatic) ($t = -1·1$, d.f. = 128, $P = 0·29$). Within group matched

t-test analyses for patient knowledge of warning signs of stroke showed a statistically significant yet small increase in the mean score for the CCPD group from 12·0 at baseline to 13·2 at follow-up ($t = -4·0$, d.f. = 60, $P < 0·001$). For the control group, the increase was not as great and was not

S. Middleton et al.

statistically significant (11·2–11·6) ($t = -1·1$, d.f. $= 63$, $P = 0·29$).

Linear regression analysis demonstrated that the improvement in patients' knowledge of stroke warning signs from baseline to follow-up was statistically significantly greater for the CCPD group ($P = 0·002$).

Knowledge of conditions that make it more likely for somebody to have a stroke

There was a small though non-significant increase in the mean score for patient knowledge of conditions that make it more likely for somebody to have a stroke for the control group (4·3–5·0) ($t = -2·0$, d.f. $= 65$, $P = 0·06$). There was no change at all for this outcome for the CCPD group (5·4–5·4) ($t = -0·0$, d.f. $= 62$, $P = 1·0$) and no statistically significant between group effect for changes between baseline and follow-up ($P = 0·46$). At follow-up, the most frequently identified condition was 'high blood pressure' ($n = 118$, 88·7%) followed by 'high cholesterol' ($n = 103$, 77·4%). 'Stress' was incorrectly identified as a condition that makes it more likely for someone to have a stroke by 90 (67·7%) patients.

Knowledge about stroke

Stroke was reported to be either 'moderately' or 'totally' preventable by 70·5% of patients in the CCPD group at baseline and 68·9% of patients in this group at follow-up, a non-significant change (McNemar's $\chi^2 = 0·0$, d.f. $= 1$, $P = 1·0$). Among the control group there was a modest thought non-significant increase in the per cent reporting stroke to be 'moderately' or 'totally' preventable from 52·5% to 59·0% (McNemar's $\chi^2 = 0·5$, d.f. $= 1$, $P = 0·5$). Repeated measures analysis also failed to find a statistically significant difference between the groups for changes in the perceived preventability of stroke ($\chi^2 = 0·9$, d.f. $= 1$, $P = 0·35$).

Stroke response

When asked what they would do if someone they were with 'looked like' they were having a stroke, patients in the CCPD group demonstrated a non-significant increase in the percentage of correct responses from baseline (91·9%) to follow-up (96·8%) ($\chi^2 = 0·8$, d.f. $= 1$, $P = 0·40$). Similarly, the control group showed a non-significant increase in the proportion of correct responses from baseline (92·1%) to follow-up (93·7%) ($\chi^2 = 0·0$, d.f. $= 1$, $P = 1·0$). There was no statistically significant difference between the groups at follow-up ($\chi^2 = 0·5$, d.f. $= 1$, $P = 0·47$).

Patient perceptions of their stroke risk

When asked their level of concern about risk of stroke during the next 12 months, the proportion of patients in the CCPD group rating their concern as low ('not at all' or 'rarely') increased statistically significantly from 34·9% at baseline to 60·3% at follow-up (McNemar's $\chi^2 = 8·0$, d.f. $= 1$, $P = 0·005$). In the control group, the proportion also increased statistically significantly (35·4% at baseline to 58·5% at follow-up) (McNemar's $\chi^2 = 7·8$, d.f. $= 1$, $P = 0·005$). There was no significant difference between the groups at follow-up however ($\chi^2 = 0·1$, d.f. $= 1$, $P = 0·83$).

Similarly, there was a statistically significant increase for both groups from baseline to follow-up in the proportion of patients who rated their risk of having a stroke over the next 12 months as being 'low'. In the CCPD group, the percentage rating their risk as low increased significantly from 29·5% at baseline to 54·1% at follow-up (McNemar's $\chi^2 = 7·3$, d.f. $= 1$, $P = 0·007$) while in the control group these figures increased from 24·2% at baseline to 61·3% at follow-up (McNemar's $\chi^2 = 16·7$, d.f. $= 1$, $P < 0·0001$). However, repeated measures analysis showed that there was no statistically significant difference between the groups for this outcome at follow-up ($\chi^2 = 1·4$, d.f. $= 1$, $P = 0·25$).

Written information read after CEA

Almost all patients from the CCPD Group ($n = 62$, 98%) reported having received written information about stroke following their CEA. Of those who did, a majority reported that this information was 'very useful' or 'useful' ($n = 57$, 91·9%) and the amount 'about right' (95·2%). Less than a quarter of patients from the control group ($n = 15$, 22·4%) reported receiving written information post-CEA. Statistically significantly fewer patients in the control group considered the amount of information received to be 'about right' when compared with the CCPD group (66·7% vs. 95·2%) ($\chi^2 = 11·3$, d.f. $= 1$, $P = 0·001$).

Verbal information received after CEA

Recollection of verbal information about stroke received from a health practitioner after CEA differed statistically significantly between groups (60·3% CCPD group vs. 40·0% control group) ($\chi^2 = 5·07$, d.f. $= 1$, $P = 0·02$).

Discussion

Advocacy for new models of nursing should be made 'on the basis of rigorous evaluation and evidence rather than on

---

What is already known about this topic

- There is little rigorous evaluation of nursing-led, co-ordinated care postdischarge models.
- No studies have evaluated nursing-led, co-ordinated care postdischarge models in vascular surgery.

What this paper adds

- Nursing-led, co-ordinated care after discharge statistically significantly improved patient knowledge of stroke warning signs.
- Nursing-led, co-ordinated care after discharge resulted in statistically significant improvements to patients' self-reported changes to lifestyle to decrease stroke risk, particularly diet modification.
- Use of telephone contact can aid co-ordination of care for patients after carotid endarterectomy.

opinion or vested interests' (Spitzer 1976, p. 212). Informing the development of better nursing services through the generation of rigorously acquired evidence from studies such as ours is imperative. Our study demonstrated statistically significant short-term benefits for patients provided with structured education and clinician liaison after CEA by a RN. This result is in keeping with positive findings supporting the effect of nursing-led, CCPD in the four previously-mentioned randomized controlled trials (DeBusk *et al.* 1994, Naylor *et al.* 1999, Escobar *et al.* 2001, Riegel *et al.* 2002). First, patient knowledge of stroke warning signs improved statistically significantly following CCPD. In addition, patients who received CCPD were statistically significantly more likely to report making lifestyle changes to decrease their stroke risk following their CEA. A statistically significantly higher number of patients from the CCPD group reported making changes to their diet at follow-up when compared with patients from the control group. Patients in the control group were statistically significantly more likely to state that they had not received any written information about stroke and or stroke risk factors since their CEA when compared with the CCPD group. For patients who indicated that they had received some written information about stroke since their CEA, those from the CCPD group were statistically significantly more likely to state that the amount of written information received was 'about right' when compared with the control group. Patients in the CCPD group were statistically significantly more likely to state that since their operation, a health professional had discussed stroke and stroke risk factors with them.

Co-ordinated care postdischarge did not improve patient knowledge of conditions that make it more likely for

somebody to have a stroke, however. Baseline level of knowledge for this question was high, with more than half of the patients identifying five of the six known conditions. Stress was incorrectly identified as a condition that makes it more likely for someone to have a stroke by over two-thirds of patients both at baseline and follow-up and this figure is higher than that obtained by Sug Yoon *et al.* (2001), indicating public misconceptions of the relationship between stress and stroke. This misunderstanding persisted from baseline to follow-up even in the CCPD group (67·7% identifying stress at baseline and also at follow-up).

Statistically significant improvements were detected from baseline to follow-up for both groups for current health status, time spent per week in physical activity, concern about having a stroke in the next 12 months and perception of this risk. While there were no between-group differences for these variables, the statistically significant within-group improvements suggest that the CEA operation itself may have been a catalyst for improved patient outcomes. Statistically significant improvements were found from baseline to follow-up within the CCPD group only for patients rating of their current general health status and sufficient time and sessions per week spent in physical activity.

Baseline data showed that 22·6% of patients were current smokers. This figure is comparable with a recent Australian audit in general practice (Sturm *et al.* 2002). Smoking cessation advice had not achieved the desired outcome for patients in our trial. There were no statistically significant changes in the prevalence of current smokers from baseline to follow-up between the two groups, although numbers were small.

The short duration of follow-up precluded determining if the intervention had any long-term effect on decreasing patient cholesterol, blood pressure, smoking and stroke rates. In addition, the study results relied on patient self-report, with no validation by GPs or determination of GP attitudes to the intervention; this was precluded because of financial and time constraints. The study was also limited by its small sample size. Recruitment depended on the number of patients admitted for CEA by participating surgeons which, despite an 8-month recruitment period, was only moderate.

Patient acceptability of the postoperative nursing-led intervention was high, with 92% of eligible patients agreeing to participate. The excellent response rates for both the baseline (100%) and follow-up surveys (98%) were also positive methodological indicators.

Conclusions

Nurses are well-placed to deliver preventive care advice within the healthcare system. Education of patients about

S. Middleton et al.

stroke, transient ischaemic attack warning signs and risk factor modification in this trial required extensive clinical knowledge. It is possible that patient acceptance of this intervention, demonstrated by the high patient participation rate, may be due to the nursing-led nature of the intervention.

While case managers exist within many hospital settings, they focus largely on co-ordination of inpatient care, with little postoperative liaison with primary care (Lyon 1993). Our results suggest that the use of telephone contact with patients in the postoperative period to aid co-ordinated care may be a useful approach. They also suggest that nursing-led, co-ordinated care after discharge can positively influence patient outcomes.

Acknowledgements

The authors thank all patients and surgeons for agreeing to participate in this study. Sandy Middleton would like to thank the National Health and Medical Research Council of Australia for awarding her a Public Health Research Scholarship to undertake this work (RegKey:# 142617).

Author contributions

JW was responsible for the study conception and design. SM performed the data collection and drafted the manuscript. SM and ND performed the data analysis. ND, JH and JW made critical revisions to the paper. ND provided statistical expertise. JH provided administrative support. JW supervised.

References

Armitage P. & Berry G. (1994) *Statistical Methods in Medical Research*, 3rd edn. Blackwell Scientific Publications, Oxford.

Armstrong T., Bauman A. & Davies J. (2000) *Physical Activity Patterns of Australian Adults. Results of the 1999 National Physical Activity Survey*, Cat no CVD 10. Australian Institute of Health and Welfare, Canberra.

Campbell M., Grimshaw J. & Steen N. (2000) Sample size calculations for cluster randomised trials. *Journal of Health Services & Research Policy* 5, 12–16.

Chambers B.R., You R.X. & Donnan G.A. (2000) Carotid endarterectomy for asymptomatic carotid stenosis. *The Cochrane Database of Systematic Reviews* 1999, Issue 4. Art. No.: CD001923. DOI: 10.1002/14651858.CD001923.

Cina C.S., Clase C.M. & Haynes R.B. (1999) Carotid endarterectomy for symptomatic carotid stenosis. *The Cochrane Database of Systematic Reviews* 1999, Issue 3. Art. No.: CD001081. DOI: 10.1002/14651858.CD001081.

De Busk R.F., Houston Miller N., Superko R., Dennis C.A., Thomas R.J., Lew H.T., Berger W.E., Heller R.S., Rompf J., Gee D.,

Kraemer H.C., Bandura A., Ghandour G., Clark M., Shah R.V., Fisher L. & Taylor C.B. (1994) A case-management system for coronary risk factor modification after acute myocardial infarction. *Annals of Internal Medicine* 120, 721–729.

Edwards P., Roberts I., Clarke M., DiGuiseppi C., Pratap S., Wentz R. & Kwan I. (2002) Increasing response rates to postal questionnaires: systematic review. *BMJ* 324, 1183–1193.

Escobar G.J., Braveman P.A., Ackerson L., Odouli R., Coleman-Phox K., Capra A.M., Wong C. & Lieu T.A. (2001) A randomized comparison of home visits and hospital-based group follow-up visits after early postpartum discharge. *Pediatrics* 108, 719–727.

Griffiths P.D., Edwards M.E., Forbes A., Harris R.L. & Ritchie G. (2002) Intermediate care in nursing-led in-patient units: effects on health care outcomes and resources (Cochrane Review). In *The Cochrane Library*, Issue 4. Update Software, Oxford.

James S. (2001) *The Heart Foundation Cookbook*. R & R Publications Marketing Pty Ltd on behalf of the National Heart Foundation, Melbourne.

Lyon J.C. (1993) Models of nursing care delivery and case management: clarification of terms. *Nursing Economics* 11, 163–169.

Middleton S. & Donnelly N. (2002) Outcomes of carotid endarterectomy: how does the Australian state of New South Wales compare with international benchmarks? *Journal of Vascular Surgery* 36, 62–69.

Middleton S., Harris J., Lusby R. & Ward J. (2003) Vascular disease risk factor management four years after carotid endarterectomy: are opportunities missed? *ANZ Journal of Surgery* 73, 225–231.

Moher D., Schulz K.F. & Altman D.G., for the CONSORT Group (2001) The CONSORT statement: revised recommendations for improving the quality of reports of parallel-group randomized trials. *Lancet* 357, 1191–1194.

Murray C.P. & Lopez A.D. (1997) Mortality by cause for eight regions of the world: Global Burden of Disease Study. *Lancet* 349, 1269–1276.

National Health and Medical Research Council (1997a) *Prevention of Stroke. The role of Anticoagulants, Antiplatelet Agents and Carotid Endarterectomy. Clinical Practice Guidelines*. Australian Government Publishing Service, Canberra. Available at http://www.nhmrc.gov.au/publications/synopses/cp45to47syn.htm.

National Health and Medical Research Council (1997b) *Prevention of Stroke. A Consumer's Guide*. Australian Government Publishing Service, Canberra.

National Stroke Foundation (1997) *National Stroke Strategy*. National Stroke Foundation, Victoria.

National Stroke Foundation (2000) *Stroke Attacks the Brain. Answers to the Top Ten Questions About Stroke*. National Stroke Foundation, Melbourne.

Naylor M., Brooten D., Campbell R., Jacobsen B., Mezey M., Pauly M. & Schwartz J. (1999) Comprehensive discharge planning and home follow-up of hospitalized elders. *Journal of the American Medical Association* 281, 613–620.

Norusis M.J. (1999) *SPSS Inc. SPSS Professional Statistics*, Version 9.0.1. SPSS, Chicago.

Phillips C.Y. (1993) Post-discharge follow-up care: effect on patient outcomes. *Journal of Nursing Care Quality* 7(4), 64–72.

Riegel B., Carlson B., Kopp Z., LePetri B., Glaser D. & Unger A. (2002) Effect of a standardized nurse case-management telephone intervention on resource use in patients with chronic heart failure. *Archives of Internal Medicine* **162**, 705–712.

SAS Institute Inc (1999) *SAS/STAT Users Guide*, Version 8. SAS Institute Inc., Cary, NC, USA.

Spitzer W.O. (1976) Evidence that justifies the introduction of new health professionals. In *The Professions and Public Policy* (Slaytor P. & Trebilcock M., eds), University of Toronto Press, Toronto. pp. 211–236.

Sturm J.W., Davis M., O'Sullivan J.G., Vedadhaghi M.E. & Donnan G. (2002) The Avoid Stroke as Soon as Possible (ASAP) general practice stroke audit. *Medical Journal of Australia* **176**, 312–316.

Sug Yoon S., Heller R., Levi C., Wiggers J. & Fitzgerald P.E. (2001) Knowledge of stroke risk factors, warning symptoms and treatment among an Australian urban population. *Stroke* **32**, 1926–1930.

Vickers A.J. & Altman D.G. (2001) Analysing controlled trials with baseline and follow up measurements. *BMJ* **323**, 1123–1124.

Zwarenstein M., Stephenson B. & Johnston L. (2002) *Case Management: Effects on Professional Practice and Health Care Outcomes*. Update Software, Oxford.

Data analysis

Adequate information is provided in the tables and narrative about the tests used. Non-parametric tests were used to determine differences between groups. Parametric tests were used for interval-scaled variables to measure within group changes. For binary outcome variables, McNemar's test for paired proportions was calculated within each group to (a) assess changes in the proportion reporting the attribute of interest, and (b) to determine whether there was a difference between groups in the percentage reporting change in the attribute of interest. For interval-scaled variables, within-group changes were conducted to determine whether the groups differed in their mean post-scores.

Findings

There were statistically significant short-term benefits for the CCPD intervention group. This result is supported by the positive findings in the four American studies. In the CCPD group there was a statistically significant improvement in knowledge of stroke warning signs and also reported lifestyle and dietary changes. However, CCPD did not improve patient knowledge about the conditions that would increase the incidence of stroke. The majority of the patients incorrectly identified stress at both baseline and follow-up as contributing to stroke. There were no statistically significant changes in smoking habits between the groups. The authors suggested that (a) telephone contact in the postoperative period to aid co-ordinated care may be useful, and (b) nursing-led co-ordinated care post discharge can positively enhance patient outcomes. Further research into nursing-led co-ordinated care for vascular surgery patients was recommended.

Limitations

The short duration of follow-up prevented determination of any long-term effect on decreasing cholesterol, blood pressure, smok-

ing and stroke rates. In addition, results relied on patient self-report with no validation by GPs. Another limitation was the small sample size despite an 8-month recruitment timeframe. However, positive aspects of the trial were evidenced by patient acceptability of the nursing-led intervention and of the high participation rate. An omission is the lack of information about how power analysis was used to determine sample size.

> **Evidence-based practice tip**
> - A randomised controlled trial is an experimental method used to determine the effects of a treatment or intervention on individuals randomly assigned to either a control or intervention group and does not state hypotheses.
> - Randomisation is a key issue impacting on the validity of a study.

> **Points to ponder**
> ► Should findings that do not support the research hypothesis be reported?
> ► How does the absence of study limitations affect the generalisability of the findings?

Summary

Research consumers need to have a clear understanding of the research process and major research approaches. Also required is the ability to read critically in order to objectively interpret and determine the usefulness and implications of a study for practice change. Critical reading involves reading for the levels of *understanding*. These are: preliminary, comprehensive, analysis, and synthesis understanding. Separate guidelines have been developed to assist in the critique of qualitative and quantitative studies. These guidelines provide a format for asking questions about the study and are useful in structuring a critical reading of qualitative and quantitative research studies.

K EY POINTS

- The best way to become an intelligent research consumer is to have a clear understanding of the research process and the major research approaches.

- The goal of synthesis understanding is to combine the parts of a research study into a whole. During this final stage the reader determines how each step relates to all the steps of the research, how well the study meets the criteria used to critique the study, and the usefulness of the study for practice.

- Critical reading involves active interpretation and objective assessment of an article, looking for key concepts, ideas and justification.

- The most important point when analysing statistical procedures in a study is the relationship of the statistics used to the research question, design and method.

- Clues to the appropriate statistical test to be used by the researcher should stem from the researcher's hypothesis.

- Ethical issues in qualitative research involve issues related to the naturalistic setting, emergent nature of the design, research–participant interaction and the 'researcher as instrument'.

Learning activities

1. To be able to critically read research articles is important for nurses and midwives because:
   (a) all nurses and midwives should conduct research
   (b) all nurses and midwives should understand the research process
   (c) the knowledge will enhance their practice
   (d) they will be able to base their practice on research evidence and improve patient care.

2. When planning your research study, a literature search is undertaken:
   (a) to identify gaps and limitations in the published research
   (b) to find a research topic
   (c) because it is important to read many articles
   (d) to learn how to read critically.

3. Synthesis understanding refers to:
   (a) preliminary understanding
   (b) seeing parts of the study in relation to the whole
   (c) combining parts into a complex whole
   (d) breaking the content into parts or sections.

4. Understanding a research article and seeing the terms in relation to the context relates to:
   (a) preliminary understanding
   (b) comprehensive understanding
   (c) analysis understanding
   (d) synthesis understanding.

5. The highest level of evidence for a therapy question is:
   (a) a randomised controlled trial
   (b) a descriptive design
   (c) a correlational design
   (d) a qualitative approach.

6. Ethical clearance from an HREC is necessary before commencing a study because:
   (a) the HREC wants to know what your research is about
   (b) the HREC wants to know when you intend to begin your research
   (c) participants in the study can be assured ethical treatment if your study has been passed by a human research ethics committee
   (d) participants want to tell their friends that they are taking part in a study.

7. Evidence-based practice is a quality improvement process because:
   (a) you have critically analysed many research articles
   (b) you have learned how to skim when reading research articles
   (c) trial and error is still important in clinical practice
   (d) evidence-based practice is a key factor contributing to accountability and benchmarking.

8. Stating recommendations for further research is important because:
   (a) it indicates that you understand that further research would enhance the knowledge base of nursing or midwifery in that area
   (b) it shows that you recognise the limitations of your research study
   (c) readers like to get ideas about topics from research studies
   (d) readers will think your research design was poor.

9. Writing about the implications of your study for healthcare is important because:
   (a) readers like to know about health problems in the community
   (b) a well-planned nursing or midwifery research study should have implications for healthcare
   (c) it indicates lack of careful planning before conducting the research
   (d) people need to know what healthcare is about.

10. Providing an audit trail when analysing data is important because:
    (a) it shows that you can audit your research
    (b) it is useful to provide a trail for readers to follow
    (c) it gives the reader information about the method by which data were analysed
    (d) it makes the study more interesting.

Additional resources

Duffy J R 2005 Critically appraising quantitative research. *Nursing and Health Sciences* 7:281–3

Sandelowski M 2004 Using qualitative research. *Qualitative Health Research* 14(10):1366–86

Sandelowski M, Barroso J 2002 Finding the findings in qualitative studies. *Journal of Nursing Scholarship* 34(3):213–19

—— 2003 Classifying the findings in qualitative studies. *Qualitative Health Research* 13(7):905–23

Saunders L D, Soomro G M, Buckingham J, Jamtvedt G, Raina P 2003 Assessing the methodological quality of non-randomised intervention studies. *Western Journal of Nursing Research* 25(2):223–37

References

Arthur D, Drury J, Sy-Sinda M T, et al. 2005 A primary health care curriculum in action: the lived experience of primary health care nurses in a school of nursing in the Philippines: a phenomenological study. *International Journal of Nursing Studies* 43:107–12

Campbell M, Torrance C 2005 Coronary angioplasty: impact on risk factors and patients' understanding of the severity of their condition. *Australian Journal of Advanced Nursing* 22(4):26–31

DiCenso A, Ciliska D, Cullum N, et al. 2004 *Evidence-based nursing: a guide to clinical practice.* Mosby, St Louis

Dunning T, Manias E 2004 Medication knowledge and self-management by people with type 2 diabetes. *Australian Journal of Advanced Nursing* 23(1):7–13

Fenwick J, Hauck Y, Downie J, et al. 2004 The childbirth expectations of a self-selected cohort of Western Australian women. *Midwifery* 21:23–35

Kvale S 1996 *InterViews. An introduction to Qualitative Research Interviewing.* Sage Publications, Thousand Oaks, California

Middleton S, Donnelly N, Harris J, et al. 2005 Nursing intervention after carotid endarterectomy: a randomised trial of Co-ordinated Care Post-Discharge (CCPD). *Journal of Advanced Nursing* 52(3):250–61

Paul R, Elder L 2001 *Critical thinking: tools for taking charge of your learning and your life.* Prentice-Hall, Englewood, New Jersey

—— 2003 *The thinker's guide on how to read a paragraph.* Foundation for Critical Thinking, Dillon Beach, California

Pravikoff D S, Tanner A B, Pierce S T 2005 Readiness of US Nurses for Evidence-Based Practice. *American Journal of Nursing* 105(9):40–51

Simpson M, Parsons M, Greenwood J, et al. 2001 Raspberry Leaf in Pregnancy: its safety and efficacy in labor. *Journal of Midwifery & Women's Health* 46(2):51–9

Webster J, Lloyd W C, Pritchard M A, et al. 1999 Development of evidence-based guidelines in midwifery and gynaecology nursing. *Midwifery* 15:2–5

Answers

TT Tutorial trigger 1

1. **Preliminary understanding**
   Skimming or lightly reading an article enables the reader to get a feel or a general sense of the content. The title and abstract are read carefully and introduce the reader to the main variables under review. Content, such as reading the introduction, major headings and one or two sentences under each heading, and the conclusion are skimmed.

2. **Comprehensive understanding**
   The purpose of this activity is to comprehend (understand) the parts (the main ideas or themes) of the study in relation to the whole; that is, show the relationship or connection of each part to the whole.

3. **Analysis understanding**
   To analyse is to break the content into essential features/sections in order to discover meaning. Examine how accurately the research study meets the criteria for each stage. You should be able to summarise each section into your own words and decide which level of evidence fits the study.

4. **Synthesis understanding**
   The process of combining the parts into a cohesive whole. At this stage determinations are made about how well the study met the criteria, its contribution to nursing and healthcare, and its practical utility. The strengths, weaknesses (limitations) and recommendations should be clear to the research consumer.

TT Tutorial trigger 2

1. Decide on the clinical area and topic she wants to investigate.
2. Discuss topic with theatre manager re practicality, feasibility, support, availability of resources and time. It is also important to establish the nurse's level of research capability and knowledge of the clinical area. When these matters are resolved, the nurse should undertake a search of the literature.
3. The nurse should search refereed journals to discover what has been published in the area.
4. Articles should be downloaded or photocopied and critically analysed in terms of sample, method, research approach, data collection methods and data analysis.
5. Identify gaps, inconsistencies and limitations in the articles. Attach an analysis of each article to the article.
6. Discuss her literature search with the theatre manager and decide on a topic, design and method.
7. Write a clear description of what she plans to do, taking account of the issues discussed in point 2.
8. If the proposed research involves patients, a hospital proposal and ethics form will have to be completed for presentation to the hospital HREC. The contents of the proposal will depend upon the design and method and elaboration of ethical issues.
9. If the proposed research involves procedures (e.g. washing hands, wearing face mask appropriately), the proposal may not have to be submitted to the hospital HREC, but instead to the Nursing Division.
10. Once approval for the research has been received, the project can commence.

TT Tutorial trigger 3

While all of us have completed the same research units, only some of us will embark on a nursing or midwifery research career. We won't all be conducting research although we may well be expected, in the clinical area, to be part of, or assist in, a research project. For example, we may be asked to collect certain data (e.g. urine samples, blood pressure readings, temperature readings) for inclusion in a clinical medical, nursing or midwifery study.

The emphasis on evidence-based practice, that is, using the best available evidence to provide quality patient care, necessitates a good understanding of the research process (which we obtained in our research unit), and the ability to critically read and evaluate research articles in order to apply the findings to our particular clinical area. So it isn't a question of some of us not intending to conduct research because our interests are elsewhere; it is a question of understanding the content (design, method, sample, data collection and analysis methods) of research articles in order to make decisions about our practice. Every nurse and midwife should be a competent research consumer.

Once we accept the responsibility of providing best practice in our nursing and midwifery care, we become accountable for the quality of care we administer. Critical reading of research articles then becomes paramount; we need to be in a position of knowledge in order to discuss which evidence relates best to our particular practices. Our knowledge of our clinical area and the research process, and the decisions we make (which include an understanding of patient preferences, needs and values) provide us with the best tools we need to offer our patients the best possible care.

Critical reading requires skilled reading, writing and reasoning abilities. And these skills can be learned — the more we practice, the more competent we become. Reading critically involves four levels of understanding: preliminary understanding (gained through a light reading), comprehensive understanding (identifying core concepts and recognising relationships between the different parts), analysis understanding (breaking the article into parts in order to gain a deeper understanding of each part), and synthesis understanding (putting the parts together again into a complex whole).

When we have mastered the critical reading technique we will be able to read articles more fluently, with greater understanding and enjoyment.

Learning activities

1. d	**2.** a	**3.** c	**4.** b
5. a	**6.** c	**7.** d	**8.** a
9. b	**10.** c		

Evidence-based practice and practice development

BRIDIE KENT AND BRENDAN MCCORMACK

Learning outcomes

After reading this chapter, you should be able to:

- outline what is meant by the terms 'evidence-based practice' and 'practice development'
- understand the relationship between evidence-based practice and practice development — in particular the relationships between evidence, practice, context and the facilitation of change
- discuss how nurses and midwives might influence their own clinical practice through practice development and evidence-based practice
- describe the five 'steps' involved in evidence-based practice
- describe the relationship between evidence-based practice and clinical research
- understand the systems and processes that underpin different models of practice development
- identify strategies for facilitating the development of practice
- outline the role of organisations, such as the Cochrane Collaboration and the Joanna Briggs Institute, in evidence synthesis and utilisation
- locate internet websites that provide useful evidence-based practice and practice development resources.

Introduction

The introduction of evidence-based practice (EBP), in the mid-1990s, marked a significant shift from care based on routine and ritual, to that based on what works best to achieve the desired outcomes. Subsequently, practice development (PD) and EBP have become familiar terms to nurses, midwives and other health professionals during the past decade. Webster et al. (1999) argue that these concepts have become acceptable to clinicians because they are intuitively 'sensible'. When used together, PD and EBP are strong and powerful mechanisms for the ongoing development of skills in practice and practice change (see Chapter 18). Competence needs to be, wherever possible, based on best available evidence derived from a variety of sources. Decision-making underpins EBP which incorporates experiential knowledge of health professionals, patient preferences and the best available empirical evidence, considered within the reality of limited resources.

Fineout-Overholt et al. (2004) comment that EBP has become a driving force for problem-solving, to improve clinical practice, and cost-effectiveness of care. Many healthcare organisations have invested heavily in strategies to increase the likelihood that all clinical practice is evidence-based wherever possible. In Australia, the National Institute for Clinical Studies (NICS) has been established for this purpose. In New Zealand, the closest comparator is the New Zealand Guidelines Group (NZGG). Also in Australia and New Zealand, regulatory authorities for health professionals use self-reflective competency frameworks to maximise client safety. For instance, New Zealand has enacted the *Health Practitioners Competency Assurance Act*, which requires evidence of clinical and theoretical competency in the form of evidence portfolios, for all registered health professionals (Ministry of Health 2003).

This chapter introduces the processes of PD and EBP, as well as identifying additional resources for further information. It complements the following chapter (Chapter 18) which deals with related issues of using research to change practice. This chapter contextualises the relationship between PD and EBP in order to engender greater awareness. In turn, this reveals the strategies being used internationally to integrate knowledge, research and practice, within the complexity of today's healthcare settings. Overviews of the history of PD and EBP are provided, including identification of the processes involved in both concepts. You will read in other texts about evidence-based nursing, evidence-based midwifery, evidence-based medicine and the like. In essence, however, whether EBP is being undertaken by a nurse, a midwife, a doctor or another health professional, the skills required are the same. Where differences occur, they do so from the types of questions being asked, rather than the methods used to answer them. The methodology of emancipatory practice development (EPD) is outlined and the processes involved considered. Linkages between evidence, the context in which it is implemented and the processes involved in facilitating its use in practice, will be considered by referring to the PARIHS project (Kitson et al. 1998; Rycroft-Malone et al. 2002). Particular approaches to facilitating developments in practice are also described and applied to practice.

Defining practice development and evidence-based practice

The terms knowledge, evidence or research utilisation are often used interchangeably. They have become widely discussed in the literature, as are the models developed to guide these processes. Stetler (1994), Kitson et al. (1998) and Estabrooks (1999) originally moved the boundaries, in beginning to make explicit the links between evidence-based practice (EBP) and practice development (PD). McCormack et al. (1999) highlighted the need for practice development as a primary mechanism for creating work environments that sustain evidence-based, person-centred practice — thus providing a framework and collection of methods for making EBP a reality. The links are also captured by the Promoting Action on Research Implementation in Health Services (PARIHS) project (Rycroft-Malone 2004). This project acknowledges the principle that successful implementation of evidence into practice, by clinicians, is more likely if a systematic, explicit and context-specific approach to facilitation is adopted. The PARIHS framework proposes that evidence, context and facilitation are interrelated and influence the success of evidence utilisation in practice. It is used to assist practice change in many countries world-wide, including Australia and New Zealand. Closely linked to the work of the PARIHS project, the methodology of PD is used to gain an in-depth understanding of practice context so that the most appropriate facilitative approach to using and generating evidence in and from practice is adopted.

Practice development definition

Practice development has been described as meaning many things to different people (Harrison 2005). However, the definition developed by Garbett and McCormack (2002; 2004) is used here. It is (2002 p 88):

> a continuous process of improvement towards increased effectiveness in patient-centred care. This is brought about by helping health care teams to develop their knowledge and skills and to transform the culture and context of care. It is enabled and supported by facilitators committed to systematic rigorous continuous processes of emancipatory change that reflect the perspectives of service users and service providers.

Central to this process is achieving increased effectiveness in patient-centred care, which requires appreciation, knowledge and implementation of evidence — each of which are complex issues in themselves.

● Evidence-based practice tip

Practice development and evidence-based practice have a synergistic relationship with the mutual intention of 'effectiveness' in practice.

Evidence-based practice definition

Evidence-based practice also holds a number of different meanings within and between healthcare professions, due largely to the history of contemporary EBP. One widely accepted definition is that first proffered by

the medical professional Sackett and his colleagues, who believe EBP involves the conscientious use of current best evidence when making decisions about patient care (Sackett et al. 2000). Another definition is that generated by DiCenso et al. (1998) who, as nurses, suggest that it is a process within which clinical decisions are made by practitioners using the best available research evidence, their clinical expertise and patient preferences, with consideration also of available and finite resources. Similarly, for midwifery, Fullerton and Thompson (2005 p 2) state that:

> evidence-based practice should be characterised by the use of best practices derived from rigorous research, combined with and balanced by client perspectives and the expert judgment based on the critical thinking of the clinician.

Stewart (2001), however, in a qualitative study of midwives, obstetricians and a research nurse, found that the concept of EBP was not 'value-free'; stating that definitions of evidence varied widely between the participants and disciplines. Practitioners should be mindful of this and clear about evidence-based concepts before proceeding with the practice development process. The following discussion should help to clarify these points.

The practice development process

As noted previously, Garbett and McCormack (2004) articulate the interconnected relationships between the development of knowledge, facilitation and skills. They also identify the relatedness of systematic, rigorous and continuous processes of emancipatory change, in order to achieve the ultimate purpose of evidence-based person-centred care. The key elements of this process are:

- increasing effectiveness in patient-centred care
- transforming the contexts and cultures in which nursing care takes place
- the importance of employing a systematic approach to effect changes in practice
- the continuous nature of PD activity
- the nature of the facilitation required for change to take place.

> ● **Evidence-based practice tip**
>
> There are a number of practice development definitions available in the literature. However, the key elements of the definition outlined here encompass the elements of other definitions — which tend to focus on specific aspects of practice rather than the culture and context of practice, as implied here.

Manley and McCormack (2004) articulate the elements of PD in a model called 'emancipatory practice development' (EPD — see following paragraph), drawing on previous theoretical developments in action research (see Chapter 15) (Grundy 1982). With EPD, the emphasis extends beyond the changing of specific aspects of practice, such as changing the way nurses or midwives undertake drug administration. This is, instead, what Manley and McCormack (2004) call 'technical practice development' (TPD), which relies on acquiring technical knowledge to improve technical skills (or competence). In TPD, best practice is universally defined and the assumption that, if practitioners know the evidence, then their (technical) practice will be effective, is central. Technical practice development, in many respects, resembles more traditional passive approaches to research utilisation whereby, promoting awareness of deficiencies in practitioners' practice and subsequently educating them on what constitutes 'best practice', practice change naturally follows on. However, research has suggested otherwise and critiques of technical approaches to helping people using knowledge in practice (e.g. a teaching session about improving pain management) have highlighted the naivety of assuming that acquired knowledge will automatically lead to a change in practice (Kitson et al. 1998).

T_T Tutorial trigger 1

Can you identify particular knowledge that you acquired in university but which you have been unable to transfer into your practice? What issues prevent you from using this knowledge in practice?

Emancipatory practice development (EPD) emphasises that, in order to bring about sustained development of practice, healthcare teams need to be enabled to transform the culture and context of practice. Thus it is a broad view of practice development and it focuses on both getting research into practice and creating a culture of innovation and clinical effectiveness. Facilitating these processes involves cycles of reflective learning and action, so that practitioners develop awareness of the need for change. This accompanies the identification of contradictions between what is espoused about practice and the realities of practice. The process therefore takes action to change practice and refine action through reflection.

Facilitated processes help practitioners remove barriers to action and enable cultures of effectiveness to be developed. Whilst evidence is important to EPD, best practice is locally defined and contextually bound. So for evidence to be understood and used, it has to be placed in a local context that makes sense to the immediacy of practice experience. Thus, evidence in this context, comes from a variety of sources (empirical evidence, practitioner experience and user preferences) (after Rycroft-Malone et al. 2004b) and is acquired through reflective engagement with collective practice experience. In terms of evaluating effectiveness, therefore, the emphasis is on both the outcomes achieved from the developments in practice and on the processes used to achieve those outcomes. Through developing a thorough understanding of the processes used to achieve particular outcomes, these processes can be transferred to other contexts and thus create cultures of continuous improvement that are committed to increasing effectiveness in patient-centred care. Figure 17.1 presents a model of EPD developed by Garbett and McCormack (2002).

The key processes of EPD are consistent with and operationalise the PARIHS framework. They are summarised in this figure as:

1. Clarifying values and beliefs about the particular development focus.
2. Identifying the existence of these values and beliefs in practice.
3. Identifying the 'gap' that exists between the espoused and the real values through processes of inquiry and evaluation.
4. Systematic approaches to developing practice are negotiated and action plans put in place to develop practice.
5. The model of facilitation that is negotiated with key stakeholders includes a sustainable commitment to learning from the processes, via reflective learning strategies, such as action learning (McGill & Brockbank 2004) and supported reflective practice (Johns 1998).

FIGURE 17.1 Practice development model

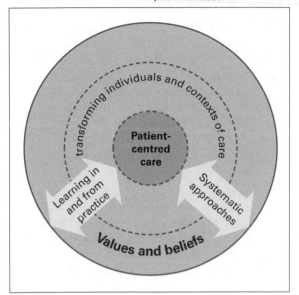

(Source: Garbett & McCormack 2002)

The evidence-based practice process

Evidence-based practice evolved from concerns expressed by Dr Archie Cochrane, in the early 1970s, about the medical profession's reliance on practices that were not substantiated by rigorous evidence reviews. The subsequent debate resulted in the formation of the Cochrane Collaboration in 1993 to facilitate practitioners' decision-making through the preparation, maintenance and updating of systematic reviews and their dissemination and application to influence service provision and clinical practice (Australasian Cochrane Centre 2005). In the southern hemisphere, Australasia's Cochrane Centre was founded in 1994, with branches now in New Zealand, Singapore and South Asia. Another related organisation contributing to EBP is the Joanna Briggs Institute (JBI), which became fully operational in 1996 and is based in South Australia. It has a number of collaborating centres around the world, with one of these being based at New Zealand's University of Auckland. The JBI pioneers recognised the need for health professionals to make decisions based on evidence derived from a range of sources, including experience, expertise and all forms of rigorous research — in addition to randomised controlled trials which are strongly

advocated by the Cochrane Collaboration (Joanna Briggs Institute 2005).

The process or steps involved in EBP still closely resemble those first proffered by Sackett et al. (2000). Adaptations to the process, however, have taken place with the wider inclusion of evidence generated through different means. Evidence-based practice is not a static process, but rather it reflects the best available evidence at that time. Therefore, whenever clinical decisions are made, it is important that current evidence is used to inform that process wherever possible. Evidence changes over time as new research becomes available, policies and governments change, users become more informed and practitioners increase their expertise. Similarly, models of evidence-based practice have also changed. There is less emphasis on the more simplistic models of research utilisation, and more on frameworks that are multifaceted, such as PARIHS, due in part to the complexity of contemporary healthcare. Implementing evidence into practice and achieving sustained practice change requires a wide range of knowledge, skills and resources, including problem-solving, evaluation and feedback.

The steps for evidence-based practice

The five steps universally accepted as being necessary for EBP are presented in Table 17.1, based on the findings of Sackett et al. (2000) and Jackson et al. (2006).

Jackson et al. (2006) have taken these steps further and designed an innovative approach to evidence appraisal called GATE: Graphical Approach to Teaching EBP (see Figure 17.2). They found that students' understanding

TABLE 17.1 Steps in evidence-based practice

1. Ask a focused question.
2. Assess appropriate evidence.
3. Appraise evidence for validity, impact and precision.
4. Apply evidence accounting for patient values/ preferences, clinical and policy issues.
5. Audit your practice/personal skills.

(Source: Jackson et al. 2006; Sackett et al. 2000)

FIGURE 17.2 The GATE

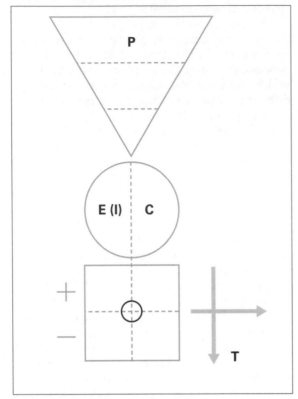

(Source: Jackson et al. 2006)

could be enhanced by 'hanging the study and numbers on the GATE frame' and therefore this approach takes practitioners through critical appraisal, using graphics to illustrate what information is needed to be retrieved from the evidence being appraised (Jackson et al. 2006 p 35).

(For more information on Figure 17.2 see: http://www.epiq.co.nz.)

Creating a clinical question

The first step of EBP requires a clinical question to be formulated to direct the subsequent phases of EBP (see Chapter 5). Although nurses and midwives ask questions every day in their practice, the development of a searchable, answerable question is a skill that must be practised and mastered to ensure the success of EBP (Green & Ruff 2005). Table 17.2 includes examples of clinical questions. The triggers for these may be discomfort or uncertainty related to an aspect of practice, coupled with the desire for greater

understanding — or as Fineout-Overholt et al. (2005) denote, a sustained spirit of inquiry.

Many involved in teaching EBP use a standard format for formulating clinical questions: these being PECOT or PICOT.

> Population,
> Exposure/Intervention of interest,
> Comparison of interest,
> Outcome of interest, and
> Timeframe.
>
> (Jackson et al. 2006; Fineout-Overholt et al. 2005)

Nurses, midwives and others need to be able to locate evidence in a timely fashion. Therefore learning an approach, such as PICOT, that complements questioning skills, helps clinicians to proceed more quickly towards searching for the best evidence.

TT Tutorial trigger 2

There are three different intravenous fluid infusions that are used to prepare equipment used for interventional radiology. How would you formulate a clinical question for this practice issue?

Searching for the best evidence

What constitutes as 'evidence' and how this should be used in practice present healthcare professionals with challenges. Rycroft-Malone et al. (2004b) conclude that effective practice can only be achieved through the use of several sources of evidence; these being research, clinical experience, patient experience and information from the local context. Each one of these need to be critically examined, using scientific and intuitive approaches, for effective person-centred evidence-based care delivery to be realised.

Locating sources of evidence is less of a problem for health professionals, or their clients, since many electronic databases and internet search engines are now easily accessible. The most commonly used databases for nursing and midwifery-related research evidence are CINAHL, Medline, MIDIRS, PubMed, PsycINFO and the Cochrane Library (see Chapter 3). In Australia and New Zealand, healthcare providers pay for access to these sources and, for health professionals employed by such organisations, this has facilitated easy access to information — even in clinical arenas. Similarly, agreements made by the Australian and New Zealand governments have enabled free access for all to the Cochrane Library.

There are many guides available to assist practitioners in their search for evidence. They do this by allowing the formulation of a search strategy, narrowing the search years of publication, the language, and evidence type. The type of research-related question will often dictate the database that is best suited for searching, as indicated in Table 17.2 (Fineout-Overholt et al. 2005).

Levels of evidence

Internationally, the following methods of determining the strength of evidence are used.

- Cook et al.'s (1995) levels and grading of evidence, which ranks evidence at one of five levels (see Table 17.3).

TABLE 17.2 EBP questions and suggested databases in which to find evidence

Questions	Potential databases
Therapy: Inpatients living in a long-term facility who are at risk for decubiti, what is the effect of an ongoing pressure ulcer prevention programme compared to the standard of care (e.g. turning every two hours) on signs of emerging decubiti?	Medline, CINAHL, Cochrane Database of Systematic Reviews (CDSR), Abstracts of Reviews of Effects (DARE), Cochrane Central Register of Controlled Trials (CCRCT)
Aetiology: Are older mothers more at risk of postpartum depression compared to younger mothers?	MIDIRS, Medline, CINAHL, PsycINFO
Diagnosis or diagnostic test: Is D-dimer assay more accurate in diagnosing deep vein thrombosis compared to ultrasound?	Medline, CINAHL, Cochrane Database of Systematic Reviews (CDSR), Abstracts of Reviews of Effects (DARE), Cochrane Central Register of Controlled Trials (CCRCT)
Prevention: For labouring women, is the prevention of oral intake necessary to reduce the risk of potential aspiration of gastric contents where general anaesthetic may be required?	MIDIRS, Medline, CINAHL, Cochrane Database of Systematic Reviews (CDSR), Abstracts of Reviews of Effects (DARE), Cochrane Central Register of Controlled Trials (CCRCT)
Prognosis: Does dietary carbohydrate intake influence healthy weight maintenance (BMI<25) in patients who have family history of obesity (BMI>30)?	Medline, CINAHL
Meaning: How do middle-aged women with fibromyalgia perceive loss of motor function?	Medline, CINAHL, PsycINFO

(Source: Fineout-Overholt et al. 2005)

TABLE 17.3 Levels of evidence and grades of recommendations for therapy

Level of evidence	Grade of recommendation
Level I: Randomised trials or meta-analyses in which the lower limit of the confidence interval for the treatment effect exceeds the minimal clinically important benefit.	Grade A
Level II: Randomised trials or meta-analyses in which the lower limit of the confidence interval for the treatment effect overlaps the minimal clinically important benefit.	Grade B
Level III: Non-randomised concurrent cohort comparisons between contemporaneous patients who did and did not receive the therapy.	Grade C
Level IV: Non-randomised historical cohort comparisons between current patients who did receive therapy and former patients who did not (from same institution or from the literature).	Grade C
Level V: Case series without controls.	Grade C

(Source: Cook et al. 1995)

TABLE 17.4 NZGG's grading structure for evidence-based guidelines

Study design	Level of evidence		Grading of recommendation	
• Systematic review • Randomised controlled trial • Cohort study • Case control study • Case series • Cost study	+	No major flaws	A	The recommendation is supported by GOOD (strong) evidence
	~	Potential flaws, but these are unlikely to substantially alter the results	B	The recommendation is supported by FAIR (reasonable evidence, but there may be minimal inconsistency, or uncertainty)
	X	Major flaws	C	The recommendation is supported by EXPERT opinion (published) only
			I	There is INSUFFICIENT evidence to make a recommendation
			✓	GOOD PRACTICE POINT (in the opinion of the guideline development group)

(Source: NZGG 2003; Lethaby 2005)

- New Zealand Guidelines Group's revised grading system and grades of recommendation (NZGG 2003; Lethaby 2005) (see Table 17.4).
- National Health and Medical Research Council (NHMRC) (1999, 2000) levels of evidence (see Table 17.5). The Joanna Briggs Institute (JBI) and its collaborating centres use these levels of evidence after altering the Level IV definition to 'evidence obtained from case series, either post-test or pre-test and post-test' (Joanna Briggs Institute 2005). The JBI grades the recommendations in its Best Practice Information Sheets, using the Grading of Recommendations in Table 17.6

Critical appraisal

When making decisions for nursing or midwifery practice, a judgment call must be made about the robustness of the evidence underpinning that intervention or action. As Bick's (2006 p 94) *Midwifery* editorial informs us:

> ... it is recommended that complex evidence is subject to critical evaluation and effect ... fully gauged before practice is changed overnight. Evidence is crucial, but we have to be mindful that, although it can be used as a powerful force to improve [client's] rights, it may also inform inappropriate change.

A range of tools and guides are, therefore, available to assist evidence appraisal (see 'Evidence-based practice tip' opposite). All facilitate the examination of both the quality of the evidence and the applicability for practice.

Evidence-based practice tip

A range of tools and guides assist with evidence appraisal. For example:
- the National Institute of Clinical Studies (NICS) is a useful resource for critical appraisal tools, links and guides (see http://wherestheevidence.nicsl.com.au/home.aspx)
- guides for evidence appraisal have been published by the *Journal of the American Medical Association* (JAMA) see http://www.usersguides.org/
- GATE can be accessed from http://www.epiq.co.nz

TABLE 17.5 NHMRC levels of evidence

I	Evidence obtained from a systematic review of all relevant randomised controlled trials.
II	Evidence obtained from at least one properly designed randomised controlled trial.
III-1	Evidence obtained from well-designed pseudo-randomised controlled trials (alternate allocation or some other method).
III-2	Evidence obtained from comparative studies (including systematic reviews of such studies) with concurrent controls and allocation not randomised, cohort studies, case-control studies, or interrupted time series with a control group.
III-3	Evidence obtained from comparative studies with historical control, two or more single arm studies, or interrupted time series without a parallel control group.
IV	Evidence obtained from case series, either post-test or pre-test/post-test.

(Source: NHMRC 1999)

TABLE 17.6 JBI grades of recommendation

Grade of recommendation	Feasibility	Appropriateness	Meaningfulness	Effectiveness
A	Immediately practicable.	Ethically acceptable and justifiable.	Provides a strong rationale for practice change.	Effectiveness established to a degree that merits application.
B	Practicable with limited training and/or modest additional resources.	Ethical acceptance is unclear.	Provides a moderate rationale for practice change.	Effectiveness established to a degree that suggests application.
C	Practicable with significant additional training and/or resources.	Conflicts to some extent with ethical principles.	Provides limited rationale for practice change.	Effectiveness established to a degree that warrants consideration of applying the findings.
D	Practicable with extensive additional training and/or resources.	Conflicts considerably with ethical principles.	Provides minimal rationale for advocating change.	Effectiveness established to a limited degree.
E	Impracticable.	Ethically unacceptable.	There is no rationale to support practice change.	Effectiveness not established.

(Copyright permission from Joanna Briggs Institute 2004)

Critical appraisal requires knowledge and skill that, once acquired, need to be practised (see Chapter 16). A basic understanding of research methods, statistical inference and effect measures (Sheldon 2000; Ciliska et al. 2001) is needed to enable the individual as an evidence (research) consumer. According to Duffy (2005), three key questions need answering when appraising any type of quantitative or qualitative study:

1. Were the results obtained via sound scientific methods?
2. Will the study results have sufficient influence on practice — clinically and/or statistically (if appropriate)?
3. Can the results be applied to and in a specific clinical setting?

There is a need to make visible the ongoing credibility, transferability and theoretical potential of qualitative evidence (Pearson 2004) — for which further guidance is provided by Russell and Gregory (2003). When considering the results of a quantitative study, it is important to judge the clinical significance because a study (especially if the sample size is large) might generate results that are statistically significant, but which have little clinical meaning. Conversely, and

more commonly for nursing and midwifery studies, results might not achieve statistical significance and yet, clinically, the differences found between study groups indicate that the evidence may be meaningful for clinical practice. It is for such reasons that the use of effect measures, such as absolute risk reduction (ARR) and numbers needed to treat (NNT; the number of patients that need to be treated with the experimental intervention to prevent one additional bad outcome), are replacing statistical inference in clinical research (DiCenso 2001).

Issues relating to the applicability of research findings to clinical practice have received much attention in recent years due, in part, to the recognition that using evidence in practice is crucial to achieving evidence-based practice (Rycroft-Malone 2004; Rycroft-Malone et al. 2004a, 2004b). Therefore it is important to ask 'are my patients so different from those in the study that the results don't apply?' (Ciliska et al. 2001).

Tutorial trigger 3

What questions do you need to ask to help you decide if the results from a research study can be applied to your practice setting?

Evidence implementation

Evidence alone does not change practice and the persistent barriers to implementing EBP, in both acute and primary healthcare settings, pose significant challenges (Fineout-Overholt et al. 2004, 2005). Lack of time (Retsas 2000) is one barrier, whilst others include lack of skills and knowledge (Pravikoff et al. 2005). Mentoring and facilitation are mechanisms that have been successfully used to assist practitioners to develop EBP. The importance of facilitation is explored by Harvey et al. (2002), who proposed a range of variable activities from discrete task-focused interventions to enabling individuals, teams and organisations. A similar approach to evidence implementation, 'Read, think, do', has been developed in Australia (Winch et al. 2005). It assists practitioners to consider the evidence, the value to practice and contextual issues pertinent to the practice setting when deciding strategies for changing practice. For this to be effective, collaboration, planning and evaluation involving all members of the clinical team and a facilitator are needed. The key components of the approach are:

- Read: accessing and reading the literature
- Think: judicious use of evidence in a specific organisational context
- Do: facilitating practice change (Winch et al. 2005).

Practice development is a key element of this Australian approach and, although progress can sometimes be slow, the authors concluded that the rewards can be substantial for practitioners and patients.

A review of concepts for knowledge-transfer highlights five roles that are commonly referred to in the EBP/knowledge-transfer literature (Thompson et al. 2006). These are: opinion leader, facilitator, champion, linking-agent and change-agent. These roles are related to each other and 'operate under the premise that interpersonal contact improves the likelihood of behavioural change, when introducing new innovations into the healthcare sector' (p 98). The importance of facilitation processes, as opposed to facilitation roles, is emphasised in this review and reiterates the centrality of these processes in developing practice and improving decision-making.

Research in brief

Greenhalgh et al. (2004, 2005) undertook a systematic review of the literature concerned with innovations in healthcare. This review explored the ways in which knowledge/evidence was translated and used in health service organisations. The authors concluded that 'simple' approaches to knowledge use were unhelpful and that if organisations are to be expected to embrace a variety of evidence, then participatory methodologies are needed — as well as evaluation approaches that embrace the complexity of healthcare teams and systems. This type of research outcome is influencing contemporary thinking about strategies to enable EBP and clinical effectiveness.

Facilitating evidence-based practice through practice development

Practice development is consistent with many of the principles proposed by Greenhalgh et al. (2004, 2005; see 'Research in brief' above). The key to practice development is facilitation. Facilitation refers to a process of enabling individuals and groups to understand what they have to go through to change aspects of their behaviour or attitudes to themselves, their work or other individuals (Marshall & McLean 1988). A similar interpretation is apparent in some approaches to practice-based learning in healthcare (Barrows & Tamblyn 1980; Titchen 1987; Johns & Butcher 1993), with the aim being to challenge existing practice and support the development of new ways of working. Heron (1989) describes a facilitator as a person who has the role of helping participants to learn in an experiential group. An effective facilitator, who wants to provide conditions for the development of autonomous learning, moves between three political modes: making decisions for learners (hierarchy), making decisions with learners (co-operation), and delegating decisions to learners (autonomy). Heron emphasises the facilitator's role in addressing issues of feelings within the group, confronting resistance and giving meaning to group discussions, as well as in planning and structuring group tasks.

Styles of facilitation

The purpose of the proposed facilitation should influence the style adopted. Harvey et al. (2002) suggest that this can vary from providing help and support to achieve a specific goal or task (technical facilitation), to enabling individuals and teams to analyse, reflect and change their own attitudes, behaviour and ways of working (holistic facilitation). These are not mutually exclusive and can be seen as extreme points on a continuum of facilitation — moving from 'doing for others' to 'enabling others' (see Figure 17.3). As the approach moves to the right of the continuum (towards holism), facilitation is increasingly concerned with addressing the whole situation and the whole process.

FIGURE 17.3 The facilitation continuum

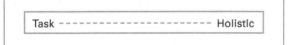

Just as there are two types of practice development (technical and emancipatory) (Manley & McCormack 2004), facilitation styles can also be distinguished in the same way.

The task (technical) approach

The aim of the task approach is to achieve a goal or task. Technical interest is about gaining technical knowledge that will enable greater skill and mastery over a technical work activity (e.g. wound care; continence promotion; breastfeeding promotion; managing intravenous access). In terms of PD, an example may be a nurse's or midwife's concern for improving the care provided to a person who is depressed. Practitioners may draw on technical knowledge derived from systematic reviews of evidence, or meta-analysis based on randomised control trials, which correlate the interventions with the outcomes of continence management strategies (see Chapter 4). Technical knowledge is therefore important in many PD contexts.

When operating in the task mode of facilitation, the facilitator is perceived as an expert authority figure. They know what has to be done, to what standard, and the criteria for success pre-exists in their mind. For example, this may equate to the implementation of clinical guidelines to ensure more effective care within a care setting or developing the competence of practitioners, in some new aspect of care, to reduce waiting times. Staff will be viewed as instruments through which the outcome is to be achieved and therefore through which practice is to be improved. The danger here is that staff may merely exist as 'pawns' that are unconsciously manipulated for the facilitator's or organisation's ends (Grundy 1982). For the purpose of elaboration, consider the following two examples (one a specific practice issue and the other an organisational issue) of technical facilitation at work.

Example 1 — developing and implementing a protocol on the use of protective gloves

The approach used to develop the protocol was deductive (i.e. the knowledge used was derived from external sources, such as empirical research or systematic reviews of published evidence) (Kitson et al. 1996). Implementation focused on informing staff about the specifics of the protocol in relation to their practice. This approach included presenting formal sessions where the protocol and evidence base underpinning it were outlined — thus attempting to develop practitioners' knowledge about what is and isn't effective. This was followed by the development and monitoring of the use of the protocol through audit.

Example 2 — developing health professionals' understanding of 'professional accountability'

The role of the facilitator was to develop a program of information and training on 'professional accountability'. Packs of relevant information were developed and a cascade approach was adopted across clinical areas; that is, where lead staff were trained in the use of the materials and then informed others about the issue in their specific clinical settings. Despite accountability being a complex concept, this approach treated it like a technical task and thus the emphasis was on increasing individual competence in performing a specific task.

Knowledge and skills acquired may not be realised in practice for a number of reasons, such as where the practice culture may not be conducive. Although staff may identify with and plan to implement interventions, on a study day or in a meeting, often when they return to their clinical areas, a host of barriers frustrate them. Not least of these are that they likely may find themselves facing the constraint of routine day-to-day care provision which, in turn, provides little opportunity to practise newfound skills. As Grundy (1982) highlights, when working with staff in this way and depending on the facilitator's skill in inspiring, enthusing and gaining commitment from staff and expertise in the area, staff may take one of three actions:

1. reject the idea of the facilitator and refuse to work for its realisation
2. consent to work towards the goal
3. adopt the idea as their own.

Task-orientated facilitation may succeed in getting theoretical knowledge used in practice, however this requires the facilitator to have a lot of expertise in facilitation (Kitson et al. 1998) as well as technical knowledge associated with the focus of facilitation. Knowledge expertise alone is inadequate because, even if staff claim ownership of the ideas, it is still the facilitator who is ultimately responsible for success or failure of the initiative being translated into practice.

The skills used in task-orientated facilitation are narrow and focus on:
- sourcing information
- assessing the relevance and adequacy of that information
- translating the information into differing formats (e.g. protocols, guidelines, information sheets)
- developing training programs
- training
- information giving
- audit and monitoring.

The focus of evaluation in task-based facilitation is measurement and this assumes correlation between independent (intervention) and dependent (outcomes) variables, regardless of context. A facilitator, using a task approach, may record the number of people trained and the number of sites implementing a particular initiative. Furthermore, they may evaluate using a variety of tools, leading to specific outcomes associated with an intervention (e.g. incontinence pads used, pressure sore rates, delivery times, caesarean rates, length of hospital stay, job satisfaction).

> ● **Evidence-based practice tip**
> Technical (task) facilitation depends on a strong facilitator who is able to drive a change in practice. Thus the power lies with the facilitator. Creating ownership among the wider group of practitioners is not a strong aspect of this type of facilitation — thus responsibility for ensuring the sustainability of the agreed processes lies with external drivers such as audit, quality monitoring and risk assessment.

The holistic (emancipatory) approach

In contrast with the technical approach, the overall aim of the holistic approach is to enable individuals and teams to become empowered to develop a transformational culture in their individual and collective service (Manley & McCormack 2004). This activity can then nurture and sustain the development of a particular goal or task. Although the overall approach may encompass elements of technical facilitation, as discussed earlier, it is important (if not essential) to recognise that technical facilitation can be integrated into holistic approaches. This needs to occur if the different needs of stakeholders are to be adequately met. The works of Wilson et al. (2005) and Barrett et al. (2005) provide useful examples, from an Australian context, of facilitators moving between differing roles and styles of facilitation.

With a holistic approach, the focus is on the social system as well as individual/group's own practice. Facilitators help participants become aware of and freed from taken-for-granted aspects of their practice and the organisational systems constraining them. They foster a climate of critical inquiry through reflective discussion involving various 'ideas' of group members and assist the group's enlightenment through nurturing a culture, which enables individuals and groups to act. Responsibility for action, therefore, does rest with the practitioners/group (Kemmis 2006). By considering the external climate and broader social system in which practitioners work, collective insight, understanding and ownership develops through practitioners' own actions, rather than the actions of others. The facilitator is responsible for enabling a culture to develop where such enlightenment is possible — a culture of critique if you will (McCormack 2003). Importantly, the facilitator may have technical expertise to share, but their contribution is of no greater or lesser importance than that of other group members. Thus the essential skills of the holistic facilitator are:

- working with values, beliefs and assumptions
- challenging contradictions
- developing moral awareness
- focusing on the impact of the context on practice, as well as practice itself
- using self-reflection and fostering reflection in others
- enabling others to 'see the possibilities'
- fostering widening participation and collaboration by all involved
- changing practices.

Manley (2001) suggests that working with holistic facilitation in PD achieves the following outcomes:

- a workplace culture which is person-centred, evidence-based and is also a learning culture
- the development of individuals and interdisciplinary teams who are able to take responsibility for quality
- continuous evaluation of services and effectiveness
- the development of evidence from practice
- integration of policy with practice and greater ability to influence policy from practice.

Evaluation may encompass the same approaches as technical facilitation but additionally would focus on personal/collective enlightenment, empowerment and emancipation. Evaluation of the culture considers the attributes of a transformational culture (Manley 2001). It is a culture where change is a way of life, is accompanied with a proactive stance to meeting changing needs, and where all key stakeholders have been involved in developing criteria for the evaluation. In this case, evaluation processes are transparent and underpinned by explicit values and beliefs in recognition that different types of knowledge are interwoven with the people they serve.

Harvey et al. (2002) suggest that the operationalisation of the facilitator role depends upon the underlying purpose and interpretation of the facilitation concept. Recent works by Walsh et al. (2005) and Lawless and Walsh (2005), in New Zealand, illustrate the use of a decision-support framework (the BEET; building effective management techniques) to identify the type of facilitation needed in particular practice development contexts.

> The BEET is divided into four sections each consisting of exercises to tease out the key message:
>
> 1. Puzzles and purpose — identifying the question to be answered and the reasons behind the engagement
> 2. Evidence — assessing the strength of the proposal for engagement
> 3. Context — considering the environment and people within which engagement will occur and identifying who else needs to be involved
> 4. Facilitation — how to bring people together constructively.
>
> (Source: Lawless & Walsh 2005)

Research in brief

Barrett et al.'s (2005) study operationalises an over-arching action research framework in a cardiothoracic surgical unit within a large teaching hospital. The outcomes from the program of work included increased participation among staff in practice development work, the implementation of a range of clinical practice changes to improve patient-centred care (e.g. pain assessment and management, medication prescribing, patient education and patient involvement in decision-making) and the creation of a workplace culture that was cognisant of the 'emotional labour' of practice.

Essential skills in facilitation

Being skilled as a facilitator is a constant state of 'becoming', in that there is always more learning to be done about being effective. As Rogers (1983) argues time and again, the authentic expert facilitator is one who treats the process as one of 'self-learning', whereby each facilitation experience is an opportunity for further learning and refinement of skills. These skills can be summarised as:

- clarity of the intent of the facilitation and the facilitator style adopted
- clarity of communication through listening and attending
- reflecting back and questioning
- giving and receiving feedback and help group members avoid collusion (e.g. not engaging in 'group think' or 'pairing')
- time management
- sourcing evidence (empirical, professional opinion and patient perspectives)
- working with individual and group feelings
- creating a milieu of trust where individuals and/or group members can 'be themselves'
- create a culture of creativity and experiment
- be assertive when consensus is needed
- empathise with individual and group perspectives (i.e. see issues through the eyes of participants)
- adopt flexible facilitation interventions (i.e. be able to draw upon more than one approach in dealing with a particular situation)
- help group members to trust their own experiences
- enable the agreed processes to happen
- evaluate the processes and outcomes of the group.

(Source: University of Ulster 2006)

Clearly, effective facilitation does not happen by 'chance' and is a deliberate process that requires a commitment to continuous learning and development.

Summary

Practice development and EBP challenge practitioners to question existing practice and are therefore agents for practice change. With increasing demands for improved patient outcomes, greater accountability and enhanced patient safety, nurses and midwives must embrace and embed EBP into the healthcare culture. The processes associated with EBP, such as critical appraisal, are useful and powerful mechanisms through which practitioners can deliver services based on the best available evidence at the time. These provide direction to the development of clinical practice, which changes as more evidence is generated and synthesised. Practice development provides a dynamic systematic approach for unravelling the 'haystack' of the context of practice; that is, the settings where practice takes place. Practice settings are complex environments so evidence needs to be contextualised if it is to be of relevance to clinicians. The use of a variety of forms of evidence is the key to successful PD and thus there is a synergistic relationship between EBP and practice development. As hinted at earlier, both EBP and PD are grounded in the formulation, implementation and evaluation of research-orientated practice change. The following chapter expands this notion.

ⓀEY POINTS

- Evidence-based practice (EBP) and practice development (PD) have differing origins but, together, they bring about systematic changes in the culture and context of practice.

- The key relationship between EBP and PD is that of knowledge use and knowledge generation. EBP is primarily concerned with increasing practice effectiveness through the use of evidence. PD is concerned with utilising the most effective methods of engaging practitioners in reflecting on and critiquing their practice and the evidence upon which they base their practice (be it from research, clinical experience, patients, clients or carers).

- EBP follows a series of steps of analysis in order to determine the most appropriate evidence to use in particular practice contexts and to inform clinical effectiveness.

- PD is a continuous process of improvement towards increased effectiveness in patient-centred care. It is brought about by helping healthcare teams to develop their knowledge and skills and to transform the culture and context of care. It is enabled and supported by facilitators committed to systematic rigorous continuous processes of emancipatory change that reflect the perspectives of service users and service providers.

Learning activities

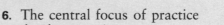

1. What are the three components of the PARIHS framework?
   (a) evidence, cost and implementation
   (b) evidence, patients and evaluation
   (c) evidence, context and facilitation
   (d) evidence, practice and facilitation

2. Which database is best for sourcing mental health related evidence?
   (a) CINAHL
   (b) Medline
   (c) PsycINFO
   (d) DARE.

3. A clinical question should be:
   (a) ethical
   (b) searchable and answerable
   (c) affordable
   (d) able to be statistically analysed.

4. Which statistic is the most clinically significant?
   (a) p
   (b) NNT
   (c) ARR
   (d) RR.

5. The founder of the EBP movement was:
   (a) Dorothy Orem
   (b) David Sackett
   (c) Bruce Willis
   (d) Archie Cochrane.

6. The central focus of practice development is:
   (a) competent practitioners
   (b) staff development
   (c) patient-centred care
   (d) organisational change.

7. Which of these activities could be described as 'technical practice development'?
   (a) changing the way that intravenous fluids are administered through a staff training program
   (b) developing a shared vision for practice among a team of intensive care nurses
   (c) introducing a best practice statement developed by the Joanna Briggs Institute through workshops and clinical audit
   (d) implementing a new national policy for pressure damage prevention through onsite teaching by clinical educators.

8. If your team had developed a shared vision for practice, which of the following facilitation processes would reflect an emancipatory PD approach to the implementation of the shared vision?

(a) engaging in reflective activities with staff in order to understand the factors that hindered them from practising according to their espoused vision

(b) teaching staff about the importance of effectiveness in practice and using the vision as a benchmark to evaluate progress with implementing changes in practice that are consistent with the shared vision

(c) as a facilitator, working alongside staff in practice and asking reflective questions

(d) all of the above.

9. Heron (1989) suggests that for a facilitator to be effective they should operate in which of the following modes?
   (a) hierarchical
   (b) co-operative and autonomous
   (c) autonomous only
   (d) a combination of hierarchical, co-operative and autonomous.

10. Which of the following are key skills to use in holistic facilitation?
    (a) reflective questioning
    (b) giving and receiving feedback
    (c) developing action plans with staff
    (d) feedback from evaluation
    (e) all of the above.

Additional resources

Australasian Cochrane Centre. Online. Available: http://www.cochrane.org.au/

Australian Centre for Evidence-Based Clinical Practice. Online. Available: http://www.acebcp.org.au/

Children's Hospital at Westmead, Nursing research and practice development unit. Online. Available: http://www.chw.edu.au/research/groups/nursing_research_and_practice_development_unit.htm

Core Library of Evidence Based Practice. Online. Available: http://www.shef.ac.uk/scharr/ir/core.html

Effective Healthcare Australia. Online. Available: http://www.eha.usyd.edu.au/

Fitzgerald M, Armitage D 2005 Clinical research: The potential of practice development. *Practice Development in Health Care* 4:150–9

Jackson R, Ameratunga S, Broad J, et al. 2006 The GATE frame: Critical appraisal with pictures. *Evidence-Based Medicine* 11:35–8. Online. Available: http://www.health.auckland.ac.nz/population-health/epidemiology-biostats/epiq/updatedGATESicily.pdf

National Institute of Clinical Studies. Online. Available: http://www.nicsl.com.au/

Royal College of Nursing (UK) Practice development website: http://www.rcn.org.uk/resources/practicedevelopment/

Stevens K R 2001 Systematic reviews: The heart of evidence-based practice. *AACN Clinical Issues Advanced Practice in Acute and Critical Care* 12:529–38

University of Bournemouth Centre for Practice Development. Online. Available: http://www.bournemouth.ac.uk/ihcs/practicedevelopment.html

References

Australasian Cochrane Centre 2005 *Role of the centre.* Online. Available: http://www.cochrane.org.au/about_us/about_us.htm [accessed 24 January 2005]

Barrett C, Angel J, Gilbert M, et al. 2005 Systematic processes for successful, sustainable practice development. *Practice Development in Health Care* 4:5–13

Barrows H S, Tamblyn R M 1980 *Problem-based learning: An approach to medical education.* Springer, New York

Bick D 2006 Editorial — The politics of evidence as the basis for change. *Midwifery* 22:93–4

Ciliska D, Cullum N, Marks S 2001 Evaluation of systematic reviews of treatment or prevention interventions. *Evidence Based Nursing* 4:100–4

Cook D J, Guyatt G H, Laupacis A, et al. 1995 Clinical recommendations using levels of evidence for antithrombotic agents. *CHEST* 108:227–30

Dewing J, Traynor V 2005 Admiral nursing competency project: Practice development and action research. *Journal of Clinical Nursing* 14:695–703

DiCenso A 2001 Clinically useful measures of the effects of treatment. *Evidence Based Nursing* 4:36–9

DiCenso A, Cullum N, Ciliska D 1998 Implementing evidence-based nursing: Some misconceptions. *Evidence Based Nursing* 1:38–9

Duffy M E 2005 Resources for critically appraising quantitative research evidence for nursing practice. *Clinical Nurse Specialist* 19:233–5

Estabrooks C A 1999 The conceptual structure of research utilisation. *Research in Nursing and Health* 22:203–16

Fineout-Overholt E, Hofstetter S, Shell L, et al. 2005 Teaching EBP: Getting to the gold: How to search for the best evidence. *Worldviews on Evidence-Based Nursing* 2:207–11

Fineout-Overholt E, Levin R F, Melnyk B M 2004 Strategies for advancing evidence-based practice in clinical settings. *Journal of the New York State Nurses Association* 35:28–32

Fullerton J T, Thompson J B 2005 Examining the evidence for the International Confederation of

Midwives' essential competencies for midwifery practice. *Midwifery* 21:2–13

Garbett R, McCormack B 2002 A concept analysis of practice development. *NT Research* 7:87–100

—— 2004 A concept analysis of practice development. In: McCormack B, Manley K, Garbett R (eds) *Practice development in nursing*. Blackwell Publishing, Oxford

Green M, Ruff T 2005 Why do residents fail to answer their clinical questions? A qualitative study of barriers to practicing evidence-based medicine. *Academic Medicine* 80:176–82

Greenhalgh T, Robert G, Bate P, et al. 2004 *How to spread good ideas: a systematic review of the literature on diffusion, dissemination and sustainability of innovations in health service delivery and organisation*. Report for the National Co-ordinating Centre for NHS Service Delivery and Organisation R&D (NCCSDO). Online. Available: http://www.sdo.lshtm.ac.uk/pdf/changemanagement_greenhalgh_report.pdf

Greenhalgh T, Robert G, Bate P, et al. 2005 *Diffusion of innovations in health service organisations: A systematic literature review*. Blackwell, Oxford

Grundy S 1982 Three modes of action research. *Curriculum Perspectives* 2:23 34

Harrison M 2005 Resource review: Practice development in nursing. *Evidence Based Nursing* 8:40

Harvey G, Loftus-Hills A, Rycroft-Malone J, et al. Kitson A, McCormack B, Seers K 2002 Getting evidence into practice: the role and function of facilitation. *Journal of Advanced Nursing* 37:577–88

Heron J 1989 *The facilitators handbook*. Kogan Page, London

Higgs J, Titchen A 2001 *Practice knowledge and expertise in the health professions*. Butterworth-Heinemann, Oxford

Jackson R, Ameratunga S, Broad J, et al. Robb G, Wells S, Glasziou P, Heneghan C 2006 The GATE frame: Critical appraisal with pictures. *Evidence-Based Medicine* 11:35–8

Joanna Briggs Institute 2004 *Systematic reviews — the review process. Levels of evidence*. Online. Available: http://www.joannabriggs.edu.au/pubs/approach.php [accessed 8 January 2007]

—— 2005 *Introduction to JBI*. Online. Available: http://www.joannabriggs.edu.au/about/about.php [accessed 26 May 2006]

Johns C, Butcher K 1993 Learning through supervision: A case study of respite care. *Journal of Clinical Nursing* 2:89–93

Johns C 1998 Opening the doors of perception. In: Johns C, Freshwater D (eds) *Transforming nursing through reflective practice*. Blackwell Science, Oxford

Kemmis M 2006 Participatory Action Research and the Public Sphere. *Educational Action Research* 14(4):459–76

Kerner J, Rimer B, Emmons K 2005 Introduction to the special section on dissemination. Dissemination research and research dissemination: How can we close the gap? *Health Psychology* 24:443–6

Kitson A, Harvey G, McCormack B 1998 Approaches to implementing research in practice. *Quality in Health Care* 7:149–59

Kitson A, Harvey G, Seers K, et al. 1996 From research to practice; one organisational model for promoting research based practice. *Journal of Advanced Nursing* 23:430–40

Lawless J, Walsh K 2005 *The BEET — Building Effective Engagement Techniques, A guide to bringing people together co-operatively to find sustainable solutions* (version 2). Nursing Research and Development Unit, Bryant Education Centre, Waikato Hospital, Hamilton, New Zealand, pp 1–20

Lethaby A 2005 *Grading for evidence-based guidelines: a simple system for a complex task?* New Zealand Guidelines Group. Online. Available: http://www.nzgg.org.nz/download/files/051215Grading.pdf [accessed 6 June 2006]

Manley K 2001 *Consultant nurse: Concept, processes, outcome*. Unpublished PhD thesis, Manchester University/RCN Institute London. London

Manley K, McCormack B 2004 Practice development: purpose, methodology, facilitation and evaluation. In: McCormack B, Manley K, Garbett R (eds) *Practice development in nursing*. Blackwell Publishing, Oxford

Marshall J, McLean A 1988. In: Reason P (ed.) *Human inquiry in action: Developments in new paradigm research*. Sage, London

McCormack B 2003 Knowing and acting: A strategic practitioner-focused approach to nursing research and practice development. *NT Research* 8:86–100

McCormack B, Manley K, Titchen A, et al. 1999 Towards practice development: A vision in reality or a reality without vision. *Journal of Nursing Management* 7:255–64

McGill I, Brockbank A 2004 *The action learning handbook: powerful techniques for education, professional development and training*. Kogan Page, London

McSherry R 2004 Practice development and health care governance: A recipe for modernisation. *Journal of Nursing Management* 12:137–46

Ministry of Health, New Zealand 2002 *Towards clinical excellence: an introduction to clinical audit, peer review and other clinical practice improvement activities*. Ministry of Health, Wellington

National Health and Medical Research Council (NHMRC) 1999 *A Guide to the development, implementation and evaluation of clinical practice guidelines*. NHMRC, Canberra

—— 2000 *How to use the evidence: assessment and application of scientific evidence*. Handbook series on preparing clinical practice guidelines. NHMRC, Canberra

NZGG 2003 *Handbook for the preparation of explicit evidence-based clinical practice guidelines*. Online. Available: http://www.nzgg.org.nz [accessed 26 May 2006]

Pearson A 2004 Balancing the evidence: incorporating the synthesis of qualitative data into systematic reviews. *JBI Reports* 2(2):45–64

Pravikoff D S, Tanner A B, Pierce S T 2005 Readiness of US nurses for evidence-based practice: Many don't understand or value research and have had little or no training to help them find evidence on which to base their practice. *American Journal of Nursing* 105:40–52

Retsas A 2000 Barriers to using research evidence in nursing practice. *Journal of Advanced Nursing* 31:599–606

Rogers C R 1983 *Freedom to learn for the 80s*. Columbus, Ohio

Russell C K, Gregory D M 2003 EBN users' guide. Evaluation of qualitative research studies. *Evidence Based Nursing* 6:36–40

Rycroft-Malone J 2004 The PARIHS framework — a framework for guiding the implementation of evidence-based practice. Promoting action on research implementation in health services. *Journal of Nursing Care Quality* 19:297–304

Rycroft-Malone J, Harvey G, Seers K, Kitson A, McCormack B, Titchen A 2004a An exploration of the factors that influence the implementation of evidence into practice. *Journal of Clinical Nursing* 13:913–24

Rycroft-Malone J, Kitson A, Harvey G, et al. 2002 Ingredients for change: Revisiting a conceptual framework. *Quality and Safety in Health Care* 11:174–80

Rycroft-Malone J, Seers K, Titchen A, et al. 2004b What counts as evidence in evidence-based practice? *Journal of Advanced Nursing* 47:81–90

Sackett D L, Richardson W S, Rosenberg W M, et al. 2000 *Evidence based medicine: how to practice and teach EBM* (2nd edn). Churchill-Livingstone, Edinburgh

Sheldon T 2000 Estimating treatment effects: real or the result of chance? *Evidence Based Nursing* 3:36–9

Stetler C B 1994 Refinement of the Stetler/Marram model for application of research findings to practice. *Nursing Outlook* 42:15–25

Stewart M 2001 Whose evidence counts? An exploration of health professionals' perceptions of evidence-based practice, focusing on the maternity services. *Midwifery* 17:279–88

Thompson G N, Estabrooks C A, Degner L F 2006 Clarifying the concepts in knowledge transfer: A literature review. *Journal of Advanced Nursing* 53:691–701

Titchen A 1987 The design and implementation of a problem-based, continuing education programme: a guide for clinical physiotherapists. *Physiotherapy* 73:318–23

University of Ulster 2006 *Postgraduate Certificate in Lifelong Learning (Facilitating Learning and Development) — Lecture 7: facilitation styles, skills and qualities*. Institute of Lifelong Learning, University of Ulster, Northern Ireland

Walsh K, Lawless J, Moss C, et al. 2005 The development of an engagement tool for practice development. *Practice Development in Health Care* 4:124–30

Ward C, McCormack B 2000 Creating an Adult learning Culture Through Practice development. *Nurse Education Today* 20:259–66

Webster J, Lloyd W C, Pritchard M A, et al. 1999 Development of evidence-based guidelines in midwifery and gynaecology nursing. *Midwifery* 15:2–5

Wilson V, McCormack B, Ives G 2005 Understanding the workplace culture of a special care nursery. *Journal of Advanced Nursing* 50:27–38

Winch S, Henderson A, Creedy D 2005 Read, think, do!: a method for fitting research evidence into practice. *Journal of Advanced Nursing* 50:20–6

Wright J, McCormack B 2001 Practice Development: individualised care. *Nursing Standard* 15(36):37–42

Answers

TT Tutorial trigger 1

You may have thought about a particular aspect of your clinical practice, such as knowledge to do with record keeping, nutrition, promotion of sleep and managing pain (we are sure you will have thought of many others, but these may just serve to trigger your thoughts), or knowledge about team working, healthcare systems/ organisations and professional standards.

When thinking about some of these examples, you may have thought about particular challenges to you working in the way the 'best evidence' would suggest and that perhaps these challenges resulted in you working differently to that stated in the evidence or you needing to adjust your practice in ways that might be inconsistent with the best evidence. Many of these challenges arise from issues that are referred to as 'contextual'; that is, characteristics of the practice setting that either enable or hinder your effectiveness — issues such as the effectiveness of the leadership in the area, the ways in which work is organised (i.e. is it task-oriented or focused on the specific needs of patients), staff attitudes, power relationships (e.g. the relationship between doctors and nurses or midwives) and the beliefs and stated wants/needs of patients. These issues are all everyday challenges faced by practitioners and ones that we need to consider when thinking about using evidence in our practice.

TT Tutorial trigger 2

Here you might want to consider the evidence available regarding the options that are available to you. You should consider reading this evidence or systematic reviews of the evidence in order to establish its validity, reliability, credibility and transferability. Consider your own practice/ practice setting and issues that would need to be addressed in order to use the evidence in practice. Think of PECOT/PICOT and reflect on each of the steps in this model and issues it raises in developing your question.

TT Tutorial trigger 3

You may have thought about questions such as:
- What is the quality of the evidence?
- Is there a systematic review of this and/or related evidence available?

- Has the evidence been translated (e.g. by Cochrane or the Joanna Briggs Institute) and is the outcome of the translation effort available to me (e.g. in the form of a clinical guideline)?
- Is the evidence relevant to my practice or my practice setting?
- What do we do currently that is consistent with this evidence and what is different about our practice?
- How might the evidence be received by others?
- If I change my own practice what effect will that have on the rest of the team and/or the processes in place for delivering care?
- What barriers to using this evidence might I have to consider?
- Are there particular enabling factors that can help me implement this evidence?
- What strategies might I use to implement this evidence in my own practice and/or others' practice?
- If I use this evidence what impact on my/ others' practice might I expect?
- How will I evaluate the impact of implementing this evidence into practice?
- How can I reflect on the experience of implementing this evidence into practice?
- What approach could I adopt to translate this learning (from my reflection) to other evidence implementation projects?
- How will I share my learning with others?

Learning activities

1. c	2. c	3. b	4. b
5. d	6. c	7. c	8. d
9. c	10. c		

18

Changing practice through research

DEAN WHITEHEAD AND PAUL ARBON

Learning outcomes

After reading this chapter, you should be able to:

- identify the theoretical and practical constructs and processes that underpin the translation, application and utilisation of research into practice
- examine the intentions, effects and outcomes of research projects when they are effectively applied in practice
- cite specific examples of effective 'translating research into practice' (TRIP) research projects from the literature
- explore the benefits and limitations of research project activity for nurses and midwives in practice settings.

Introduction

The implementing of evidence-based practice change is normally associated with nurses and midwives trained/training at the postgraduate level. Undergraduate nurses and midwives, however, are not exempt or excluded from being involved in such processes. They are actively encouraged to participate where they can and, at the very least, should be conversant with the theoretical and philosophical positions that underpin evidence-based practice-change initiatives and interventions. In fact, nurses and midwives starting out in their career often provide the impetus for practice change through their insight and enthusiasm as new members of their profession. (See Bail et al.'s 'Research in brief' box, later in this chapter.) It is for these reasons that a research text, such as this, devotes a whole chapter to this concept.

Improving healthcare outcomes requires a sustained effort to ensure that the findings of high quality research influence the daily practice of health professionals. Health professionals can no longer rely on tacit or experiential knowledge and/or personal expertise or motivation alone, but must build their practice on an integration of best available evidence — aligned with a wide body of clinical expertise and multidisciplinary networking. As already stated, such skills will normally be associated with nurses and midwives trained at the postgraduate level. Students are encouraged however, throughout this book, to become conversant with the principles of research utilisation and practice change. This facilitates the move from a position of research awareness, through to research consumerism and, eventually, research application. The gap between what we know in terms of research and what we use in practice is at the heart of the research utilisation debate (Dufault 2004). Helpfully though, many examples now exist that investigate this phenomenon, in an attempt to clarify the situation for research utilisation and practice change, in clinical settings (Edwards et al. 2002; Jones 2003; Olade 2003; Veeramah 2004; Olade 2004; French 2005a; Cleary & Freeman 2005).

This chapter complements the preceding chapter (Chapter 17) on practice development (PD) and evidence-based practice (EBP). To all intents and purposes, these practices are underpinned by the research utilisation and practice-change debates and strategies. This chapter, however, draws on specific and ongoing Australasian examples to highlight research processes as they apply to certain projects. The projects are well known to the authors. It is hoped that, in offering such examples, both undergraduate and postgraduate nurses and midwives can benefit from understanding the activities that constitute concerted practice-change projects. This is as they prepare themselves to either observe or become involved in the skills of research translation and utilisation (research transition).

Efforts to understand the difficulties associated with implementing research findings, into clinical practice, have mainly concentrated on identification of limitations, constraints, contexts and barriers (Hutchinson & Johnston 2004; Roxburgh 2006; French 2005b). Four major categories of barrier have been identified in Australian research: accessibility of research findings; anticipated outcomes of using research; organisational support to use research; and support from others to use research (Retsas 2000). Similarly, research conducted in both New Zealand and Australia has identified that several strategies are still needed to improve research utilisation in practice, these being:

- a more concerted generation of interest, ownership and capacity at the clinical level
- reducing the prevailing culture of resistance in the area of evidence generation
- more strategies to target change agents at the local clinical level
- a more co-ordinated and systematic approach to implementing clinical evidence
- a better understanding of the conceptual construction of effective research utilisation
- and the deployment of multiple strategies targeting clinical change at the individual, organisational and cultural levels (Kitson 2001).

Research in brief

French (2005b) studied a group of clinical nurse specialists to develop evidence-based guidelines for nursing practice and policy formulation. The main contextual factors, arising from the study that influenced the extent to which research would be acknowledged and used for practice change were: translation of evidence to practice, research preferences, working practices of multiple stakeholders, organisational complexity, and the extent of inter-organisational and inter-agency working.

Research in brief

Webster et al. (1999) report on their research project aimed at developing practice guidelines for both midwives and gynaecology nurses, based in Brisbane. The guidelines emerged as a result of using an EBP approach as the focus of their Continuous Improvement Based on Evidence and Research (CIBER) project. They conclude that the project has resulted in an increased interest and ownership of research activity, a commitment to change based on scientific evidence, and a contribution to hospital-wide quality improvement.

Understanding the barriers to research use is critical in understanding how to implement research in practice. However, studies that help to identify the processes and frameworks needed to implement effective research are more important, especially given the paucity in the nursing and midwifery research literature. Also important is consideration of how systematic and structured organisational approaches can enhance use of evidence in practice. Building on proactive approaches, this chapter aims to provide examples for research implementation in the practice setting. In this chapter we will consider examples that focus on changing practice at the level of client care and examples of research implementation, aimed at changing systems of care. Such projects frequently combine the application of existing research evidence into practice and, through data collection and analysis, the development and application of new understandings about care.

T_T Tutorial trigger 1

Do you agree with the following statement: 'The findings of nursing and midwifery research are largely relevant in my daily clinical practice or when, as a student, I am on a clinical placement'? If not, why might this be?

Key factors to consider when translating and applying research into practice

At the individual level, several factors influence the successful implementation of research and the application of research evidence in clinical settings. Practitioners developing a research and evidence-based approach to healthcare delivery require a number of skills, including:

- An understanding of the concepts of effectiveness, safety and acceptability to ensure that the intervention being assessed achieves the desired patient outcomes.
- The ability to access and assess the quality and generalisability of the clinical evidence presented. This includes access to resources such as databases and journals and the capacity to critically read and interpret published research. For most health professionals, both at the undergraduate and postgraduate level, the searching for and critical understanding and translation of the existing empirical research literature constitutes the first step in promoting evidence-based practice and sound practice-change principles (see Chapters 3, 4 and 16).
- The ability to assess the applicability of the findings to the local population follows on from the critical searching and reviewing of the literature. Published research will have usually already been undertaken in populations with varying degrees of similarity to the local population of interest. Assessing local applicability will help determine if the population and context are similar enough for immediate use or if further primary or translational research in the target population is required.
- The capacity and skills to effect practice change. Nurses working to change practice and apply evidence in practice situations

Research in brief

Halcomb et al. (2006) conducted an extensive review of the evidence contained within the literature pertaining to the role of the practice nurse services in Australia. While their investigation did not directly change practice, it indirectly serves as a springboard for change. Their findings highlight existing exploratory, descriptive research that could inform future strategic decision-making for professional development, policy and further research into the practice nurse services.

require a working knowledge of research practices (good research awareness through to research consumerism) and at least beginning leadership skills. This will exclude the novice undergraduate student, as they come to terms with developing research awareness and where they are also learning beginning clinical skills. It does not, however, exclude the undergraduate nursing student altogether. Involvement in practice change, for undergraduate students, is more likely in the final stages of training, as they make the transition to qualified practitioner. Students at this stage, and beyond, have a professional duty to make the transition from that of a research consumer to that of a practitioner who is capable of effective research application (although still under supervision).

The abovementioned skills alone, however, do not ensure that research findings will ultimately be adopted. Health professionals must also ensure that they work in environments where they receive support from their peers for the application of evidence into practice, where the culture is supportive of such practice, and where adequate resources are in place to effect practice change. This can be achieved by either striving to work within an environment where this capacity is already known to exist, or actively working to change an existing environment to incorporate such practices — both at the individual and collective level.

A broad understanding of factors influencing practice change, beyond characteristics of the individual, needs to be addressed. Rycroft-

Malone et al. (2004) suggest that practice change requires consideration of three key elements: evidence, context and facilitation. For example, there may be little primary research evidence to guide a clinical decision, and therefore clinicians predominantly use their clinical experience and feedback from past patients in determining how to care for the patient. Clinicians should be wary, however, of changing practice where insufficient research evidence exists. Parsons' (2004) study demonstrates that, in the absence of conclusive research evidence and where midwives were divided on the issue, the management of oral intake for labouring women was variable at best.

Sometimes existing evidence has been developed in another context of care and must be assessed for its suitability and application. This requires further 'translational' research whereby the existing evidence is interpreted or investigated to match against a different clinical context. Context refers to the environment in which the proposed change is to be implemented. Organisations with a questioning, learning environment and a commitment to staff empowerment are more likely to support evidence-based practice. Thus, the ideal environment for practice change is one where there are clear roles and responsibilities, effective teams, an organisational structure that supports change and leaders, and one that encourages innovation through all levels of staff. Facilitation recognises that, in order to change, people may require help to delineate what needs changing and how they can facilitate the achievement of whatever is the desired outcome. This is especially so with beginning and newly qualified practitioners and could be so for undergraduates. Successful facilitators of practice change are therefore supportive of others, approachable, reliable and confident, and have the ability to think innovatively and to listen to the perspectives of others.

T_T Tutorial trigger 2

Consider the following statement: 'My current unit or placement is supportive and accepting of practice change'. Support your position with examples of innovative, evidence-based practice changes that you observe in your current clinical experience. Where this is not the case, list what practice-change innovations you think would benefit where you are currently working, learning or studying?

A process for applying practice change

As with research itself, and many other nursing and midwifery-related procedures, a systematic process is needed for the effective application of practice-change strategy. This is especially at the organisational level. Useful examples of such processes can be found in the literature (e.g. Redfern & Christian 2003; Redfern et al. 2003). Various strategies exist, such as the following adapted ten-step process. This process was developed from the experience of the Peter MacCallum Cancer Institute Mucositis Project (Aranda & Pollard 2003).

1. identify the need for change
2. make current tacit knowledge explicit
3. identify and involve key stakeholders
4. develop an answerable question
5. gather, appraise and synthesise the evidence
6. compare the evidence to current practice and determine what, if anything, needs to change
7. plan for the practice change
8. implement and evaluate the change
9. sustain the change
10. share findings and disseminate what was learnt.

Structured approaches such as this consider EBP change as a research activity — albeit one derived from existing primary research and overlapping with other quality improvement activities. Some readers may also note the similarities of the above-stated process, as it relates to the change process of action research (see Chapter 15). Walsgrove and Fulbrook (2005), in their study on nurse practitioners in an organisational context, present their practice development action research as a successful project that adhered to similar structured and systematic process.

Essential to the practice-change process is an acknowledgment that EBP change is a rigorous, systematic and purpose-driven activity that requires a clear audit trail to enable evaluation and replication of the process. Considering that most nursing and midwifery research is qualitative in nature, it is important that it too is seen to adhere to rigorous process within the paradigm of evidence-based practice (Barbour 2000; Tripp-Reimer & Doebbeling 2004; Jack 2006).

Research in brief

Lindholm et al. (2006) identify 'clinical application research', in the context of using an interpretive qualitative hermeneutical approach (see Chapter 7), as a process of applying clinical research. It should be noted, however, that this is just one interpretation of how 'clinical application research' can be applied. The cornerstones of their specific process are identified as ontology, context, appropriation, under-standing, interpretation, and application.

Translating research into practice (TRIP)

There are many examples of projects that focus on practice change and are underpinned by the desire to apply evidence to and within practice. For instance, at the ward or unit level, projects might test the introduction of new devices or procedures for care. They may apply existing research evidence to the efficacy of the device or procedure, but also test their application in a specific location of care (context). Sometimes this form of investigation is referred to as 'translational research'. This is a process that seeks to translate more theoretical knowledge into the constructs of the clinical practice (Titler 2004; Dawson 2004; Kirchoff 2004).

Not all research immediately reaches the heart of the clinical problem and then resolves or overturns the situation there and then. Careful exploratory research is often the first step in the process, but should be conducted knowing that, with evidence in hand of the necessity to change practice, the next step (as separate research) will be to action change. Visentin et al. (2006) conducted a preliminary investigation into the experiences of South Australian adolescents with type 1 diabetes, as they transferred from children's to adult-based diabetes services. They noted that the required transition services of preparation, formal transition and evaluation, were not properly implemented. The authors state that, as a result of the preliminary study, the 'scene has been set' to follow through with developing a multidisciplinary working party that will work collaboratively across agencies, to develop effective transition pathways and programs.

● **Evidence-based practice tip**

Where undergraduate students may find it difficult to get actively involved in full-scale research projects, they may find it easier if they target earlier preliminary, exploratory studies — leading to full-scale projects.

Examples of Australasian practice-change projects

In this section, two Australian examples of projects, designed to facilitate practice change and to investigate the impact of new practices, are discussed. They are examples of projects that adhere to the principles of 'translating research into practice' (TRIP). Such projects utilise existing research evidence and subsequently require the development of new approaches to care through active translation of research knowledge into clinical practice settings, situations and contexts.

● **Evidence-based practice tip**

As you read through these examples consider if and how the ten-step process of Aranda and Pollard (2003), referred to previously in this chapter, has been applied in each project.

The Aged-Care Nurse Practitioner Pilot Project (ACNPPP) — changing practice systems

At times, practice-change projects set out to demonstrate the applicability of evidence to the local population. They require the establishment of interdisciplinary teams, monitoring by stakeholder groups and steering committees and high-level support from management or government. These projects may test interventions that involve fundamental changes to the way in which healthcare is delivered to consumers. Currently one of the emerging changes to the provision of healthcare that

challenges previously established approaches is the nurse practitioner role.

The Aged-Care Nurse Practitioner Pilot Project (ACNPPP) (ACT Health 2005) is an example of an extensive and inter-disciplinary evaluation of the potential role of nurse practitioners in aged-care. The project aims were to investigate the impact of the nurse practitioner role in health service delivery for the ACT aged-care population, and to provide information about the impact of the role on selected outcomes.

The ACNPPP project was a mixed-methods study using multiple data sources (see Chapter 15). Aged-care student nurse practitioners (SNPs) were examined across the continuum of care in acute, community and residential aged-care settings. It is useful to note that this project actively included students in its scope, albeit that they were postgraduate 'Masters' students who, as with all postgraduate and advanced nurses, would be expected to take a keen interest in practice improvement and be empowered to make practice changes. The potential role of the nurse practitioner in these areas was evaluated qualitatively and quantitatively. This was to identify a model of care that would enhance the delivery of efficient and effective healthcare and produce improved outcomes in each venue.

Because this project considered the potential impact of this new role, across the traditional boundaries of acute, community and residential aged care, three human research ethics committees were required to approve the project. This in itself is a substantial undertaking requiring experience and skill from the project team. A governance framework was developed to support the project (see Figure 18.1). A clinical support team (CST) provided clinical oversight, approved recommended clinical interventions and mentored the SNPs, the research and investigating teams (RITs) performed data collection and analysis respectively, and a central clinical co-ordinating committee (CCCC) provided direction and troubleshooting for the project. This included the approval of pilot clinical practice guidelines and a steering committee composed of key stakeholders. Peak bodies and consumer representatives provided a venue for broad consultation. Membership of each of these project groups was interdisciplinary involving nurses, medical practitioners and allied health clinicians.

FIGURE 18.1 Governance framework for the Aged-Care Nurse Practitioner Pilot Project (ACNPPP)

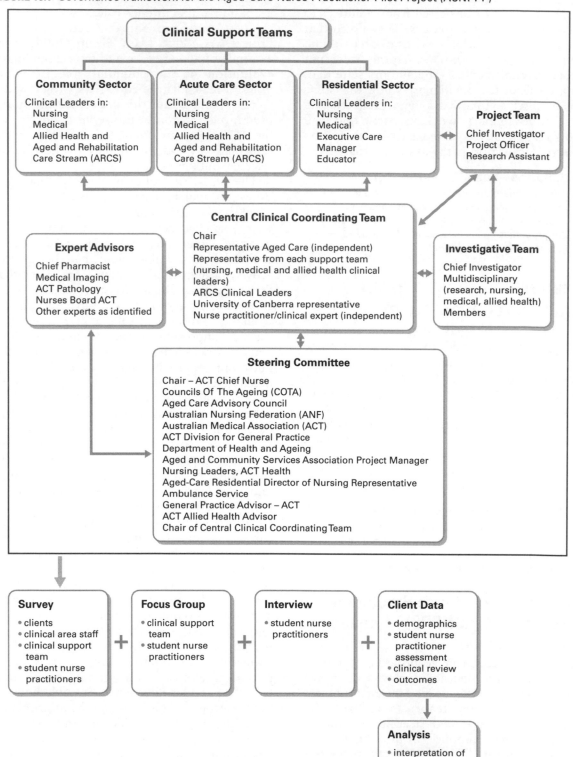

Research in brief

McCallin (2006) conducted a grounded theory study into how, as organisational structures changed and practices altered, multidisciplinary teams managed practice-based problems. In this study, the changing research context, the meaning of interdisciplinary working, collaboration and competence, and inter-professional learning opportunities are explored. It concludes that, although potentially complex and risky, interdisciplinary research offers health professionals the opportunity for professional growth, development, and research work satisfaction.

For the ACNPPP project, data were collected from a wide variety of sources to provide a comprehensive assessment of the potential impact of a nurse practitioner in aged-care. Different sources and stakeholder groups dictate that a variety of methods were implemented so as to gather rich and varied feedback for comparison and contrast. Different sources of data included those listed below.

Student nurse practitioners
- *Generic data*, including demographic detail for each client enrolled in the project.
- *Consultation details for each visit*, including reason for visit/return, presenting issue, possible diagnosis, recommended pathology, X-rays, other tests, medication, interventions, referrals, and rationale for these recommendations.
- *Clinical review of SNP recommendations by the clinical support team*, including presenting issue, provisional assessment, tests recommended, care plan, clinical review comment by support team members and clinical management plan.
- *Clinical outcome data*, including expected outcomes, medication management and improvement in function.
- *Student nurse practitioner interviews*. These were fortnightly semi-structured in-depth interviews reflecting positive experiences, difficulties, challenges, CST interactions, client responses, coping strategies and learning experiences.

- *Focus groups*. These were semi-structured focus groups covering positive experiences, difficulties, challenges, CST interactions, client responses, coping strategies, learning experiences, shared experiences on transition and integration of role.

Clinical support team data
- *Survey data*. This was a survey of the contribution of SNPs to aged-care, strengths and weaknesses of role, autonomy and clinical leadership.
- *Focus groups*. These semi-structured focus groups covered the same areas mentioned above.

Service area staff
- *Survey data*. This was a survey of staff location and role, their views on the value of SNPs, the multidisciplinary relationships, the disadvantages/advantages for the healthcare team and for patient care, and how care was applied prior to SNPs intervention.

Clients
- *Satisfaction surveys*. These included patient awareness of services, ratings of the services, satisfaction levels, whether they would access services again and service likes/dislikes.

Research in brief

As in the ACNPPP example cited above, Gardner et al. (2006) investigated nurse practitioner competency standards across New Zealand and Australia. Using a multi-methods approach, the researchers interviewed nurse practitioners and reviewed curricula and policy sources. Findings identified three generic standards for practice; namely dynamic practice, professional efficacy and clinical leadership. The researchers hope that the formulation of such standards, against a practice-change context, will support a standardised approach and mutual recognition of nurse practitioners' scope of practice across the two countries. Klardie et al. (2004) also report on the application of clinical practice guidelines as they relate to nurse practitioner interventions on patient outcomes.

The ACNPPP project involved comprehensive data collection and triangulation across data sources (see Chapter 15). Importantly, an over-arching governance framework ensured that key stakeholders were engaged and that communication about the trial was maintained throughout the project. In addition to regular communication with the steering committee, the project team maintained a newsletter and web page accessible to healthcare professionals and consumers. Numerous forums and meetings with interested organisations were attended to update on and disseminate findings as they occurred (see Chapter 21).

The Pressure Injury Prevention (PIP) project — changing clinical practice

The Pressure Injury Prevention (PIP) project (Dunk & Trevitt 2005) is an example of an Australian project designed to apply existing research knowledge, concerning the evaluation of risk and prevention of pressure injury to practice settings. The project facilitated the implementation of the Australian Wound Management Association's Clinical Practice Guidelines for Prediction and Prevention of Pressure Ulcers. Furthermore, it provided an analysis of the effect of this intervention on the prevalence of pressure injury within healthcare settings in the Australian Capital Territory

(ACT). The project utilised a relatively simple pre-test, intervention and post-test design (see Chapter 10). Nonetheless, the planning, implementation, analysis of data and reporting of the project were carefully planned and extended over a period of three years.

The pre-test phase focused on current practice and consumer outcomes and involved the identification of baseline data. Data collected included information about current risk assessment practices, the use of pressure relieving devices and a pressure ulcer prevalence study (ACT Health 2004). The intervention phase involved the development and provision of a tiered education program, aimed at providing nurses with knowledge and skills associated with the clinical practice guidelines. Principal among these was the adoption of a standard predictive tool (the Waterlow Scale) for assessing client risk of pressure injury. The final stage involved a follow-up evaluation of prevalence to assess the impact of the education program on prevalence rates across clinical settings, evaluation of the education program, and identification of resources that would be required to sustain any improvement in the management of pressure injury. Figure 18.2 outlines the project.

The PIP project provides an example of an evidence-based practice-change project. Projects like these can be straightforward, but rely on good research knowledge and

FIGURE 18.2 PIP project

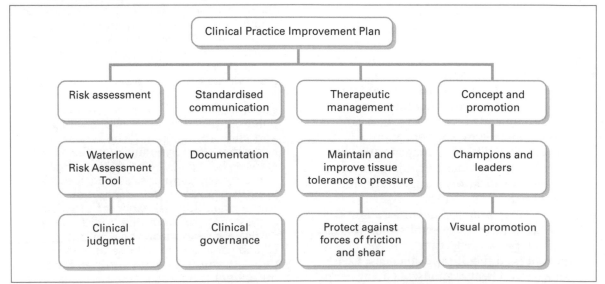

(Source: ACT Health 2004)

skill, excellent communication strategies and effective collaboration with stakeholders. The project involves collaboration between healthcare units in two hospitals and across the community health service. A systematic and structured approach has been used and substantial effort has been required to develop the research and educational tools required to successfully implement the project.

Sustaining any improvement in patient outcomes arising from practice-change projects relies on clinical leaders working alongside and developing nurses at all levels for similar future roles. Once projects have been concluded and the intervention has proven to have a positive effect, it is then up to both beginning and experienced practitioners to maintain and extend new approaches to care. For example, the PIP project found that a significant challenge to the provision of effective pressure injury prevention was the availability of pressure relieving devices within healthcare venues. The issue of sustainable pressure injury prevention would need to be addressed in the future with a range of research and evidence-based-related activities.

What makes research project activity in practice settings effective and successful?

It is useful to consider the intentions, effects and outcomes of research projects when they are effectively applied in practice. At a superficial level, the application of a rigorous and systematic process to the development of a project is expected to result in positive and predictable changes in practice. The intention, therefore, is to influence practice change and the effect is to apply evidence in practice. However, this systematic activity has other effects which are often not recognised — or at least not immediately. Successful clinical research projects also act to enhance future collaboration between researchers and clinicians, between disciplines and between departments. This helps in building confidence amongst staff within clinical areas, makes it easier to conduct future projects, and facilitates the development of an evidence-based culture in practice. Each successful project builds a stronger foundation for future work.

Research in brief

Webster et al. (1999) report on their research project aimed at developing practice guidelines for both midwives and gynaecology nurses, based in Brisbane. The guidelines emerged as a result of using an EBP approach as the focus of their Continuous Improvement Based on Evidence and Research (CIBER) project. Findings have ensured changes in practice — such as a reduction in babies routinely suctioned at delivery. Also noted is a major cost-saving move from 'date-related' practices, of determining the shelf-life of sterile articles, towards 'event-based' practices.

Point to ponder

▶ Practice change is rarely a one-off strategy. Successful practice change usually has a 'domino effect' whereby other areas of practice seek to align with change activity and services/organisations offer further support and resources to extend the scope of change.

Projects applying research to practice require a team approach combining research and evaluation expertise with clinical and health service management expertise. These projects are overlaid with competing opinions about the future development of care, political and financial concerns and implications, and require teams capable of managing through the project. Such teams must be capable of providing expert clinical input and come equipped with strong research experience. Again, this may appear to exclude novice researchers (students or otherwise), but there are many different levels of practice change and intervention that contribute to make 'wholesale' change. It is the overall

---

Evidence-based practice tip

Certain underpinning constructs must be in place to facilitate effective practice-change strategies and projects. The most important ones include a strong research evidence base to support establishment of projects, effective team working that draws upon and utilises the strengths of participants/supporters, careful and detailed data collection, analysis and evaluation, and achievable and realistic outcome-based recommendations for practice.

management of wholesale organisational or large project change that requires a high level of experience and expertise. Part of this management responsibility is to realise and nurture contributions from those with varying degrees of research ability. Henderson et al. (2005) describe how the nursing executive of a Queensland-based tertiary referral facility reviewed their management structures and, subsequently, created an improved, sustainable infrastructure for synthesising clinical and educational research activity. This, in turn, collectively improved organisational research services at all levels — from novice to skilled practitioner.

Evidence-based practice tip

Practice development takes the evidence, locates it in a particular context, and systematically evaluates the 'readiness' of that context for moving towards a different way of practising. It also facilitates step-by-step emancipatory processes to bring about changes in practice and the context in which that happens.

Research in brief

In her New Zealand-based study, McCallin (2006) reports on the changing context of clinical research — namely issues centred on interdisciplinary learning, working, collaboration, integration and competence. She concludes that, while many health professional researchers are well trained and experienced, their skills need to be extended to developing active roles as interdisciplinary research leaders, innovators and managers.

𝑇𝑇 Tutorial trigger 3

If you or your tutorial group were to effect practice change through an evidence-based research project activity what, to you, are the most important issues/features/factors that have to be in place to facilitate this?

As much as it is possible to identify the factors which facilitate effective practice-change project strategies, in the nursing and midwifery literature, the barriers too are noted. Hutchinson and Johnston (2004), in their Melbourne-based survey, involving 761 nurses and using the Barriers to Research Utilisation Scale, state the main barriers. These are: lack of research awareness and evidence base, inadequate skills in critical appraisal of existing research, lack of time, insufficient authority to change practice, and lack of support to implement change. Pravikoff et al. (2005) stress that, above all, a lack of time to develop or conduct research is the biggest barrier of all for all clinicians. Where such situations exist, with little or no attempt to overcome them, practice-change strategies are unlikely to emerge or, where they do, are less likely to succeed. Professional bodies are in a position to overcome research barriers where they dictate, enhance and support practice change. Fullerton and Thompson (2005), for instance, report the fact that the International Confederation of Midwives (ICM) *Essential Competencies for Midwifery Practice (2002)* are derived from EBP and strongly advocate the implementation of EBP and practice-change competencies.

Research in brief

Using a survey design, Phillips (2005) investigated the barriers and supports for research for mental health nurses, in two New Zealand District Health Boards. Questionnaires were sent to 285 mental health nurses: 108 nurses responded. Results showed that the main support areas needed to implement research in practice were: time-out to participate in research, more research knowledge/training, research mentoring, general support, feeling valued, and resource access. In rank order (highest to lowest) the main barriers were reported as; high workload, no relief, lack of knowledge, lack of support, lack of resources, no interest in research, and research not been valued.

Conventional barriers to practice change are there to be overcome. Successful practice-change projects require that many factors are considered and put in place to ensure maximum impact and outcome. Such factors are likely to be:

• Before beginning a practice-change initiative, it is important to have an understanding of the organisation, in terms of the level of the culture of learning and innovation, openness to change, and willingness to change.

- Practitioners are more likely to collaborate with practice-change initiatives when their expertise is acknowledged and overt criticism of their current practice is avoided. Where expertise is lacking, a commitment to support and development is equally vital.

- Measuring current staff's understanding of concepts related to evidence-based practice and practice change, as well as evaluation of current research awareness and uptake of research evidence in the workplace (Banning 2005; McSherry et al. 2006).

- Approach a practice-change initiative like any other research process. A structured approach and meticulous planning will help ensure success.

- Project success will be enhanced if funding and other resources are available to support project work. Projects undertaken in addition to clinical responsibilities will take longer and may lose momentum.

- Identify and involve stakeholders early. This can be facilitated by mapping out the likely progress of the full project and considering who will need to be consulted at each step.

- Practice change must be clearly justifiable and confined to those aspects of care where evidence indicates a need for change that is achievable and sustainable.

- Select a pilot site and patient group where opportunities for success are high (local staff expertise, local staff commitment, effective research training, support and development).

- Disseminate information about the project and its progress through targeted consultation, open forums and ongoing discussion that encourage expressions of resistance, identification of problems and alternative ideas (see Chapter 21).

- Involvement of unit-based staff as near-peer facilitators of the change may reduce local resistance and overcome feelings of being overburdened by change demands.

Point to ponder

▶ Nursing and midwifery students often bring a theoretically sound and up-to-date 'critical eye' to practice situations. From this point of view, barriers can appear more as opportunities. Where students might lack practical research experience to change practice, they are certainly a valuable resource in helping at least to initiate projects — alongside this critical perspective. Furthermore, students are often likely to possess unclouded persistence stamina and motivation to see projects through. The following 'Research in brief' is a useful example of this.

Research in brief

Bail et al.'s (in press) study is an examination of the effectiveness of hospital nursing policies as agents of support and/or control of current nursing practice. As a new graduate nurse, Bail was puzzled by the disparity between what nurses did, and what the policies said they did (or should do). She wanted to investigate the manifestation and latent functions of a diverse range of hospital nursing policies, through an analysis of those policies' representations of nursing knowledge. Through the Research Centre for Nursing Practice, at the Canberra-based hospital in which she was working, a team was set up to write a funding proposal for the graduate nurse to perform the research. In this case, the graduate nurse describes how she was able to learn and conduct clinical research in a safe and supported environment. The new graduate's instigation and drive of the research was well informed — but supported by the more experienced researchers' skills and experience. Bail et al. (in press) hope that through this study the knowledge derived from the research findings will inform development of organisational nursing policies that enable and support hospital nurses to undertake autonomous practice, based on current best evidence.

Magnet Hospitals

It is important to mention the emerging influence of 'Magnet Hospitals' in developing and sustaining an environment where nursing- and midwifery-related evidence-based practice and practice change are more likely to occur. The over-arching premise of a Magnet Hospital is to create a whole-hospital environment whereby it is easier to recruit and retain high quality staff. The more conducive the working environment is, the higher the likelihood of this occurring becomes. Magnet Hospitals, alongside a whole raft of broad outcomes, aim to provide a commitment to staff development and training, effective systems for implementing and evaluating quality-based treatment and care, and sustainable long-term resourcing. These activities are facilitated, in turn, by enabling effective systems of support. This support is manifested in ongoing and appropriate practice change, flexible working systems, proactive recruitment and retention schemes, devolved and shared management structures, and sustainable collaboration across disciplines, agencies and settings.

The Magnet Hospital concept is now well developed and its application is increasing in both New Zealand and Australia. Clark (2006) reports that evidence-based practices are a cornerstone of Magnet Hospital programs, as well as a naturally occurring phenomenon within such programs. Parsons et al. (2006) note that the Magnet principles — of shared leadership and change management — are underpinned by attempts to educate nursing personnel at all levels in EBP. This activity includes utilising recognised evidence-based models of care and involving staff in measuring practice-change outcomes. Practitioners who feel valued, who observe and have the time and resources to offer high quality care, are far more likely to be receptive to and perform EBP. More and more studies are validating the place of Magnet Hospitals in terms of practice change, organisational change and their ability to directly translate and apply appropriate research findings (Baker et al. 2004; Robinson 2006; Caramanica & Small 2006).

Innovative approaches to practice change

Innovations are occurring within nursing and midwifery research, in terms of research practice-change translation and utilisation. This is to ensure that frameworks and processes are evolving and are robust. Recently, for instance, Lindholm et al. (2006) adapted a participatory action research design to incorporate an alternative research 'clinical application research' approach. Darbyshire et al. (2005) draw on the context of 'entrepreneurialism' as another innovative research approach for practice change. The search for alternative research approaches is necessary where increasing research competition calls for different research approaches — as health practitioners compete to secure the support needed to turn their clinical project ideas into reality. The practitioners also need to look to develop and utilise new approaches for evidencing practice change. This situation remains, given the existing concerns of authors who feel that many health professionals do not understand or value research findings, nor are training or trained to incorporate clinical findings to effect practice change (Pravikoff et al. 2005).

Summary

Challenges to the successful implementation of practice change are many and varied. They may include difficulty in establishing a local network of clinicians who possess the range of research and clinical skills required to complete the project. Further limitations may be imposed by the more immediate needs of the clinical area. These are likely to be issues around staffing or funding work within the unit or setting, and a lack of active support for research work, where a culture of innovation and quality improvement does not already exist. These challenges can be linked to the need for effective facilitation of practice-change evidence, referred to earlier in this chapter. These referred-to processes of evidence, research project implementation and practice change, provide a template for success and demonstrate that the rewards are substantial.

(K)EY POINTS

- Using research processes to change practice is an approach that is intrinsically allied with the processes of evidence-based practice (EBP) and practice development (PD) (see Chapter 17).

- Translating and applying practice changes, within the clinical setting, adhere to specific processes that need to be acknowledged, implemented and evaluated to ensure successful outcomes.

- Effective practice change occurs usually within the context of wholesale organisational change, where adequate research support, resources and development are in place; that is, Magnet Hospitals.

Learning activities

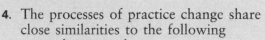

1. The main thrust of the 'research utilisation' debate is:
   (a) Why do nurses and midwives need to use research?
   (b) What exactly is research?
   (c) What do we know and what do we practice?
   (d) Who should conduct research?

2. What are the four major categories of barrier identified in Australian research according to Retsas (2000):
   (a) accessibility of research findings; anticipated outcomes of using research; organisational support to use research; and support from others to use research
   (b) accessibility of research findings; implementation of research; organisational support to use research; and lack of time
   (c) lack of time; evaluation of research; organisational support to use research; and support from others to use research
   (d) not trusting research findings; anticipated outcomes of using research; not understanding research; and support from others to use research.

3. Practice change requires consideration of three key elements. These being:
   (a) interdisciplinary effort, knowledge base, commitment
   (b) time, effort, cost
   (c) evidence, context and facilitation
   (d) assessment, evaluation, team working.

4. The processes of practice change share close similarities to the following research approach:
   (c) ethnography
   (b) action research
   (c) grounded theory
   (d) experimental.

5. Strategies needed to improve research utilisation in practice would most likely include:
   (a) ownership and capacity at the clinical level, reducing the prevailing culture of resistance in the area of evidence generation, more strategies to target change agents at the local clinical level, a more co-ordinated and systematic approach to implementing clinical evidence
   (b) having a good job, feeling valued at work, more resources to support research, good career prospects
   (c) sharing research, working closely with others, good research aims, effective time management
   (d) commitment to changing practice, supportive managers, co-operative clients, effective research outcomes.

6. Practice change is most likely to occur where:
   (a) respect for other professionals is witnessed
   (b) whole service or organisation change is witnessed
   (c) resources are made available
   (d) leaders support evidence-based practice.

7. Essential to the practice-change process is an acknowledgment that evidence-based practice change is:
   (a) workable in practice
   (b) consistent with the aims of the clients and practitioners that it affects
   (c) presented in a way that makes it meaningful to practitioners
   (d) a rigorous, systematic and purpose-driven activity that requires a clear audit trail to enable evaluation and replication of the process.

8. TRIP stands for:
   (a) translating rigour into practice
   (b) testing rigour in practice
   (c) translating research into practice
   (d) testing research in practice.

9. Practitioners are more likely to collaborate with practice-change initiatives when:
   (a) their expertise is acknowledged and overt criticism of their current practice is avoided
   (b) they are given time aside to train, in-house, for research
   (c) they undertake postgraduate research papers
   (d) they see that their colleagues are also conducting research.

10. Magnet Hospitals aim to create a whole-hospital environment where it is:
    (a) more transparent how staff and clients are treated
    (b) easier to train staff to perform to the common goal of the organisation
    (c) easier to offer in-service training
    (d) easier to recruit and retain high quality staff.

Additional resources

Bucknall T K 2004 Implementation of research evidence into practice: international perpsectives and initiatives. *Worldviews on Evidence-Based Nursing* 1:234–6

Clifford C, Murray S 2001 Pre- and post-test evaluation of a project to facilitate research development in practice in a hospital setting. *Journal of Advanced Nursing* 36:685–95

Department of Human Services and Health Victoria Australia 2002 Victorian public hospital websites. Online. Available: http:/www.health.gov.au/hospitals/pubwebs.htm

Donaldson N E, Rutledge D N, Ashley J 2004 Outcomes of adoption: measuring evidence uptake by individuals and organisations. *Worldviews on Evidence-Based Nursing* 1:S41–S51

Dykes P C 2003 Practice guidelines and measurement: state-of-the-science. *Nursing Outlook* 41:65–9

References

ACT Health 2004 *Establishment of sustainable processes for pressure injury management in the Australian Capital Territory*. Project Report. ACT Health, ACT, August, p 14

—— 2005 *The Aged-Care Nurse Practitioner Pilot Project (ACNPPP): Final report to the Australian Government*. ACT Health, ACT

Aranda S, Pollard A 2003 Implementing research into practice. In: Schneider Z, Elliott D, LoBiondo-Wood G, Haber J (eds) *Nursing Research: Methods, Critical Appraisal and Utilisation*, 2nd edn. Mosby, Sydney

Bail K, Gardner A, Cook R (in press) Confusion within hospital nursing policies: a discourse analysis. *Nursing Inquiry*

Baker C M, Bingle J M, Hajewski C J et al. 2004 Advancing the Magnet Recognition Program in master's education through service-learning. *Nursing Outlook* 52:134–41

Banning M 2005 Conceptions of evidence, evidence-based medicine, evidence-based practice and their use in nursing: independent nurse prescribers' views. *Journal of Clinical Nursing* 14:411–17

Barbour R S 2000 The role of qualitative research in broadening the 'evidence base' for clinical practice. *Journal of Evaluation in Clinical Practice* 6:75–106

Caramanica L, Small D 2006 Seeding the growth of professional nursing practice with the MAGNET Forces. *Nurse Leader* 4:56–61

Clark M L 2006 The Magnet Recognition Program and evidence-based practice. *Journal of PeriAnesthesia Nursing* 21:186–9

Cleary M, Freeman A 2005 Facilitating research within clinical settings: the development of a beginner's guide. *International Journal of Mental Health* 14:202–8

Darbyshire P, Downes M, Collins C, et al. 2005 Moving from institutional dependence to entrepreneurialism. Creating and funding a collaborative research and practice development position. *Journal of Clinical Nursing* 14:926–34

Dawson J D 2004 Quantitative analytical methods in translation research. *Worldviews on Evidence-Based Nursing* 1:S60–S64

Dufault M 2004 Testing a collaborative research utilisation model to translate best practices in pain management. *Worldviews on Evidence-Based Nursing* 1(S.1):S26–S32

Dunk A M, Trevitt T 2005 How the AWMA Clinical Practice Guidelines for the Prediction and Prevention of Pressure Ulcers are being used across the ACT. *Primary Intention* 13.121

Edwards H, Chapman H, Davis L M 2002 Utilisation of research evidence by nurses. *Nursing and Health Sciences* 4:89–95

French B 2005a The process of research use in nursing. *Journal of Advanced Nursing* 49:125–34

—— 2005b Contextual factors influencing research use in nursing. *Worldviews on Evidence-Based Nursing* 2:172–83

Fullerton J T, Thompson J B 2005 Examining the evidence for the International Confederation of Midwives' essential competencies for midwifery practice. *Midwifery* 21:2–13

Gardner G, Carryer J, Gardner A, Dunn S 2006 Nurse practitioner competency standards: findings from collaborative Australian and New Zealand research. *International Journal of Nursing Studies* 43:601–10

Halcomb E J, Patterson E, Davidson P M 2006 Evolution of practice nursing in Australia. *Journal of Advanced Nursing* 55:376–90

Henderson A, Winch S, Henney R, et al. 2005 'Working from the inside': an infrastructure for the continuing development of nurses' professional practice. *Journal of Nursing Management* 13:106–10

Hutchinson A M, Johnston L 2004 Bridging the divide: a survey of nurses' opinions regarding barriers to, and facilitators of, research utilisation in the practice setting. *Journal of Clinical Nursing* 13:304–15

Jack S M 2006 Utility of qualitative research findings in evidence-based public health research. *Public Health Nursing* 23:277–83

Jones J 2003 Performance improvement through clinical research utilisation: the linkage model. *Journal of Nursing Care Quality* 15:49–54

Kirchoff K T 2004 State of the science of translational research: from demonstration projects to intervention testing. *Worldviews on Evidence-Based Nursing* 1:S6–S12

Kitson A 2001 Approaches used to implement research findings into nursing practice: report of a study tour to Australia and New Zealand. *International Journal of Nursing Practice* 7:392–405

Klardie K A, Johnson J, McNaughton M A, et al. 2004 Integrating the principles of evidence-based practice into clinical practice. *Journal of the American Academy of Nurse Practitioners* 16:98–105

Lindholm L, Nieminen A-L, Mäkelä C, et al. 2006 Clinical application research: a hermeneutical approach to the appropriation of caring sciences. *Qualitative Health Research* 16:137–50

McCallin A M 2006 Interdisciplinary researching: exploring the opportunities and risks of working together. *Nursing and Health Sciences* 8:88–94

McSherry R, Artley A, Holloran J 2006 Research awareness: an important factor for evidence-based practice? *Worldviews on Evidence-Based Nursing* 3:103–15

Olade R A 2003 Attitudes and factors affecting research utilisation. *Nursing Forum* 38:5–15

—— 2004 Evidence-based practice and research utilisation activities among rural nurses. *Journal of Nursing Scholarship* 36:220–5

Parsons M 2004 A midwifery practice dichotomy on oral intake in labour. *Midwifery* 20:72–81

Parsons M L, Cornett P A, Golightly-Jenkins C 2006 Creating healthy workplaces. *Nurse Leader* 4:34–9

Phillips B N 2005 A survey of mental health nurses' opinion of barriers and supports for research. *Nursing Praxis in New Zealand* 21:24–32

Pravikoff D S, Tanner A B, Pierce S T 2005 Readiness of US Nurses for Evidence-Based Practice. *American Journal of Nursing* 105:40–51

Redfern S, Christian S 2003 Achieving change in health care practice. *Journal of Evaluation in Clinical Practice* 9:225–38

Redfern S, Christian S, Norman I 2003 Evaluating change in healthcare practice: lessons from three studies. *Journal of Evaluation in Clinical Practice* 9:239–49

Retsas A 2000 Barriers to using research evidence in nursing practice. *Journal of Advanced Nursing* 31:599–606

Robinson C 2006 From magnet and beyond. *Nurse Leader* 4:23–7

Roxburgh M 2006 An exploration of factors which constrain nurses from research participation. *Journal of Clinical Nursing* 15(5):535–45

Rycroft-Malone J, Harvey G, Seers K, et al. 2004 An exploration of the factors that influence the implementation of evidence into practice. *Journal of Clinical Nursing* 13:913–24

Titler M G 2004 Methods in translation science. *Worldviews on Evidence-Based Nursing* 1:38–48

Tripp-Reimer T, Doebbeling B 2004 Qualitative perspectives in translational research. *Worldviews on Evidence-Based Nursing* 1:S63–S72

Veeramah V 2004 Utilisation of research findings by graduate nurses and midwives. *Journal of Advanced Nursing* 47:183–91

Visentin K, Koch T, Kralik D 2006 Adolescents with type 1 diabetes: transition between diabetes services. *Journal of Clinical Nursing* 15:761–9

Walsgrove H, Fulbrook P 2005 Advancing the clinical perspective: a practice development project to develop the nurse practitioner role in an acute hospital trust. *Journal of Clinical Nursing* 14:444–55

Webster J, Lloyd W C, Pritchard M A, et al. 1999 Development of evidence-based guidelines in midwifery and gynaecology nursing. *Midwifery* 15:2–5

Answers

TT Tutorial trigger 1

You may not agree with the statement because:
1. research may not be visible — even if it is happening
2. research may be conducted by those others than nurses and midwives
3. clinical practice may be based on task, routine and/or traditional practices
4. research may not be understood or known that it is research
5. cultures of hierarchy, suppression and lack of information, professional protectionism, mistrust, lack of collaboration and change resistance may exist
6. there may be a general lack of time and resources to support research.

TT Tutorial trigger 2

Personal observation/experience exercise, not requiring suggested answers.

TT Tutorial trigger 3

- Before beginning a practice-change initiative it is important to have an understanding of the organisation, in terms of the level of the culture of learning and innovation, openness to change, and willingness to change.
- Practitioners are more likely to collaborate with practice-change initiatives when their expertise is acknowledged and overt criticism of their current practice is avoided.
- Approach a practice-change initiative like any other research process. A structured approach and meticulous planning will help ensure success.
- Project success will be enhanced if funding and other resources are available to support project work. Projects undertaken in addition to clinical responsibilities will take longer and may lose momentum.
- Identify and involve stakeholders early. This can be facilitated by mapping out the likely progress of the full project and considering who will need to be consulted at each step.
- Practice change must be clearly justifiable and confined to those aspects of care where evidence indicates a need for change.
- Select a pilot site and patient group where opportunities for success are high (local staff expertise, local staff commitment).
- Disseminate information about the project and its progress through targeted consultation, open forums and ongoing discussion that encourage expressions of resistance, identification of problems and alternative ideas.
- Involvement of unit-based staff as near-peer facilitators of the change may reduce local resistance and overcome feelings of being overburdened by change demands.

Learning activities
1. c
2. a
3. c
4. b
5. a
6. b
7. d
8. c
9. a
10. d

Conducting
primary research

Writing proposals and grant applications

Zevia Schneider

Learning outcomes

After reading this chapter, you should be able to:

- describe the structure and content of a research proposal
- outline the process for preparing and submitting a research proposal
- identify the statement of the problem in research studies
- identify funding agencies appropriate for nursing or midwifery projects
- prepare a draft research proposal according to a specified format.

Introduction

Nursing and midwifery are disciplines engaged in both *art* and *science*. This assertion applies equally to proposal writing. The *art* implied refers to writing style, coherence, knowledge of the research problem/question, clarity and readability. The *science* refers to the techniques and rigour involved in writing a proposal. The research proposal, be it for course requirements, a higher degree or a submission for funding, is the initial and major means of communicating with the relevant research committee and human research ethics committee (HREC) of health services or universities or funding agencies. For students seeking to gain approval for their proposal, the essence of success is in writing a clear and cogent argument about the need for, and feasibility of, the research project they are proposing.

This chapter describes the major components and processes involved in developing a research proposal. The stages for preparing and submitting a research proposal are presented in a way that will facilitate familiarity with the information required by institutional ethics committees and funding agencies. Information regarding appropriate funding agencies for nursing and midwifery is also provided.

What is a research proposal?

A proposal is a plan or blueprint for an investigation of some kind. A research proposal then is a plan that details a reasoned, rigorous and systematic inquiry into a topic to justify the need for the study and to gain a clearer understanding of the area. The format of the proposal is influenced by the specific purpose of the research and by the audience for whom it is intended. A research proposal may be written for any of the following reasons:

- gaining approval of a higher degrees committee in a university to undertake a student research project
- for an ethics committee requesting permission to conduct research, including a pilot study, using human subjects or animals
- the purpose of gaining approval of a relevant committee to undertake an academic activity not related to a research higher degree; for example, a minor thesis that may require a literature review, or a meta-analysis of the literature
- applying to a funding agency requesting financial support to conduct a research study.

Regardless of the audience, the proposal must demonstrate that:

- the investigator is competent to undertake the research
- the topic is important and that the findings will be of benefit to, for example, patients, a particular group, advancing new knowledge
- the design, method and timeframe are feasible and appropriate
- the risk–benefit for participants is acceptable
- participant privacy and safety are protected
- if the proposal is submitted as part of a higher degree, assurance from the head of department that the student will have appropriate supervision and access to the required facilities.

Planning a project

As with any project, planning is an important preliminary element. This stage involves:

- reading the relevant literature in your area of interest (see Chapter 4)
- identifying and clarifying a researchable topic (see Chapter 5)
- a description of the beneficiaries and benefits of the project
- applying a research approach to address the research question or objective (see methods chapters in Section 2)
- identifying the requirements for submission to a particular HREC
- consulting resource personnel available to advise on the development and submission of the proposal (e.g. academic colleagues, clinical staff, ethics office staff).

Choosing a topic

Sometimes a student has a clear idea of what to research, but equally at times, there are students who are not sure what to research. There are many places where research ideas can be found: the clinical area in which you work; conference presentations; networking at conferences and elsewhere with people who have a similar interest; reading the literature; the internet; colleagues and other people you may meet. The clinical area, nursing management and nursing education provide unlimited opportunities for nurses and midwives to identify problems and challenges (e.g. nursing care, nursing rituals, communication with patients, family and colleagues, patients' understanding of their medical condition, reading habits of graduate nurses, the concerns of first-time mothers on leaving hospital).

When considering a topic for a research project, the purpose of the proposal — that is, whether the proposal is for a higher degree, applying for an external grant, or some other academic exercise — will be an important factor. If you are enrolled in a higher degree or fulfilling the research requirement for an undergraduate program, your supervisor will tell you what the research objectives and goals are in the faculty's strategic plan. Recognition of faculty goals or research priorities is important, particularly if you are seeking funding from the department/faculty or university, or even from an external agency. A head of department or dean will more likely agree to fund a project that is congruent with faculty goals. An academic supervisor or the faculty in which you are enrolled may encourage research in a particular area; for example, two or three students may develop projects related to the same topic area from different standpoints. If the proposal is directed to a funding agency, it may be that certain research priorities and criteria have been stipulated and these criteria may impact on your choice of topic and design. It may also be that you have been given a certain amount of freedom in choosing the area you wish to research.

Faculty resources are also important to consider during planning, including appropriate supervision by academics who have the interest and knowledge to guide you, and facilities (e.g. equipment, computers, space). Most universities offer postgraduate support grants. The amount of the grant may differ, but the purpose is generally to assist students with various costs related to the research being undertaken (e.g. data collection, consumables, conference attendance, use of office equipment, special materials). Information about intellectual property (discussed later in this chapter), may be obtained from your supervisor, head of school, the intellectual property office or the university solicitor. It is most important that the prospective student understands exactly what these conditions mean. Issues surrounding intellectual property are important when applying for external funding and it is the researcher's responsibility to seek clarification before embarking on writing a proposal.

Nurses and midwives considering higher degrees should bear in mind that they are not expected to write a proposal without any assistance. Providing skilled guidance for students writing proposals is part of an academic's teaching role, and thus includes issues about interpersonal relationships between students and academics (Phillips & Pugh 1994). This guidance becomes more obvious when one considers that it is the responsibility of the academic to inform the student about the feasibility, appropriateness, and potential value of the research, availability of resources in the department/university, and availability and appropriateness of adequate supervision should the proposal lead to a higher degree by research.

In the university or hospital, appropriately qualified staff are there to assist students,

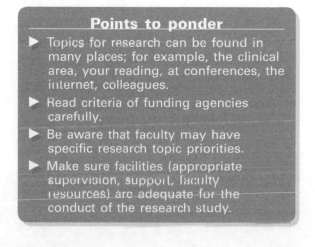

Points to ponder

▶ Topics for research can be found in many places; for example, the clinical area, your reading, at conferences, the internet, colleagues.

▶ Read criteria of funding agencies carefully.

▶ Be aware that faculty may have specific research topic priorities.

▶ Make sure facilities (appropriate supervision, support, faculty resources) are adequate for the conduct of the research study.

however, some strategies may be helpful when considering a project. It may be useful to write a draft of the significance of the project (this may be in a particular discipline in nursing e.g. palliative care, neonatal intensive care, the clinical area, or community health). This activity may form part of the application process for higher degree candidature or applying for funding.

Format requirements for the proposal

Most academic institutions use a standard format for writing proposals. A separate standard form requiring different information may be required by a hospital human ethics committee. These forms may differ from those used by funding agencies who usually provide their own application forms. Also, the funding agency's criteria will certainly be different, as will the specific areas they are committed to funding. Most academic institutions also require a plain language statement about the research topic. This requirement is necessary for the review panel, which may include academics outside of the student's particular discipline, to understand clearly what the research is about.

Intellectual property

A contentious issue for health professionals planning a research project is the question of intellectual property. What constitutes a student's rights regarding intellectual property is an important concern; specific meanings and interpretation are available (Australian Research Council et al. 2001; Australian Vice-Chancellors' Committee 2002). Most universities provide students with a copy of 'acceptance of conditions of offer for higher degree candidature' to read and sign, which sets out, inter alia, conditions regarding candidature, intellectual property and commercial agreements, and information about maintaining contact with your supervisor(s).

As a student, it is important to understand your rights and obligations should your research have the potential to result in patentable inventions or any other discoveries that have commercial value. Such innovations or discoveries may arise out of research

conducted by higher degree students in departments of biomedical science, toxicology and animal research. Students engaged in research that may result in discoveries are usually included as one of a number with senior academic researchers undertaking funded research of a commercial nature. These students would be informed about the nature of the research project.

The pilot study

Often, a pilot study is undertaken to test the feasibility of conducting a larger study, or may be a requirement for a research unit, and may be advised for students enrolled in a Doctor of Philosophy (PhD), Doctor of Nursing (DN) or Doctor of Midwifery (DM) program. A research proposal may be required for this initial and independent small-scale study, or the pilot study may form a component of a larger project and proposal. A pilot study tests the feasibility of the procedure or proposed instrument. For example, if new protocols or procedures were being introduced into a clinical area, it is important that the clinical nurses or midwives are familiar with the new procedures and understand what is required of them. A pilot study would highlight any ambiguities or misunderstandings the staff may have. When new procedures are understood, their implementation in the clinical area is likely to result in less stress for the nursing staff and enhance the conduct of the project. Funding agencies often expect applicants to have undertaken a pilot study.

Writing a proposal

Writing a proposal involves good writing skills, clarity, logic, and a clear understanding of the purpose for which the proposal is written. Developing drafts and discussing the proposed study with supervisors or colleagues will frequently highlight any limitations or weaknesses in the plan. It is useful to assume that the committee (e.g. hospital, grant review panels, university boards) reviewing your proposal will have a limited knowledge of your specific area. This will help you focus on writing comprehensively and clearly, with minimal jargon. Most research committees, scholarship boards and funding organisations provide a specific pro-forma or template for writing a proposal, although these are not necessarily standardised. Variations in proposals may therefore be required depending on the specific requirements (e.g. thesis, course requirement or hospital project). Application forms for different funding agencies will also vary.

Not everyone who writes a proposal adopts the same process: some individuals have a clear idea of a topic, others begin a literature search to explore a vague idea, and others may adopt a different approach. Regardless of your approach, the time and effort spent thinking about the topic is never wasted. A research proposal is evidence of the investigator's written skills. However, good writing will not necessarily lead to a good research proposal. Success in writing a research proposal may be seen as an indication of how thoroughly the researcher has understood, conceptualised, and communicated the information relating to the research topic in a well-thought-out plan (see Sections 1 and 2).

It is a good idea to write a draft about the purpose, significance and potential usefulness of the study. Identifying the aims assists in clarifying your thoughts and provides a basis for discussion with colleagues and/or lecturers. The appropriateness of the study in terms of feasibility, budget, practicality, availability of resources and facilities, and supervision, can then be considered with the benefit of enhanced clarity.

Generally, the following structure and content are required:
- the title of the research project
- the investigators
- an abstract or summary (about 300 words)
- a statement of the problem being investigated
- the significance or importance of the project
- a literature review or background of the topic
- assumptions and definitions
- the aims and objectives of the project
- the research plan (e.g. methodology, samples and sampling [selection of participants, inclusion/exclusion criteria], setting, procedure, instrumentation, data collection and data analysis)
- ethical issues (including the participant information sheet and informed consent form)

- dissemination of the findings
- the budget (including justifications for items).

A table of contents may be required for a lengthy proposal (check the submission requirements). The structure and content of a research proposal for both qualitative and quantitative proposals are basically the same, although differences are likely in the 'Research plan/method' section when writing about:
- recruitment of participants (e.g. random sample, purposive sample, snowballing)
- the kinds of relationship with participants and major tasks of the researcher (e.g. collaborator, participant observer, emancipation)
- purpose of the research (e.g. testing hypotheses, instrument development, theory building)
- data collection strategies (e.g. interventions, tests, audiotapes, field notes from memory, transcripts of conversations, audit trail)
- data analysis procedures (e.g. descriptive or inferential statistics, data reduction).

Note the specific requirements for each committee or funding body to which the proposal is being submitted. Be aware also of the different ethics formats; for example, some HRECs allow only two pages of free text for the background and research plan, while granting bodies (e.g. NHMRC) allow up to ten pages. Each component of the research proposal is now discussed in more detail.

Project title

Give your project a working title that is clear, descriptive and succinct. The title should be informative but not too long as this may result in confusion about the specific question or issue. Similar to a journal article title, the proposal title should include the study participants, concept or variable/s being studied, the research approach, and the intervention used (if any). Keywords (significant words) are commonly used to be explicit and unambiguous in what the research project is about. Initially, the use of a subtitle may be useful; for example, 'An investigation of hospitalised first-time mothers' experiences of learning how to breastfeed following instruction and assisted by a midwife in the immediate postpartum period'. During the course of writing a proposal, some ideas may change and it may be necessary to change the title as well. The above subtitle may well become 'Breastfeeding experiences of first-time hospitalised mothers'. However, a broad working title is acceptable and it is imprudent to cling to a title slavishly when your thinking about the research dictates otherwise.

The investigators

As noted earlier, proposal reviewers need to assess the ability of the investigators in the research team to undertake the research. Therefore, proposals require some information about the research team (e.g. name, qualifications, employment position) as a minimum. In some instances (e.g. NHMRC grants), a short biography (research track record) and publications list are necessary for each chief investigator. All authors on the research team should provide intellectual capital to the research project; that is, they must actively participate in the project and contribute to the generation of knowledge. Following some unfortunate episodes of 'honorary authorship' to persons in authority who provided no academic input to the research and related publications, there are now guidelines on authorship, sponsorship and accountability, issued by, among others, the International Committee of Medical Journal Editors (ICMJE) (Halperin et al. 2005), and the Australian Vice-Chancellors' Committee (see 'Additional resources').

Abstract

An abstract or summary is typically about 300 words and describes the aims and methods of the proposed study. It is often useful to begin the introductory paragraph with the original question. In this way the topic or key sentence provides the focus and alerts the reader from the outset to the point of the proposal. Having explained what the proposal is about, the next point is to describe how to address the issue or answer the research question. In some cases, keywords or disciplinary field codes may be required. Foundations sometimes use the abstract to make a basic determination about the worthiness of the proposal.

Different journals require different formats for abstracts e.g. *Australian Journal of Advanced Nursing* stipulates the following headings: Objectives, Design, Main Outcome Measures, Results and Conclusion.

Statement of the problem and justification for the project

This section of the proposal informs the reviewer about the need for the study. A statement, sometimes called 'the plain language statement' or 'lay person description', should provide the rationale and justification for undertaking the project. The clarity required for the plain language statement will be the same for proposals that use a quantitative or qualitative research approach. The research question should be stated and an indication given of the pragmatic value; that is, how you think the findings of the study will be useful (e.g. will it benefit patients, advance knowledge, influence protocols and policies?) and the implications of the knowledge gained for the field (e.g. theory building, expanding the knowledge base). The paucity of published research is often included as a justification for undertaking research. 'Few studies reporting the employment experiences of new graduate nurses beyond the initial orientation period' was one justification for the study by Halfer and Graf (2006) on graduate nurse perceptions of the work experience. Timelines should be included.

Literature review

A critical literature review is documented to identify the current knowledge about the topic, and place the research problem in context. Reviewing the literature helps to conceptualise the research problem (see Chapter 4, 'Reviewing the literature'). The literature review demonstrates your ability to critically evaluate the information and should convince the relevant committee that the proposed research addressing the identified omission/s is important and necessary. Reasons for undertaking the research should be based on an analysis of the shortcomings of the reviewed literature (e.g. inappropriateness of design and/or tests administered, gaps in knowledge, conflicting or inconclusive findings, and problems with the samples, such as numbers, selection or profile). It is usual to cite studies less than five years old unless they are seminal works or, if little research has been conducted in the area. Further suggestions about constructing a bibliography or reference list are available (Jamieson 1999).

Points to ponder

Student literature reviews may be compromised by (Langley 2002):

► lack of organisation

► lack of focus and cohesion

► being verbose

► poor analysis and citation of important articles

► citing irrelevant references

► dependence on secondary sources.

Aims and objectives of the project

Aims are usually broad and are a statement of purpose. Research objectives should be specific and explicit and describe the activities employed to achieve the aim(s). Both aims and objectives should be feasible, achievable and unambiguous. The purpose of the project should be very clear; that is, why the project is important in itself and what the benefits might be. In writing the proposal, the investigator must be ever-mindful of the congruency between the aims and objectives and the plan of the project within the given timeframe (see Chapter 5).

When considering the aims and objectives of the project, it is important to remember that these aims constitute the boundaries of the research. The aims guide the ways in which data are collected and analysed. For example, if the aim is to find out whether nurses coming from a night's work think as clearly as they do after a night's sleep, an objective might be to administer some kind of cognitive test which will yield results that can be measured. These issues are important because other nurses may want to replicate or repeat the design and test(s) to see whether they obtain the same results. If, on the other hand, your aim is to find out how women experience and cope with breast cancer, the design will probably include a face-to-face interview at different times (e.g. at diagnosis, following surgery and 3 months after surgery).

Research in brief

The aim in Pascoe et al.'s (2005 p 44) study was 'to describe the workforce characteristics and current responsibilities' of 222 nurses currently working in Australian general practice settings. The objective was achieved through the administration and analysis of a survey administered by telephone interview.

TT Tutorial trigger 1

Your research class is debating the importance of aims and objectives in a research proposal. Why are they important?

Assumptions and definitions

Assumptions and definitions should be clearly stated to avoid any ambiguity or confusion, and variables should be operationally defined where appropriate. For example, if the plan is to administer a self-care program to a group of patients, an assumption may be that most people want to learn how to care for themselves. Human beings may be further defined in terms of health status, education, age and cultural background. A researcher may define the concept of *self-care* as the acceptance of responsibility by individuals for their care in those activities of daily living considered appropriate for their particular health status. There may well be other definitions of self-care. However, an important point is that having chosen a particular definition considered appropriate for the project, the researcher can then decide how best to operationalise the objectives. That is, the conceptual definition is translated into a form that can be measured (see Chapter 5). Jamison (2001 p 83) defined the concept of 'wellness' as a 'dynamic state that is unique, relative, multidimensional and measurable'. Any researcher using this particular definition must decide how best to operationalise these concepts. When the empirical referents have been clearly stated by the researcher, the research consumer is able to evaluate the findings.

Research plan

Notwithstanding the importance of the literature review, the research plan is the most important section of the proposal, providing the principal description of the study — detailing the research design, method and involvement of the study participants. The method includes the design, sampling (how participants will be recruited) and sample profile (inclusion and exclusion criteria), intervention (if appropriate), measuring instruments (including reliability and validity), procedure, data gathering (describe what data will be collected and method of data collection), data analysis techniques/strategies (these should correspond with the objectives of the project), and the projected timeframe for the stages of the project. Be prepared to write several drafts of the proposal prior to submission. As with other sections of the proposal, it is important to present the design in detail; this section can be refined and shortened later if necessary. The design must be carefully explained in order to convince reviewers that the research approach and methods entailed in the proposal are the most logical and appropriate for this particular research question.

Each research approach has its own philosophy and theoretical or conceptual framework, and strategies for data collection and analysis. The main consideration is always to find the research design and approach that will best answer the research question(s) (see Chapter 2 for an overview of research approaches). Chapters 7, 8 and 9 describe some common qualitative research approaches: grounded theory, phenomenology, and ethnography. Chapters 10, 11, 12, 13 and 14 are devoted to quantitative research approaches. Appropriate articles included in the chapters illustrate how the investigators have matched their research designs to their research questions. These chapters should be carefully read and understood prior to writing a proposal. Whether a qualitative approach or quantitative design is chosen, bear in mind the feasibility of the project in terms of access to the sample(s), ethical issues and financial restraints.

Inclusion of a theoretical or conceptual framework

One issue in writing a proposal is the question of a theoretical or conceptual framework. The importance of a conceptual framework is in linking the proposed or current study to the previous knowledge base of the concept of interest — this may be through examining relationships between concepts or building on known and established theories or models. As an applied discipline, nursing can legitimately use appropriate frameworks from the social or medical sciences as well as from within the discipline.

Finding an appropriate theoretical or conceptual framework for a study appears to cause many nurses and midwives some difficulty. Some research studies benefit from specific theoretical frameworks and some do not. Some research topics may be investigated or explored from a non-theoretical standpoint. Interest in a topic may arise from the clinical area; for example, how proficient graduate nurses are in calculating drugs, or whether a labouring woman's anxiety levels are lower or higher when her partner is present. Similarly, a topic may be of social or community importance; for example, what factors influence the utilisation of the health system in 20- to 30-year-old men from a non-English speaking background? Generally, however, some kind of framework should be used to help clarify the concepts and their relationships. Students should discuss this issue with their supervisor and be guided by their advice.

> ### Points to ponder
>
> ▶ Review the institution/agency guidelines carefully before you decide on your topic; some agencies have specific topics they are prepared to fund.
>
> ▶ Ensure that you meet the respective eligibility criteria.
>
> ▶ Make sure that the amount of funding required is commensurate with what the agency is offering.
>
> ▶ Request application forms.
>
> ▶ Look at the checklist before posting your application; some agencies will not review incomplete applications.

_TT_ Tutorial trigger 2

Discuss the importance of a literature review in the development of a research proposal?

Ethical considerations

Ethical issues are concerned with the protection of human and animal subjects in research. The regulations aim to ensure the absence or minimisation of harm, trauma, anxiety and discomfort to participants, be they human or animal. Researchers must take every precaution to protect people being studied from physical or mental harm or discomfort. It is not always clear what constitutes harm or discomfort. Nurses should be aware of their role in the research process, whether functioning as researcher, caregiver (including patient advocate) or research consumer. Ethical issues must be dealt with comprehensively in the research proposal and includes a consent form and information sheet. Chapter 6 provides a comprehensive coverage of ethical and legal issues, including examples of a consent form and information sheet, and instances of unethical conduct in research.

Guidelines for the ethical conduct of research involving humans have been developed by the National Health and Medical Research Council (NHMRC) (2004). These guidelines build on the principles laid down by the Nuremberg Code and the Helsinki Declaration and provide a framework for the ethical conduct of research. The Health Research Council in New Zealand has separate guidelines for Maōri and Pacific peoples. All HRECs in Australia and New Zealand require research proposals to adhere to these guidelines (see 'Additional resources' at the end of this chapter).

In Australia, _Standards for Research for The Nursing Profession_, together with a code of ethics and a code of professional conduct for nurses, were developed by the Australian Nursing Federation (1997). These standards contain statements about the ethical conduct of research undertaken by Australian nurses and midwives. The standards and codes are important in safeguarding both individuals who participate in research and members of the nursing profession. Additional reading in ethical issues in proposal writing can be found in Cohen et al. (1993), Gitlin & Lyons (1996), Hall (1988), and Orb et al. (2001).

Protection of human rights

The term 'human rights' was outlined in the American Nurses Association (1985, currently under review) guidelines as follows:
- right to self-determination
- right to privacy and dignity
- right to anonymity or confidentiality
- right to fair treatment
- right to protection from discomfort and harm.

These rights apply to everyone — participants and team members involved in a research project.

Informed consent

Informed consent is the process by which participants who are recruited for a research study are informed, at their level of comprehension, about the nature of the study, the purpose, demands, the interventions (if required), and the risks and benefits to them. Participants should also be provided with an information sheet (a plain language statement about the project) and a consent form (see Chapter 6). Any questions raised by the participants must be answered clearly and unambiguously in order for them to make a decision about participating or not. In addition, it is desirable that consent should be obtained in writing. Information about informed consent and other ethical and legal issues can be found in Chapter 6 and NHMRC (2004).

No investigator may involve a human being as a research participant before obtaining legally effective informed consent from them or their legally authorised representative. The language of the consent form must be clear and understandable for the individual or group concerned. Subjects _must not_ be coerced into participating, nor may researchers collect data on participants who have explicitly refused to be involved in a study. An ethical violation of this principle occurred when an audit conducted in 1994 indicated that medical data on at least three dozen women were collected and analysed without authorisation, against the women's expressed wishes (Snowdon 1994).

The following points must be considered when planning a research project and care taken that they are addressed in the proposal:

- individuals should not be involved in research without asking them whether or not they wish to participate
- information should not be withheld from participants
- information provided should not be misleading
- participants should not be made to do or say things that violate their moral standards or expose participants to mental or physical stress
- anonymity and confidentiality of participants, organisations and institutions should be maintained
- privacy should not be invaded
- benefits should not be withheld from the control groups
- results should be made known to participants
- the informed consent of the participant should be gained — also consider the long-term effects of the study on the participants
- consider the welfare of laboratory animals or other animals participating in the project
- consider storage and safety of data.

This section serves only as an introduction to the concept of legal/ethical issues related to animal experimentation. Principles of protection of animal rights in research have evolved over time, as has a growing body of literature in the area (Langley 1989; NHMRC 2004; Singer 1991). Animals, unlike humans, cannot give informed consent, but conditions safeguarding their welfare must not be ignored. Nurses who encounter the use of animals in research should be alert to the rights of all animals.

T_T Tutorial trigger 3

You have been asked by the faculty higher degrees committee or funding agency to justify the research design in your proposal. What factors would you consider in your answer?

Dissemination of findings

If the research is worth doing, it is worth publishing the findings for the benefit of adding to the knowledge base of nursing and midwifery. It is sometimes said that if findings are not published, it is as though the research has not been done — certainly the research process has not been completed. The proposal application form from funding agencies requires specific information as to the proposed dissemination of findings. Examples of sources for disseminating findings are conferences, lectures, and refereed journals of nursing, midwifery, public health and education. (See Chapter 21 for information on presenting and publishing research.)

Budget

A detailed itemised account of all expenditures (e.g. personnel, equipment, travel, accommodation, printing, telephone charges, photocopying and stationery) is required by funding agencies and when applying for a grant from a nursing department or university. The university may also charge a fee for managing a research account. Some funding agencies stipulate that a university must manage the account. In this event, it is important to add the appropriate on-costs (15–25%) for this purpose. This figure should be discussed with the university research office. In their application for funding, the NHMRC (*Guidelines for Funding in 2007*) stipulate six categories/levels of Personnel Support Packages (PSP): non-graduate personnel, junior graduate research assistant, experienced graduate research assistant, experienced postdoctoral researcher, senior experienced postdoctoral researcher, and senior researcher. Formats and salary scales do vary from one funding source to another and relevant information will be provided on each form. Figure 19.1 shows an example of an abbreviated budget justification form. A useful website is the NHMRC 'Budget Mechanism for Project Grant Funding' which provides information about personnel, costs, salary loading and so forth — hhtp://www.nhmrc.gov.au/funding/apply/granttype/projects/budget.htm.

The financial remuneration is designed to cover all salary and salary on-costs (e.g. workers compensation, payroll tax, leave loading), and some additional support for minor maintenance, such as phone/fax, stationery, computer hardware and software. On-costs can also vary between research assistants, administrative and technical staff and casual employees, from one institution to another, and should be added onto the basic salary. (See Higdon & Topp 2004 in 'Additional resources' at the end of this chapter.)

FIGURE 19.1 A sample of a budget justification form

	$
PERSONNEL	
Principal Researcher	
Research Assistant Level 3 to assist with data collection for 6 months	
Salary $3,000/mo × 6 months = $18,000 + benefits	
Salary total	18,000
Consultant for statistical analyses (20 hours @ $150 ph)	3,000
Personnel TOTAL	$21,000
SUPPLIES	
Photocopy (printing of questionnaires)	300
Telephone	50
Postage (400 questionnaires @ $1.50)	600
Equipment rental (computer)	supplied by Faculty
Supplies TOTAL	$950
TRAVEL	
Conference air travel interstate (Sydney)	320
Hotel accommodation ($195 × 3 nights)	585
Meals × 3 days ($45 per day)	135
Local travel (400 kms @ 65c p km)	260
Travel TOTAL	$1,300
TOTAL	$23,250
POTENTIAL ON-COSTS FOR MANAGING THE BUDGET	
(varies between agencies — at 20%) On-costs at 20% = $4,650	$4,650
TOTAL BUDGET	$27,900

References and appendices

References should be up to date and arranged in a standard format. This is most frequently the Harvard system (author–date system e.g. Smith and Barton 2007), or Vancouver system (numbered system e.g. a numeral appears in the text which represents the author/s details which appear in full in the reference list). Whichever format is used, consistency is the key element. This book uses the APA style of referencing, which is a variant of the author–date style. Increasingly, online resources will be used as references, and the reference format must also include the date the information was accessed, as well as the other bibliographic details (see 'Additional resources').

Appendices will include a participant information sheet and related consent form, as well as other documents, such as questionnaires or an interview schedule that will be used in the research.

Letters of support

Letters of support will be required from Department Heads and external funding agencies, to verify that the research is achievable and appropriate resources are available from the department/university and/or hospital. Letters of support may also be required by external organisations or universities should the nature of the research project warrant support from particular cultural groups. For example, in ethnographic studies there are levels of entry and access to participants that have to be negotiated with the assistance of power holders within the community/organisation or an intermediary, in order to acquire consent to settings, conduct observations, and interview people (Glesne & Peshkin 1992).

Points to ponder

Common errors in proposals:
- ► misreading guidelines and criteria
- ► weak motivation for doing the study
- ► unconvincing literature review
- ► poorly expressed and written proposal
- ► budget problems; for example, lack of detail, inaccurate costings
- ► failure to demonstrate the feasibility, practicality and applicability of the proposed study.

Submitting a proposal for review

With effective planning, a suitable timeframe for proposal development, informal review and refinement will enable the completed proposal to be submitted on time. As noted earlier, check the submission requirements, particularly the frequency of meetings, due dates for submission to the ethics office; and whether online, email attachment, or paper copies of the proposals are requested.

Online submissions

Most funding agencies and universities have their application forms and guidelines for submitting research proposals online. The guidelines provide step-by-step information to ensure that you address all the requirements. A discussion of the role of research review committees and ethics research committees follows.

Research committee review and human research ethics committee review

In some institutions there are two different committees who review research proposals, namely, a research committee and a human

research ethics committee (HREC). In the first instance, the proposal is reviewed by the research committee. If approved, the proposal is then submitted to the HREC. In some institutions both committee functions are incorporated in one committee.

The membership of university and hospital research committees is generally comprised of staff from the respective institutions. However, membership of HRECs and Animal Experimentation Ethics committees are specified by government bodies. For example, the Australian Health Ethics Committee (AHEC) has 15 members representing medical research, law, philosophy, religion, public health research, social science research, clinical medical practice, nursing or allied health practices and health consumer issues (see website http://www.nhmrc.gov.au/ethics/human/ahec/overview/index.htm).

Submitted proposals are reviewed by the relevant committee (e.g. hospital, scholarship board, university, funding organisation), and discussed at a committee meeting. In general, research and ethics committee meetings are planned a year in advance. Although not common, a researcher may be invited to speak about their proposal at the committee meeting. Regardless, a written reply is sent advising the outcome of the committee's review. The proposal may be approved, or clarification or additional information may be requested, modification or amendments may be required, or the proposal may be rejected.

Following rejection of a proposal, some funding agencies permit a re-submission to give the researcher an opportunity to answer their questions. A re-submitted proposal should be written as comprehensively and clearly as the original, with all questions and requirements answered. A comprehensive re-submission is important as committee members change and the re-submitted proposal may be reviewed by new reviewers.

Funding sources

Nurses and midwives in Australia and New Zealand seeking financial assistance to pursue academic interests and funding for research projects have a number of options.
- Scholarships (bursaries) for a higher degree and funding for nursing and midwifery research projects are offered

by most universities. The Australian and New Zealand governments provide funding at selected schools for, for example, the Rural and Remote Nurse Scholarship Program, Aboriginal and Torres Strait Islander Health Scholarship, and the Commonwealth Aged Care Nursing Scholarship. Most nursing scholarships are administered by the Royal College of Nursing Australia (RCNA) National Research and Scholarship Fund (NRSF).

- Public sector funding in Australia is through the NHMRC and the Australian Research Council (ARC). Applications for research grants are highly competitive. Nurses compete for funding with other health professionals.
- In New Zealand there are professional organisations (e.g. College of Nurses Scholarships, NZ College of Mental Health Nurses, Nursing Education & Research Foundation [NERF]) who offer financial support to nurses. All public (government) sector funding in New Zealand is through the Ministry of Research, Science and Technology (MORST); www.morst.govt.nz. The Health Research Council of New Zealand (HRC) offers career development opportunities to encourage health research (e.g. Māori Health Research Awards, Summer Studentships in Māori and Pacific Health). In addition, the Accident Compensation Corporation (ACC) offers scholarships for Masters, PhD and postdoctoral candidates for research in injury prevention. ACC specifies research priorities.
- Funding from external agencies; for example, Australian government grants and non-government organisations (see relevant section below).

The Australian government has identified the following research priorities to direct specific investigator-initiated projects:
- an environmentally sustainable Australia
- promoting and maintaining good health
- frontier technologies for building and transforming Australian industries
- safeguarding Australia.

While 'promoting and maintaining good health' directly fits with nursing and midwifery research, other priority areas may also be appropriate when describing the importance of specific research topics. For example, projects examining Severe Acute Respiratory Syndrome (SARS) or Avian Influenza fits with the priority 'safeguarding Australia'.

Australian Commonwealth grants

There are many Commonwealth schemes and foundations that offer funding for specific research areas. The National Health and Medical Research Council (NHMRC) provides the majority of funding in Australia for health and medical research, while the Australian Research Council (ARC) mostly supports other science and humanities research. Funding from both the NHMRC and the ARC is highly competitive, and historically nurses and midwives have not been very successful in applying for these research grants. Hundreds of applications from various health fields are submitted but, because funds are limited, there is a cut-off point and even excellent proposals may not get funded. In addition, applicants with track records are more favourably considered. Some difficulties nurses and midwives have competing relate to 'irrelevance and/or poor quality' projects (White 2005 p 368).

Non-government organisations schemes

There are hundreds of non-government organisation (NGO) grant schemes in Australia; for example, the Australian Cancer Research Foundation, Australian Rotary Health Research Fund, Kidney Health Australia, National Breast Council Foundation, and National Heart Foundation of Australia offer 'Grants-in-Aid' for research (biomedical and education/health promotion) from which funding may be obtained. Numerous charitable organisations in New Zealand offer funding; for example, Wellcome Trust, Cancer Society and Family Planning. Many non-government organisation schemes also have specific research priorities.

Summary

Research proposals may be written for a number of reasons; for example, undertaking a higher degree, applying for financial assistance to undertake a research project, complying with nursing degree course requirements, or applying to an ethics committee for approval to conduct a research project. Research ideas can come from the clinical or administrative areas, reading the literature and networking at conferences. Grants may be available from universities, government agencies and non-government agencies. Funding agencies' research priorities must be considered when applying for funding. Faculty research priorities, appropriate supervision and facilities are important when planning a project. Each ethics committee or funding body may have specific requirements regarding application forms and format. Proposals must adhere to the standards for research for the nursing profession, the code of ethics and the code of professional conduct for nurses.

(K)EY POINTS

- A research proposal provides a detailed and reasoned explanation of the research problem, the design, participant profile, exclusion/inclusion criteria, data analysis and data collection methods.

- A proposal may be written for a higher degrees committee, a department/faculty research committee, a human ethics research committee, a hospital research committee, or a funding agency.

- Students undertaking research involved in commercial enterprises must be aware of their rights and obligations in relation to intellectual property.

- Legally effective informed consent must be obtained from each participant in the research project.

Learning activities

1. A literature review of your topic should be conducted:
    (a) when you have time
    (b) after you have written your proposal
    (c) after you have sought permission from faculty to proceed
    (d) once you have identified your research problem/topic.

2. How will a literature review support your argument that your topic should be investigated?
    (a) Nothing has been written on your proposed topic.
    (b) The literature review will identify shortcomings and limitations in published research.
    (c) The literature review will help you identify a research problem.

    (d) It will convince the committee that you have been reading the literature.

3. What does operationalising objectives mean?
    (a) Translating objectives into measurable and observable phenomena.
    (b) Defining aims and objectives.
    (c) Identifies the feasibility and potential value of a study.
    (d) Helps to identify a research problem.

4. A pilot study is done because:
    (a) it's a compulsory requirement for a larger study
    (b) you have the time to do it
    (c) it tests the feasibility of doing a larger study
    (d) you don't have to write a proposal.

5. A plain language statement is written because:
   (a) no one on the committee knows anything about your topic
   (b) it provides the rationale and justification for undertaking the project
   (c) it is an ethical requirement
   (d) the committee doesn't understand the format of a proposal.

6. A well-written literature review:
   (a) uses mainly old and well-reviewed articles
   (b) uses very few relevant articles
   (c) demonstrates your knowledge of the research problem
   (d) demonstrates good writing skills.

7. Some procedures for protecting the rights of your participants are:
   (a) assuring them that you will protect their rights
   (b) a letter of explanation, informed consent, ethics approval for the study
   (c) being friendly and honest with them
   (d) telling them that you won't disclose any information about them.

8. The funding agency needs to be persuaded that you:
   (a) enjoy writing proposals
   (b) think research is an important academic activity
   (c) are qualified to carry out your research design
   (d) can spare the time to do the research.

9. Two key preliminary steps in writing a research proposal are:
   (a) spending a lot of time reading
   (b) attending conferences and talking to colleagues
   (c) operationalising objectives
   (d) identifying a feasible research question and finding a design that will answer the research question.

10. Committees usually make decisions about proposals on the basis of:
    (a) how long they take to read them
    (b) their purpose, clarity, logic, standard and appropriateness
    (c) how much they enjoyed reading them
    (d) how relevant the research problem is to the faculty's strategic research plan.

Additional resources

Australian Directory of Philanthropy Australia (2006) lists over 370 foundations and trusts with their contact details and funding preferences. Online. Available: http://www.philanthropy.org.au/publications/directory.htm

Australian Health Ethics Committee. Online. Available: http://www.ahmrc.gov.au/ethics/human/ahec/overview/index.htm

Australian Vice-Chancellors' Committee. Online. Available: http://www.avcc.edu.au

Funding agencies — lists can be accessed through Google: http://www.google.com.au/search?hl=en&q=Australian+Funding+Foundation&btnG=

Health Research Council of New Zealand. Online. Available: http://www.hrc.govt.nz/ethigud3.htm

Higdon J, Topp R 2004 How to develop a budget for a research proposal. *Western Journal of Nursing Research* 26(8):922–9

International Committee of Medical Journal Editors (ICMJE). Online. Available: http://www.icmje.org

Langley B C 2002 How to Write a Research Proposal. Featured Article. Online. Available: http://www.meaning.ca/articles/print/writing_research_proposal_may02.htm

Lusk S L 2004 Developing an outstanding grant application. *Western Journal of Nursing Research* 26(3):367–73

Ministry of Research, Science and Technology (MORST), New Zealand. Online. Available: www.morst.govt.nz

National Health and Medical Research Council (NHMRC) Budget mechanism for Project Grant funding. Online. Available: http://www.nhmrc.gov.au/funding/apply/granttype/projects/budget.htm

—— Statement on Human Experimentation. Online. Available: http://www.health.gov.au/nhmrc/ethics/humanexp/

Penrod J 2003 Getting funded: writing a successful qualitative small-project proposal. *Qualitative Health Research* 13(6):821–32

References

American Nurses Association 1985 *Guidelines for nurses in clinical and other research*. Kansas City, ANA

Australian Nursing Federation 1997 *Standards for Research for the Nursing Profession*. Australian Nursing Federation, Melbourne

Australian Research Council (ARC), Australian Tertiary Institutions Commercial Companies Association, Australian Vice-Chancellors' Committee, Department of Education, Training & Youth Affairs, The Department of Industry Science and Resources, IP Australia, The National Health and Medical Research Council 2001 *National principles of intellectual property management for publicly funded research*. Department of Industry, Science and Resources, Canberra

Australian Vice-Chancellors' Committee 2002 Ownership of intellectual property in universities: Policy and good practice guide. AVCC. Canberra. Online. Available: http://www.avcc.edu.au/ [accessed 26 July 2006]

Cohen M Z, Knafl K, Dzurec L C 1993 Grant writing for qualitative research. *Image: Journal of Nursing Scholarship* 25(2):151

Gitlin L N, Lyons K J 1996 *Successful grant writing. Strategies for health and human service professionals.* Springer Publishing, New York

Glesne C, Peshkin A 1992 *Becoming qualitative researchers: an introduction.* Longman, New York

Halfer D, Graf E 2006 Graduate Nurse Perceptions of the Work Experience. *Nursing Economics* 24(3):150–5

Hall M 1988 *Getting funded: a complete guide to proposal writing*, 3rd edn. Continuing Education Publications, Portland, Oregon

Halperin S A, Scherfele D, Duval B, et al. 2005 Conforming to ICMJE Principles. *Canadian Medical Association Journal* 173(11):1358–9

Higdon J, Topp R 2004 How to develop a budget for a research proposal. *Western Journal of Nursing Research* 26(8):922–9

Jamieson S 1999 Writing Research Proposals. Online. Available: http://www.users.drew/edu/-sjamieso/research_proposal.html [accessed 14 November 2005]

Jamison J R 2001 Maintaining Health in Primary Care. *Guidelines for Wellness in the 21st Century.* Churchill Livingstone, London

Langley B C 2002 How to Write a Research Proposal. Featured Article. Online. Available: http://www.meaning.ca/articles/print/writing_research_proposal_may02.htm [accessed 30 November 2006]

Langley G (ed.) 1989 *Animal experimentation: consensus changes.* MacMillan Press, London

National Health and Medical Research Council (NHMRC) 1992 Statement of human experimentation and supplementary notes. Canberra. Updated 29 June 2005. Online. Available: http://www.nhmrc.gov.au/funding/types/index.htm [accessed 14 November 2005]

—— 2002 *Research Ethics Handbook*. Online. Available: www.7.health.gov.au/nhmrc/publications/hrecbook/02-ethics/01.htm [accessed 19 April 2006]

—— 2004 *The Australian Code of Practice for the Care and Use of Animals for Scientific Purposes*, 7th edn. Published by the NHMRC in conjunction with CSIRO, the Australian Research Council and the Australian Vice-Chancellors' Committee, Canberra

Orb A, Eisenhauer L, Wynaden D 2001 Ethics in qualitative research. *Journal of Nursing Scholarship* 33(1):93–6

Pascoe T, Foley E, Hutchinson R, et al. 2005 The changing face of nurses in Australian general practice. *Australian Journal of Advanced Nursing* 23(1):44–7

Phillips E M, Pugh D S 1994 *How to get a PhD: a handbook for students and their supervisors*, 2nd edn. Open University Press, London

Singer P 1991 *Practical ethics*. Cambridge University Press, London

Snowdon J 1994 Breast cancer study monitored patients against their wishes. *Houston Chronicle*, A22, December 17

White E 2005 Strengthening the nursing research endeavour. *Journal of Research in Nursing* 10(4):365–8

Answers

TT Tutorial trigger 1

Aims and objectives serve different purposes and are important in a research study. The aims of a research study are usually broad and are a statement of purpose (the reasons why the study is being done). Objectives should be specific and describe the activities employed to achieve the aims. Both aims and objectives should be feasible and achievable and there should be congruency between them. For example, the aims of a study may be to investigate whether first year nurses in hospital X consume more food on day or night duty. The aim of the investigation might be to satisfy hospital administration, parents, and the nurses themselves that they are having an adequate diet on both shifts. An objective could be that nurses keep a diary and record their daily food intake for a specified time, say 2 weeks on night duty, and 2 weeks when they return to day duty. The charts they fill in could be divided into food categories and calories for easy measurement and manipulation. These data would yield important information regarding the eating habits of the nurses.

TT Tutorial trigger 2

A critical literature review:
- a critical literature review identifies the current knowledge about your research topic and places the proposed research in context
- convinces the reviewers of the importance and relevance of your research topic
- convinces reviewers that you are able to critically analyse and evaluate the research literature (e.g. methodological problems,

vague criteria, absence of definitions and assumptions, lack of standardised measures, identifying gaps, limitations, inconclusive findings, inappropriate design)
- assists with the conceptualisation of the research problem
- identifies research projects, conceptual frameworks and designs that you may want to replicate.

TT Tutorial trigger 3

Points to consider in a qualitative research design
- Is the design/approach appropriate to address the research question? How was this determination made? For example, the goal of a phenomenological approach is to develop an understanding of a phenomenon through the human lived experience of the particular phenomenon.
- The researcher's historical background of experience, understanding and knowledge must be made explicit. Researcher bias is acknowledged.
- Selection and recruitment of participants. Phenomenological research is an interactive involvement of both the researcher (interviewer) and participant (interviewee). Participants are chosen because they are experiencing the phenomenon of interest and are able to articulate their experience.
- Inclusion/exclusion criteria.
- Ethical considerations.
- Data collection strategies would include in-depth interviewing (focus groups), tape recorded interviews, transcription of recorded material.

- Analysis of the data is usually achieved by reading and re-reading in whole, and in parts, identifying structures of meaning and themes that illuminate the meaning of the experience. There is no standard method of text analysis. There are a number of ways to analyse the data, however, in the first instance, inductive analysis is used which leads to a narrative summary and synthesis of the information

Points to consider in a quantitative research design
- Is the design appropriate to address/answer the research question? How was this determination made?
- Description and recruitment of sample. Is the design congruent with how the sample is recruited? How was the sample determined? (e.g. experimental — address issues of randomisation, control and manipulation; quasi or non-experimental designs — concepts of control and levels).
- Inclusion/exclusion criteria.
- Ethical considerations.
- Interventions e.g. tests, medications, a learning program.
- Validation and reliability of instruments.
- Data collection: questionnaires, tests.
- Data analysis: parametric tests (alpha levels) or non-parametric tests — adequacy of sample size.

Learning activities
1. d	2. b	3. a	4. c
5. b	6. c	7. b	8. c
9. d	10. b		

Managing a
research project

LEANNE AITKEN AND DOUG ELLIOTT

Learning outcomes

After reading this chapter, you should be able to:

- understand the various roles and activities of research team members in managing a research project
- develop a participant recruitment and retention strategy for a planned study
- describe the challenges in ensuring adequate representation of minority sub-groups in relevant research
- outline strategies for effective planning and ongoing management of a research budget.

Introduction

Planning a research project commonly involves formulation of an idea, examination of other work in the area through a literature review, consultation with relevant stakeholders and development of a research proposal. The development of a research proposal, usually for ethics approval and/or funding purposes, was discussed in the previous chapter. A range of issues that are normally outlined in an ethics or grant application are also discussed in this chapter in terms of implementing the proposed study. This chapter also discusses research team, data and budget management, as well as study reporting requirements. While these issues focus on the actual conduct of a research project, the content is also relevant to research consumers in enabling a broader understanding of an entire research project. Many of the components described here are often only described in minimal detail in a research report or published article, but are important in maintaining study quality and integrity.

Implementing an approved study

Strategic planning and operational management of an approved project includes organising the research team, recruitment and retention of participants, data management and budget management (if applicable). These principles apply to all projects regardless of design and method, although the specific detail of each phase may vary. Factors that influence variations in project management include:

- the position or orientation of the researcher, reflected in the subsequent design and method
- size of the research team and resources available
- number of research sites and proposed number of participants
- length, frequency and type of data collected
- the timelines and budget available.

Several forms of approval are required prior to a study moving from planning into the implementation phase, including approval from local health service managers (which may be through a local research review committee) and ethics approval from the appropriate HREC(s). While proposals to these bodies highlight all aspects of the study procedure, further detail is actually required to implement each of the steps in a project on a daily basis. A number of research team planning meetings and documents may therefore be required to finalise a clear and explicit study procedure prior to implementation. Communication with study sites and clinical staff about the timelines and processes of involvement can include staff in-service sessions and summary documents outlining the upcoming study. If the study meets the criteria for a clinical trial, it may also be necessary to register it with a clinical trials register prior to commencing the study.

Trials registries

Recently, the World Health Organization recommended standards for the registration of all clinical trials (WHO 2006) that prospectively assign human subjects to intervention and comparison groups to study the cause-and-effect relationship between a clinical intervention and a health outcome. This supports an earlier initiative undertaken by the International Committee of Medical Journal Editors (ICMJE) to publish only those studies whose study protocols are registered on specific public-domain trials registers (e.g. the Australian Clinical Trials Register (ACTR); Clinical Trials — see 'Additional resources' at the end of this chapter). At present, the Health Research Council of New Zealand encourages that country's researchers to use the ACTR. The purpose of these registers is to provide open and public disclosure of study protocols — a trial's objectives, main design features, sample size and statistics, treatments under investigation, outcomes assessed, principal investigators, and contact details for specific trial information.

> ### Point to ponder
> ▶ Access the Australian Clinical Trials Registry (http://www.actr.org.au), and search for current trials in an area of your clinical interest.

Managing a research team

A research team can range from a single investigator through to a study with a number of chief investigators, associate investigators or other project staff, research students and research assistants. The number and type of team members are dependent on the study question/s and methods. The individual and collective skills set of the team, in terms of expertise and experience, need to address all the necessary components to effectively and efficiently complete the study (see Table 20.1). As noted in the previous chapter, the track record and experience of the investigators are usually assessed during the grant application review process.

Effective organisation for the project team is therefore essential to achieve consistent, co-ordinated progress of the study. Strategies include:

- comprehensive documentation of the purpose, aims and method of the study
- documentation of all processes related to the study in a format that is readily accessed by team members — for example, position descriptions, participant

TABLE 20.1 Roles of research team members

Role*	Description
Chief (Principal) Investigator/s (CI)	Lead/s the study; developed the proposal; provides strategic direction and operational support to team members; there may be a team of CIs, with one acting as the lead investigator.
Associate Investigator/s (AI)	Provides specialist expertise or experience in a specific aspect of the study (e.g. data analysis expert), or site/participant access (e.g. senior clinician).
Postdoctoral fellow/research student (PhD, Honours)	Training program, leading specific aspects of the study (under supervision).
Project Officer/ Research Assistant	Range of activities and level of appointment, depending on required skill set and available budget (e.g. project manager, data collection, entry and management).

* Terms vary.

recruitment and follow-up procedures, data management processes, HREC approvals and reporting requirements, other report requirements, team communication strategies and budget management

- monitoring processes that enable ongoing assessment of recruitment and retention targets in relation to project timelines
- organisation of relevant documents on a computer share drive that is accessible by relevant team members
- effective communication strategies with all team members.

Staff recruitment, team communications and meetings, and researcher safety if visiting participants' homes, are discussed below.

Recruiting project staff

While some studies require minimal external support, other studies, because of the question or scope of the investigation, require additional resources such as funded project staff or research assistants to successfully conduct the research. Unfunded or 'soft-funded' studies (use of general operating funds to minimally support some aspects of a project) rely on the chief investigators and perhaps other staff to conduct a study as part of their usual duties. This is common particularly for early exploratory or pilot work, where academic and clinical staff undertake primary research in preparation for institutional or external funding (see the previous chapter).

If study funding is available for additional personnel, the specific role, tasks, scope, timeframe and funding for the position are known (Kang et al. 2005). A position description is then constructed to address the required skill set for the role. For example, the role may require a particular level of academic qualification, a clinical background, experience in conducting in-depth interviews, or previous experience in co-ordinating multiple data collection sites. (Box 20.1 illustrates an example of selection criteria.)

Team communications

As noted earlier, effective team communication processes are essential for achieving a successful project outcome, by providing all study personnel with clear guidelines regarding their

BOX 20.1 **Example of selection criteria for a Research Assistant**

Selection criteria

Essential

1. Tertiary qualifications in a relevant health discipline.
2. Demonstrated effective interpersonal skills including excellent oral and written communication skills and ability to work effectively as part of a team.
3. Demonstrated ability to work independently.
4. High level computer literacy (both word processing and database management).
5. Demonstrated ability to produce high quality reports and publications.
6. Significant experience in the conduct and management of research projects.

Desirable

1. Experience in clinical research teams
2. Experience in qualitative data analysis.
3. Postgraduate qualifications in a relevant discipline or equivalent advanced professional experience.

role and others' expectations. Communication should use various forms and cater for planning the study implementation and strategic decision-making as well as daily problem-solving activities. Communication formats may include email, websites, phone, newsletters, regular (i.e. monthly) reports, site visits and meetings or teleconferences. While ad hoc communications can be initiated by any member of the research team, routine communication (e.g. newsletters, regular reports) are usually initiated by the project manager and forwarded to all team members.

Site visits are a particularly important feature of multi-site studies and should be conducted by the project manager and sometimes the principal investigator. Site visits are beneficial at multiple time points including:

- the beginning of the study — to ascertain adequacy of the facilities, determine additional resources required and provide site-team education
- during the study — to monitor ongoing activities and adherence to the study protocol

- on completion of the study — to wind up the study activities, provide feedback and thank the on-site study team for their involvement in the study; this provides positive closure of the project and facilitates clinical support for any future research.

Depending on the complexity of the study, site visits will be at least several hours duration or may extend to 1 to 2 days. Appropriate costing for site visits are incorporated into the study budget.

Point to ponder

▶ Given the rapid development of information technology, consider how some of the more recent modes of communication, such as web discussion lists and blogs, might be used to facilitate research team communication.

Team meetings

Team meetings should occur on a regular basis, with the frequency determined by the size and complexity of the study and the number of issues that require group consideration. Depending on the geographical distribution of study sites and team members, meetings might be conducted in either face-to-face, teleconference or videoconference mode. Where study sites are geographically distant, face-to-face meetings should be encouraged on as frequent a basis as possible. In general the purposes of team meetings include:

- monitoring the progress of the study, including participant recruitment, management and retention
- examining areas of progress that are proving problematic, including discussion of possible solutions
- discussion of the management and analysis of data
- monitoring of staff issues, including need for additional staff and leave coverage
- monitoring compliance with reporting commitments.

To ensure optimal benefit from team meetings, regular reports detailing study progression and problems should be circulated prior to the meeting to allow consideration of issues and solutions. It is also essential that team meetings are chaired effectively, and an accurate record of decisions made is circulated following the meeting to ensure all team members have an ongoing record. Note that any substantive changes to study protocol that are planned may require notification to the HREC.

> ● **Evidence-based practice tip**
> When all study team members understand the purpose and protocol of a study, are aware of progress and challenges, and feel valued in the conduct of the study, adherence to study protocol and timelines is likely to be optimised.

Researcher safety

If research staff are required to work away from the study site, particularly if the research includes visits to participants' homes for data collection such as interviews or to implement any study intervention, then a researcher safety protocol is necessary. The safety protocol considers the study activities in relation to a risk assessment of participants and their home environment (Paterson et al. 1999) so that any identified hazards or risks are minimised in a systematic process. In particular the safety protocol should consider any insult or injury that could occur to the researcher and outline any strategies to minimise, prevent or respond to that risk.

A randomised controlled trial (RCT) of a home-based physical rehabilitation for survivors of a critical illness required assessors and trainers to visit participants in their homes. A researcher safety protocol was included in the HREC application, noting the following points:

1. a list of visits is held by the responsible investigator for each recruitment site with the participant's address, date, time and approximate duration of each visit
2. the assessor/trainer carry a mobile phone for researcher contact back at the study site
3. the assessor/trainer sends a text message to the investigator prior to entering the home and when the visit is complete
4. if no contact is made, the investigator phones the assessor/trainer, then the participant's home phone (if connected) (Elliott et al. 2006 p 4).

In the above example the greatest risk to the trainers and assessors was considered to be in the form of physical assault by participants or other individuals in the home. A system to ensure another member of the research team always knew when a trainer/assessor was in a participant's home was therefore established. In this way, if the trainer/assessor did not leave the participant's home as planned, timely action to contact the trainer/assessor, or in the worst case scenario to contact police support, can be undertaken.

Managing participant involvement

Recruitment and retention of sufficient participants with the relevant characteristics to meet the objectives of the study is essential to the success of the study. This section discusses participant recruitment (sampling, identifying and approaching potential participants, randomisation and blinding), strategies to optimise recruitment, and participant retention and follow-up.

Participant recruitment

An effective recruitment strategy is dependent on careful planning and development, considering the population of interest, the numbers likely to be accessed and the possible barriers to accessing or obtaining consent from potential participants. Potential participants may be involved in other current studies within the local study site. Research overload of specific groups of participants is therefore a potential problem that can be identified through discussions with other researchers in the same field, highlighted by local clinical areas or ethics committees, or searches of appropriate clinical trials registries.

For many projects, recruitment represents one of the largest components of work. Both the recruitment process and the subsequent retention of participants must be clearly documented during data management. For qualitative studies, the focus is on achieving an information-rich sample of participants. For quantitative studies, information relates to how many participants were approached for inclusion, how many were actually enrolled, how many participants were included at each of the follow-up points, and how many participants were allocated to different study groups (if appropriate). While the principles for reporting these details are the same for most study designs, the requirements for randomised trials are clearly articulated in the CONSORT statement guidelines (Altman et al. 2001). (See 'Additional resources' at the end of this chapter, and further discussion in the subsection on randomisation below.)

Sampling issues

The issues related to achieving data saturation (for qualitative studies) or adequate power to answer the question (for quantitative studies), have been discussed previously in Chapters 8 and 11, respectively. The specific implications of inadequate or inappropriate sampling vary depending on the research method but generally result in questions remaining regarding detail, depth or variations in data, or a lack of clarity as to whether a statistically insignificant result is due to absence of effect or insufficient participant numbers to detect a difference (type II error for quantitative studies). All studies, regardless of resources or budget, require planning to enable an appropriate sample of participants necessary to answer the question. It is also important to ensure that the sample size is not so large that it incorporates more participants than required, therefore wasting valuable resources including the time and effort of potential research participants.

In quantitative studies investigating the impact of a treatment the required sample size is dependent on several factors including the size of the effect produced by the intervention, the size of the outcome measurement and associated standard deviation, the desired power and the significance level of the study. As noted in earlier chapters, effect size refers to the extent of change that occurs as a result of the intervention. For example a new dressing product may result in a 2% reduction in wound infections from 7% to 5% during pilot studies. This is considered a small effect and would therefore require a large number of participants to demonstrate a significant difference in a future study. In contrast, the use of patient controlled analgesia by patients with chest trauma might result in a reduction in the incidence of inadequate pain relief from 40% to 20% of patients. This is a moderate to large effect and therefore requires less

participants to demonstrate a significant difference in future studies.

Sampling with minority groups

Recruitment of relevant minority groups is an important consideration, particularly when a study seeks to reflect the reality of a clinical population. Depending on the research question, it may be appropriate to ensure appropriate sampling for gender, age, ethnic, cultural, socioeconomic or other minority groups. While women are not minority in population terms, they have traditionally been under-represented in many studies (Wenger 1992). The principles of minority recruitment are therefore often applied to ensure an appropriate gender balance (HREC application forms request information about proposed gender balance).

Studies using questionnaires or interviews often require potential participants to have suitable English-language skills, particularly because of the need for ensuring appropriate informed consent, and the additional time and costs associated with involving culturally and linguistically diverse (CALD) populations (Ballard et al. 1993; Buist & Greenlick 1995; Adams et al. 1997). The ethical issues related to working with CALD populations have been previously described in Chapters 6 and 19. Specific strategies may be necessary to access a cultural or community group (e.g. consultation with a representative of the group, contact with professionals who work with minority groups, advertising in specific community newspapers or locations). The important aspects from a project management perspective are in relation to culturally appropriate contact with the community for approval, followed by participant engagement and empowerment within the study context.

Recruitment of participants with multiple minority characteristics (e.g. older people from a specific ethnic group), is even more challenging. Although there are no specific guidelines regarding minority representation in research samples in Australian or New Zealand settings, it is encouraged in both the National Statement on Ethical Conduct in Research Involving Humans (National Health and Medical Research Council (NHMRC) 1999) and the *Guidelines on Ethics in Health Research* (Health Research Council (HRC) 2002).

Research in brief

A study examined nutrition and physical activities of 3275 New Zealand school children from different cultural backgrounds — Māori, Pacific and European. The Māori and Pacific communities had representatives as principal investigators, advisory board members, and fieldwork researchers. Fieldworkers were trained in Māori and Pacific cultural considerations (Utter et al. 2006 p 51). The study noted that children from Māori and Pacific cultures were more physically active than children from a European background, but were more likely to skip meals or consume foods with high fat or sugar.

Where there is preliminary evidence, or physiological or cultural rationale, that minority sub-groups might experience different outcomes to the general population, recruitment should target relevant minority sub-groups using a stratified sampling approach (Bolen et al. 2006). For example, if you were investigating the adequacy and relevance of services to assist people being managed in the community with dementia, it is likely that ethnic sub-groups may have greater difficulty finding services that were linguistically and culturally sensitive. It may therefore be appropriate to incorporate different ethnic groups in the study sample. Depending on the characteristics of the minority sub-groups, appropriate representation may not be possible with recruitment from one venue only, and researchers may need to develop a multi-site collaboration to achieve the desired representation.

Identification of potential participants

Potential participants can be identified using different methods, depending on the type of study, the specialised nature of the potential participants and the number in both the desired sample and the entire population. Two broad types of participants are usually sought in healthcare research — individuals who have (or the potential to develop) a specific healthcare condition or have accessed a healthcare or community service, and healthy members of the population (including those who may participate as control participants). Participants may also include healthcare staff or other individuals of research interest. Potential participants can be identified through:

- contact with healthcare (e.g. GPs, outpatient clinics, pharmacies), or community services
- the local environment — advertising in council buildings, shopping centres, religious buildings, support groups
- public documents — telephone books or electoral rolls
- publications — local or national newspapers, newsletters, magazines or websites (Eysenbach & Wyatt 2002)
- media — radio and television (Smith & Coyle 2006).

Use of local print publications or electronic media can be through paid advertising or invited commentary in response to press releases (Smith & Coyle 2006). Commentary has the benefit of raising the profile of the health research issue and community awareness of the study, resulting in inquiries and recruitment. In order for recruitment strategies to be effective there is a need for sufficient response capability including free-call phone numbers and rapid replies to potential participants. Where the support of healthcare personnel is sought for recruitment, it is essential that appropriate information regarding the study is supplied. This may be in the form of educational sessions and written material, as well as regular newsletters to ensure awareness of the study remains high.

With voluntary methods of patient identification (e.g. asking participants to reply via telephone or email), the likely non-representative nature of these respondents, sometimes referred to as the 'volunteer effect' (Eysenbach & Wyatt 2002) should be considered. This 'selection bias' occurs when participants who respond to recruitment requests have different psychosocial characteristics or attitudes from those who choose not to respond.

Approaching and enrolling potential participants

The recruitment process used should consider the likelihood of success through using each of the recruitment strategies, and the cost of each alternative, in terms of both time and resources. Any ethical implications associated with each of the potential recruitment strategies must also be considered (see Chapter 6). Each strategy has associated advantages and disadvantages which suit different types of studies and populations (see Table 20.2).

Random allocation of participants

As noted in earlier chapters, randomisation is the allocation of participants to an intervention or control group in a study, either at the individual or group (cluster randomisation) level (Watson et al. 2004). The principle of 'random sampling' is to ensure that every member of an identified population has an equal chance of being selected for the study. Randomisation ('random allocation') is about ensuring that each participant has an equal chance of being allocated to a control or intervention group. This process minimises potential differences or biases between study groups.

TABLE 20.2 Recruitment strategies

Method	Description	Advantages	Disadvantages
Invitation letters	Mailed to potential participants outlining proposed research and providing contact details for more information.	• Inexpensive. • Easy contact with large numbers. • Allows participants time to think about participation. • Able to target specific sub-groups.	• Requires access to contact details. • Impersonal. • Low participation rate. • Requires participants to actively contact researchers.
Telephone contact	Contact made with all potential participants, outlining proposed research and requesting involvement.	• Provides forum to correct apprehension or misunderstandings regarding research. • Able to target specific sub-groups of sample.	• Requires access to contact details. • Time-consuming. • Many people not at home when call is made. • Relatively impersonal. • Participants might feel pressured to agree to research. • Many other unsolicited callers; therefore, calls may be screened.
Direct approach	Clinical or research staff approach potential participants directly during a healthcare episode.	• Increased ratio of screened participants agree to participate. • Provides opportunity to explain study, and answer questions. • Able to target specific sub-groups. • Able to increase or decrease rate of recruitment as needed (Smith & Coyle 2006).	• Can be too confronting for some potential participants. • Very time-consuming • Immediate concerns about current healthcare episode might be preoccupying.
Poster or newspaper advertising	Display posters or advertisements in locations likely to be visited or accessed by potential participants (e.g. clinics, newspapers, internet).	• Inexpensive for some sites. • Easy contact with relatively large numbers. • Allows potential participants to make the first contact if interested.	• Low participation rate. • Requires participant to actively contact researchers. • Impersonal. • Can be expensive for a newspaper/commercial internet site. • Reduced control of sub-group composition of sample.

(Source: adapted from Aitken L, Gallagher R, Madronio C 2003 Principles of recruitment and retention in clinical trials. *International Journal of Nursing Practice* 9:342; used with permission)

As demonstrated by Middleton et al. (2005) in their investigation of the effect of a nursing intervention after carotid endarterectomy, the effect of randomisation, in terms of known patient characteristics, should be checked prior to analysis to identify any differences between the groups (see Middleton et al. 2005, Table 2, p 256). Similarly, a study of a midwife-led counselling intervention for women self-identified as suffering a traumatic birth, compared the characteristics of the control (n = 53) and intervention (n = 50) groups. The two groups were found to be not significantly different for age group, marital status, ethnicity, education level and type of birth, except for emergency caesarean section (23% vs 40%) (Gamble et al. 2005).

Central randomisation, carried out by an independent person located away from the study site, with the group allocation communicated via either telephone or internet as required, is considered the most effective and rigorous due to the integrity of allocation concealment. Essential requirements for random allocation include:

- allocation concealment — the group allocation of the next participant must not be able to be identified (or guessed) prior to their enrolment (e.g. if group allocation is based on the days of the week, it will be clear which group a participant will be allocated to, depending on the day they are enrolled in the study)
- timing — randomisation should occur as close as possible in time to when the intervention commences, to reduce the occurrence of drop-out or cross-over between groups.

● Evidence-based practice tip

Allocation concealment is always possible in randomised studies, and should always be incorporated into a study protocol to reduce the potential bias of results.

In its simplest form, random allocation can be achieved through tossing a coin. Allocation to either group based on heads or tails is a chance event that is not related to the characteristics of the study participant. While a coin toss is simple to implement, 'chance' may result in uneven numbers in the study groups. In studies with large participant numbers and/or multiple recruitment sites, computer-generated randomisation methods

are used. 'Block randomisation' minimises the risk of uneven numbers with simple randomisation, by randomising participants in blocks of 4, 6 or 8 etc, ensuring that at the end of each block numbers are equal in each group; this is often referred to as 'permuted blocks' (Middleton et al. 2005). However, the use of one predetermined block size allows a 'guess' as to which group the last participants in each block will be allocated to; uneven block sizes are therefore frequently used.

If there is potential for an outcome to be influenced by characteristics of a sub-group (e.g. gender, age or ethnic group), then 'stratified randomisation' can be performed within each of those sub-groups or strata. This approach does increase complexity of the randomisations, and more participants are required to ensure adequate power within each stratum. Occasionally there may be justification for using 'unequal randomisation' (i.e. a ratio other than 1:1 in each of the study groups). This strategy is recommended in some settings based on cost, learning or ethical considerations, and does not have a major impact on the power of the study for ratios of 1:2 or 1:3 (Dumville et al. 2006). This approach increases the overall power of a study by:

- enrolling more participants in the control group when there is only limited funding for the most expensive (usually new treatment) arm of the study
- increasing the numbers in the control group and reducing the number of participants in the intervention group because of potential hazards associated with the new treatment
- enrolling more participants in the intervention group when there is a 'learning effect' associated with the intervention.

Blinding

An intervention study can conceal the study group allocation from participants and personnel involved in delivering the intervention and measuring the outcomes of the study. This feature is referred to as 'blinding'; not being able to 'see' the type of intervention that is delivered reduces potential bias. Blinding the investigators or outcome assessors reduces the likelihood that they will differentially measure the outcomes based on any predetermined attitude about whether they perceive the study intervention to be beneficial or not (Schulz & Grimes 2002). The purpose of blinding the study participants is to reduce the likelihood that they will report differential effects of the intervention if they are aware of receiving the study or control intervention. Blinding of either the investigators/outcome assessors or the participants is referred to as 'single blinding', while blinding of both the investigators/outcome assessors and the participants is referred to as 'double blinding'.

> ● **Evidence-based practice tip**
>
> Blinding of participants as well as investigators/ outcome assessors increases the likelihood that study findings are a true reflection of the impact of the intervention.

It is common to be able to achieve double blinding in pharmaceutical trials where the study medication and the non-active 'placebo' are not distinguishable. In contrast, behavioural studies may only be able to achieve single blinding as it is not possible to blind the participants from their intervention. It may however still be possible to ensure blinded outcome assessment. Every effort should be made to ensure at least single blinding in the study design where an intervention and outcome assessment is involved.

Research in brief

A bi-national multi-site RCT compared 4% albumin and 0.9% saline during fluid resuscitation of 6997 critically ill individuals, using 28-day mortality as the primary end-point. As the two fluids are easily identifiable by colour, 'double blinding' (of clinicians and patients) was ensured by supplying the study fluids in identical 500 mL bottles, and the use of specially designed masking cartons and intravenous administration sets (Finfer et al. 2004 p 2248). This study demonstrated that the number of deaths was equivalent between the two groups (relative risk 0.99, 95% confidence interval 0.91 – 1.09, p = 0.87).

Strategies to optimise recruitment

One aim for recruitment is to minimise the burden on participants. Despite extensive planning of a recruitment strategy, there will always remain a number of barriers that prevent otherwise eligible participants from enrolling. These barriers relate to the research site, the need for a participant to travel to the research site, sufficient and flexible time for research commitments or other miscellaneous issues such as caring responsibilities (Aitken et al. 2003). For example, an elderly lady with heart disease wanted to participate in a study about experiences of being diagnosed with heart disease later in life, but did not feel able to leave her dependent elderly husband at home by himself for 3 hours. Participation in the study required some investigations which had to be conducted within a healthcare facility.

If possible, the research team could visit a participant in their own home or in a local community venue that is easily accessible. While advantageous for recruitment and retention, the associated issues of entering a participant's home with safety, the potential for influence from other family members, and the increased travel time and costs for the research need to be considered. Challenges associated with conducting the study in community venues, such as hire costs, access to telephone, computing and operational support, also need to be examined. Flexibility in the times for interaction with participants may be necessary to facilitate study participation, by offering after hours and weekend times for data collection to work around participants' other commitments, such as caring for family members or work and study requirements.

Other challenges in recruitment include language barriers, over-exposure of potential participants to multiple study teams and the requirements and associated stress of current healthcare. Working with culturally and linguistically diverse (CALD) communities may include language translation, but cost and time requirements are usually significant. The problems associated with multiple study teams approaching patients require co-ordination between research personnel, as well as consideration by ethics committees who are aware of all research being undertaken in the local environment. Populations that tend to have multiple study teams approach them include those with chronic disease — for example, cardiac disease — and those with health problems that are perceived by the community as worthy of significant research funding contribution — for example, cancer patients. Similarly, competing interests between healthcare and research requires co-ordination and communication between the personnel involved, with recognition of the relevant priorities. Where recruitment for a study is required within a short period of time after a significant health event — for example, after cardiac surgery or intensive care admission — the feasibility and associated processes must be considered during planning.

TT Tutorial trigger 1

Develop a recruitment strategy for a study conducted within your area of practice to answer a question of interest. Consider the inclusion and exclusion criteria you would use and the recruitment strategies that would enable you to enrol the appropriate participants.

Participant retention and follow-up

Participant retention and follow-up must be effectively managed to maximise the benefit of efficient recruitment processes (Hanson 2006; Robiner 2005). Appropriate levels of retention will depend on the participant–researcher relationship, type of commitment required from participants, as well as the study timeframe. Longitudinal studies in particular, whether qualitative or quantitative, require effective ongoing engagement with participants. In some cases, a referral process may be required when a researcher identifies some potential risk for a participant in terms of physical, psychological or cultural safety. This risk may be related to their health status unrelated to the study, or related to a study intervention. Commonly, these potential events are addressed in an ethics proposal, but the actual process of referral needs to be documented and implemented as part of the project's management.

'Loss to follow-up' (also called 'study mortality') is when participants withdraw from a study for a range of reasons, obviously including illness or death. Withdrawal also occurs because participants have difficulty accommodating study commitments due to

work and lack of time, frequent or inflexible study appointments, and complicated and cumbersome treatment or record-keeping requirements (Sprague et al. 2003; Strusberg et al. 2005). A variety of strategies can be used during the trial design, recruitment and follow-up to effectively track participants and limit loss to follow-up (Aitken et al. 2003; Robiner 2005; Sprague et al. 2003) (see Table 20.3). The principles underlying effective tracking of participants include frequent and multiple different methods of contact.

While there are no specific levels at which retention is considered appropriate for quantitative studies, low retention levels (below approximately 80%) have the potential to cause bias in the study results if the participants who are lost to follow-up are systematically different from those who are retained in the study. In studies with multiple groups this problem is further exacerbated if there is a differential loss to follow-up rate in each of the study groups (Robiner 2005; Sprague et al. 2003).

TT Tutorial trigger 2

In a study currently being conducted approximately one-third of participants have been enrolled with a 30% loss to follow-up in the 6-month duration of the study. Consider some strategies that might be implemented to reduce subsequent loss to follow-up.

Regardless of the level of loss to follow-up in a study, it is essential that it is reported accurately and in detail in subsequent reports and publications (Dumville et al. 2006). Where appropriate this should be according to the CONSORT statement guidelines (Altman et al. 2001), using a flow diagram of study participation. See page 289 for an example of an RCT of a nurse-co-ordinated care intervention following carotid artery surgery (Middleton et al. 2005). Comparison of the baseline characteristics of those who completed the study compared to those who did not complete the study enables assessment for potential bias.

Managing the data

As noted earlier, while an ethics proposal outlines the study outcomes, data collection process and data analysis techniques, more details are required to operationalise the entire data management process (Brandt et al.

TABLE 20.3 Mechanisms to track study participants and reduce loss to follow-up

Mechanism	Comments
Minimising loss to follow-up	
Clearly describe study and associated burden	Explicit requirements and burden enable potential participants to make an informed decision whether to commit to the study.
Free-call number	Provide study participants with details of a contact point, preferably a free-call number, and ask that they contact the researchers if their residential/contact details change.
Multiple contact names and numbers of friends/relatives should be recorded	Subject to ethics approval, names and contact details of one or more friends or relatives can be gained from a participant on enrolment in the study. These contacts can be used when a participant is not able to be located using their initial contact details.
Obtain contact details for general practitioner (GP)	Participants may relocate within the same general location and continue to visit the same GP; participants could be located this way. GPs will not normally provide the new contact details directly, but can contact a participant on the researcher's behalf.
Ensure frequent follow-up	Frequent follow-up, preferably by phone or in person in addition to post, will remind the participant of the study, enable collection of details regarding address changes and remind the participant of the value of study involvement.
Provision of study newsletter	Providing participants with regular (e.g. 6 monthly) study newsletters provides information about the progress of the study, as well as the value of their involvement.
Facilitate follow-up commitments	Ensure flexibility in follow-up visits or telephone calls, provide multiple methods of completing study questionnaires (e.g. completing and returning in reply paid envelope or via telephone), reimburse study participants for time.
Follow-up processes	Ensure effective processes for identifying timely follow-up so that participant contact is not missed or overdue.
Locating participants considered lost to follow-up	
Registries of Births, Deaths and Marriages	Different registries have different guidelines for data access, but death registers are frequently able to be searched (after providing appropriate ethics approval and signed consent forms), a fee is sometimes required. Note that deaths are only registered in the jurisdiction where the death occurs, therefore knowledge of location or searching of multiple registries may be necessary to locate a study participant.
Electoral roll	The Australian Electoral Roll is available for viewing in electronic format at any of the Australian Electoral Commission offices. Note that not all people are registered with the Electoral Commission, and some are registered in a confidential manner. Also, address changes may not be supplied in a timely manner by many voters.
Electronic telephone books	Many telephone books are able to be searched via the internet, although this may present multiple people with the same name, particularly where a suburb of residence is not known.
Monitor admissions to clinical units	Where the study participants are patients of a specific clinical unit, establish a mechanism to monitor for re-admissions of study participants.

2006). Data collection and data analysis approaches for both qualitative and quantitative designs were discussed previously in relevant chapters. Detailed data monitoring and reporting are particularly important when there is a potential risk to study participants. This may occur when there is possibility of psychological or social risk or harm when a qualitative researcher is asking participants to recount possibly painful experiences or a field investigator is forming close personal relationships within the context of an ethnographic investigation. Similarly, the introduction of an intervention in a quantitative study may have potential risks for participants. The focus of this section is on broad operational issues, such as data storage, monitoring and auditing.

Data collection and storage

Confidential and secure storage of data is a requirement of HREC approval, as outlined by the NHMRC (see Chapter 6). As data materials can include files, audiotapes, questionnaires, videotapes or photographs, arrangements for appropriate secure storage is important. The ethics proposal will have addressed questions regarding confidentiality, storage and disposal of data, similar to those listed in Table 20.4, and procedures to reflect those statements are developed to guide all research team members.

Development of a database specific to the study requires planning, construction and testing prior to actual data entry (Brandt et al. 2006). The database can be developed using numerous software applications such as a spreadsheet, relational database, qualitative analysis or statistical analysis program. All necessary data fields need to be identified, including their form (text or numerical) and definition of any numerical codes (e.g. 1 = female, 2 = male). Ensure that copies of de-identified data are regularly backed up and stored in a separate secure location, such as a password-protected removable hard disc drive or flash drive, or your organisation's server.

Monitoring data collection

Effective management of data collected from a participant includes processes to guide accurate data entry, description of any transformations to enable data analysis, and auditing activities to ensure the quality of the data. These activities are guided by the study design and analytical approaches. Specific activities to verify the accuracy of data can include double data entry, quality checks of data entry and random data audits (Brandt et al. 2006). Regardless of the approach, a reader should be able to identify the transparency of activities used to monitor data collection and management in a confidential, ethical and rigorous manner.

Data monitoring and safety committee

For intervention studies, an independent data monitoring committee (DMC), comprising relevant experts in clinical trials, biostatistics, and the clinical specialty may be established (DAMOCLES Study Group 2005). The committee is a prospective strategy used to assess the risks and progress of a current study (Slimmer & Andersen 2004). The committee reviews unblinded data on patient characteristics, treatment compliance and study outcomes at regular intervals during the study to ensure compliance with the study protocol and that reported trial data are accurate, complete and verifiable from the source documents (DAMOCLES Study Group 2005). A DMC can also recommend the cessation of clinical trials early, particularly if serious adverse events are identified in one or both groups (Grant 2004), as may occur in drug trials.

TABLE 20.4 Data storage

Sample HREC proposal questions	Sample responses
How will the confidentiality of data (including the identity of participants) be ensured?	Participant's personal details will be kept confidential; and questionnaires will be coded with a study number. Personal details will be stored separately from study numbers and accessible only to researchers responsible for data collection. Data sheets/files will not contain any information capable of identifying an individual participant and will be stored in a locked cabinet in a locked office of the chief investigator.
How and where will data be stored, and who will have access to the data?	Hard copies of the questionnaires and computer discs containing electronic data will be stored in a locked filing cabinet in the chief investigator's office. Electronic data will be stored on a computer hard drive that is password protected.
How long will data be retained for, and how will they be disposed of?	Data will be retained for a minimum of 7 years after the study, after which hard copies of the data will be shredded and disposed. Electronic copies will be deleted from hard discs and backup copies on CD will be destroyed.

Managing the budget

Budgets to support research projects are generally limited in their capacity and are provided for specific but not all related activities. The previous chapter described the development of a grant application, including specific details related to project staff, study consumables and/ or equipment. When developing the plan for the study a detailed budget should be constructed and reviewed by an appropriate budget manager within the organisation. Components such as staff on-costs (usually approximately 25%) and research overheads charged by most universities (possibly 20–60%) need to be identified as they can account for significant proportions of a study budget. The research team manages the budget in relation to:

- the amount of funds available, including payment of instalments from the funding body
- the timeframe available for expenditure and whether mechanisms are available to roll funding over to another budget period
- the level of discretion available in spending the actual budget compared to the details specified in the grant application (e.g. can funding for staff salaries be expended on other study components such as consumables?)
- the level and frequency of budget reporting required by the funding organisation.

Budget items can include staff salaries, equipment purchases, computing hardware and software, travel costs, office supplies and printing, telephone and mail costs, fees to use any of the study material such as questionnaires, participant reimbursement costs, insurance costs, and consultancy fees for specialist advice such as a statistician. Where funding is provided in an international currency, senior level budget advice for the study contracts should be sought to safeguard against any dramatic currency shifts.

Throughout the duration of the study, mechanisms for effective budget management include:

- regular updates of budget projections as activities or costs change
- regular (e.g. monthly) monitoring of income and expenditure in relation to the planned budget

- discussion of variations in the budget with study team members
- realistic costing of proposed changes prior to implementation of any change.

In general, research funding agencies do not require intricate detail regarding budgetary processes, so long as the aim of the research is achieved and no further funding is required. Modest re-allocations of budget from one item within the study to another item, in order to more effectively carry out the study, are usually acceptable. If in doubt, check with the funding source.

Reporting requirements

Both HRECs and funding bodies require regular progress reports for the duration of the study (usually every 6 or 12 months), and further instalments of funding and continued approval may be contingent on satisfactory progress. These reports vary slightly depending on the recipient of the report, but should include an indication of progress to date, including a comment on any differences when compared to planned progression, challenges that have been encountered and how these have been overcome, a summary of any ethical issues that have arisen (individual adverse events will have been previously reported to the HREC) and a summary of the budgetary status of the study. A final more detailed report is required at the completion of the project.

Completing the study

At certain times in the project, participant recruitment and data collection will be complete, and the study activities focus more on data analysis and interpretation. At this time, the research team can consider feedback to both the study participants and the study site personnel. As participants complete their individual commitments to the study, researchers can provide a letter of appreciation and/or individual study results, noting the timeframe for the final results to be available. Progress reports and the final results for the study can also be presented to the clinical staff involved in the study, particularly in relation to translation of research evidence into clinical practice (see Chapter 18).

While completing the final reports for HRECs and funding bodies is a requirement for approval and funding, there is also an expectation that the study findings will be presented at professional conferences and submitted for publication, providing wide dissemination of the work. The following final chapter discusses the dissemination of primary research.

Summary

Managing a research project is a complex set of activities, requiring detailed planning and an eye for detail during implementation, monitoring and evaluation. Transparent decision-making processes and effective communication strategies are necessary for all team members, study participants, and other clinical or professional staff.

K EY POINTS

- A research team is developed so that the necessary skills set, expertise and experience are available to address all the requirements of a study.
- Recruitment and retention plans require detailed planning, discussion and evaluation to ensure optimal study participation.

- Recruitment of specific sub-groups of a sample may require specific strategies.
- Managing a budget requires informed and accurate estimates of likely expenses, accurate and detailed record-keeping, frequent review of actual costs compared to budget predictions, and effective communication with all team members.

Learning activities

1. Adequate sample size for an interventional study is based on:
   (a) effect size of the intervention
   (b) size and standard deviation of outcome measurement
   (c) desired power and significance of study
   (d) all of the above.

2. Which of the following is NOT a strategy to achieve effective organisation of a research team:
   (a) documentation and communication of the purpose, aims and method of the study
   (b) provision of a newsletter to past participants of the study
   (c) monitoring of processes and associated targets of recruitment and retention
   (d) regular communication with all members of the research team.

3. Site visits are beneficial to ensure:
   i. the site facilities and personnel are sufficient and able to conduct the study

   ii. the research team is thanked for their efforts by the study site staff
   iii. the study protocol is being adhered to.
   (a) i and ii
   (b) i and iii
   (c) ii and iii
   (d) i, ii and iii.

4. Which of the following is NOT considered when planning a recruitment strategy:
   (a) should minority representation be incorporated into the study
   (b) are there any language requirements, for example English literacy, necessary for study participants
   (c) designing a researcher safety protocol
   (d) the likely number of study participants who will meet the enrolment criteria.

5. Team meetings are used to address:
   i. monitoring participant recruitment, management and retention, and management and analysis of data
   ii. examining areas of the study progress that are proving problematic
   iii. monitoring of staff issues, including need for additional staff and leave coverage
   iv. monitoring compliance with reporting commitments.
   (a) i, ii and iii
   (b) i, ii and iv
   (c) ii, iii and iv
   (d) i, ii, iii and iv.

6. The role of an associate investigator in a research team is to provide:
   (a) strategic direction and operational support
   (b) specialist expertise or experience
   (c) input into specific aspects of a study as part of a training program
   (d) study site project management.

7. The advantages of the direct approach for participant recruitment do not include:
   (a) providing a forum to correct misunderstandings regarding the study
   (b) able to target specific sub-groups
   (c) being inexpensive and time-efficient
   (d) being able to increase or decrease the rate of recruitment as needed.

8. The disadvantages of telephone contact for participant recruitment do not include:
   (a) time-consuming
   (b) requires participants to contact researchers
   (c) many people not at home when a call is made
   (d) many other unsolicited callers; therefore, calls may be screened.

9. Allocation concealment:
   (a) is where group allocation for the next participant cannot be identified prior to enrolment
   (b) is the allocation of participants to an intervention or control group by the research team
   (c) enables every member of an identified population to have an equal chance of being selected in the study
   (d) ensures that each participant has an equal chance of being allocated to a control or intervention group.

10. Reasons for study 'loss to follow-up' include:
    i. study mortality
    ii. death
    iii. relocation without providing a forwarding address
    iv. continuing respondent burden.
    (a) i, ii and iii
    (b) i, ii and iv
    (c) ii, iii and iv
    (d) i, ii, iii and iv.

Additional resources

Australian Clinical Trials Register. A resource of the NHMRC Clinical Trials Centre. Online. Available: http://www.actr.org.au

Clinical Trials. A service of the U.S. National Institutes of Health. Online. Available: http://www.clinicaltrials.gov

CONSORT (Consolidated Standards of Reporting Trials) Statement. Online. Available: http://www.consort-statement.org/

Contemporary Clinical Trials (formerly *Controlled Clinical Trials*). A journal publishing papers on design, methods and operational aspects of clinical trials

International Committee of Medical Journal Editors (ICMJE). Online. Available: http://www.icmje.org

References

Adams J, Silverman M, Musa D, et al. 1997 Recruiting older adults for clinical trials. *Controlled Clinical Trials* 18:14–26

Aitken L, Gallagher R, Madronio C 2003 Principles of recruitment and retention in clinical trials. *International Journal of Nursing Practice* 9:338–46

Altman D G, Schulz K F, Moher D, et al. 2001 The revised CONSORT statement for reporting randomized trials: explanation and elaboration. *Annals of Internal Medicine* 134:663–94

Ballard E L, Nash F, Raiford K, et al. 1993 Recruitment of black elderly for clinical research studies of dementia: the CERAD experience. *Gerontologist* 33:561–5

Bolen S, Tilburt J, Baffi C, et al. 2006 Defining 'success' in recruitment of underrepresented populations to cancer clinical trials: moving toward a more consistent approach. *Cancer* 106:1197–204

Brandt C A, Argraves S, Money R, et al. 2006 Informatics tools to improve clinical research study implementation. *Contemporary Clinical Trials* 27:112–22

Buist A S, Greenlick M R 1995 Response to 'Inclusion of women and minorities in clinical trials and the NIH Revitalization Act of 1993: the perspective of NIH clinical trialists'. *Controlled Clinical Trials* 16:296–8

Daly B J, Douglas S L, Kelley C G 2005 Benefits and challenges of developing a program of research. *Western Journal of Nursing Research* 27:364–77

DAMOCLES Study Group 2005 A proposed charter for clinical trial data monitoring committees: helping them do their job well. *Lancet* 365:711–22

Dumville J C, Hahn S, Miles J N, et al. 2006 The use of unequal randomisation ratios in clinical trials: a review. *Contemporary Clinical Trials* 27:1–12

Dumville J C, Torgerson D J, Hewitt C E 2006 Reporting attrition in randomised controlled trials. *British Medical Journal* 332(7547):969–71

Elliott D, McKinley S, Alison J A, et al. 2006 Study protocol: home-based physical rehabilitation for survivors of a critical illness. *Critical Care* 10(3): R90

Eysenbach G, Wyatt J 2002 Using the internet for surveys and health research. *Journal of Medical Internet Research* 4(2):E13

Finfer S, Bellomo R, Boyce N, et al. 2004 A comparison of albumin and saline for fluid resuscitation in the intensive care unit. *New England Journal of Medicine* 350:2247–56

Gamble J, Creedy D, Moyle W, et al. 2005 Effectiveness of a counselling intervention after a traumatic childbirth: a randomised controlled trial. *Birth* 21:11–19

Grant A 2004 Stopping clinical trials early (editorial). *British Medical Journal* 329:525–6

Hanson B P 2006 Designing, conducting and reporting clinical research: a step by step approach. *Injury, International Journal of the Care of the Injured* 37:583–94

Health Research Council (HRC) 2002 *Guidelines on Ethics in Health Research, Auckland.* Health Research Council, New Zealand

Kang D-H, Davis L, Habermann B, et al. 2005 Hiring the right people and management of research staff. *Western Journal of Nursing Research* 27:1059–66

Middleton S, Donnelly N, Harris J, et al. 2005 Nursing intervention after carotid endarterectomy: a randomized trial of co-ordinated care post-discharge (CCPD). *Journal of Advanced Nursing* 52:250–61

National Health and Medical Research Council (NHMRC) 1999 National Statement on Ethical Conduct in Research Involving Humans. Commonwealth of Australia, Canberra

Paterson B L, Gregory D, Thorne S 1999 A protocol for researcher safety. *Qualitative Health Research* 9:259–69

Robiner W N 2005 Enhancing adherence in clinical research. *Contemporary Clinical Trials* 26:59–77

Schulz K F, Grimes D A 2002 Blinding in randomised trials: hiding who got what. *Lancet* 359(9307): 696–700

Slimmer L, Andersen B 2004 Designing a data and safety monitoring plan. *Western Journal of Nursing Research* 26:797–803

Smith C A, Coyle M E 2006 Recruitment and implementation strategies in randomised controlled trials of acupuncture and herbal medicine in women's health. *Complementary Therapy and Medicine* 14:81–6

Sprague S, Leece P, Bhandari M, et al. 2003 Limiting loss to follow-up in a multicenter randomized trial in orthopedic surgery. *Controlled Clinical Trials* 24:719–25

Strusberg I, Bertoli A M, Ramos M, et al. 2005 Factors associated with patients' loss to follow-up after finishing randomized clinical trial participation. *Contemporary Clinical Trials* 26:38–44

Utter J, Scragg R, Schaaf D, et al. 2006 Nutrition and physical activity behaviours among Māori, Pacific and NZ European children: identifying opportunities for population-based interventions. *Australian and New Zealand Journal of Public Health* 30:50–6

Watson L, Small R, Brown S, et al. 2004 Mounting a community-randomized trial: sample size, matching, selection, and randomization issues in PRISM. *Controlled Clinical Trials* 25:235–50

Wenger N K 1992 Exclusion of the elderly and women from coronary trials: is their quality of care compromised? *Journal of the American Medical Association* 268:1460–1

World Health Organization (WHO) 2006 The World Health Organization announces new standards for registration of all human medical research. Online. Available: http://www.who.int/mediacentre/news/releases/2006/pr25/en/index.html [accessed 19 May 2006]

Answers

TT Tutorial trigger 1

Recruitment strategies should incorporate the following:

- Inclusion and exclusion criteria will vary depending on the research question and methodology, but should be designed to incorporate participants that will enable sufficient depth of information to answer the question or to facilitate generalisation to the broader population, as well as to answer the study in the relevant groups/sub-groups of the population.

- The locations desired for potential participants should be considered when designing the recruitment strategy; for example, there is no point advertising in the local community newspaper if the participants you are seeking live in a different geographical area or area unlikely to read the local newspaper.
- Consider whether there will be language or understanding issues that have to be overcome in the advertising and recruitment process.

TT Tutorial trigger 2

The following issues should be considered:

- Is the high loss to follow-up rate related to participants choosing to withdraw from the study or not able to be contacted by the study personnel after 6 months?
- Are the study requirements more onerous than they need to be?
- Is there an easy method for participants to contact the study personnel when desired; for example, a free-call number with an answering machine 24 hours?

- Have multiple contact details been collected from participants at the time of enrolment to overcome problems of participants moving etc?
- Does follow-up require the participant to visit a clinic or similar?
- If so are appointments flexible, is it easy to get to the clinic and find parking etc?
- Does the study require a complicated intervention?
- If so is there any way that it can be simplified?
- Has there been communication with the participants between the time of enrolment and 6-month follow-up?
- If not, consider the possibility of interim follow-up at approximately 3 months.

Learning activities

1. d	2. b	3. b	4. c
5. d	6. b	7. c	8. b
9. a	10. c		

Writing and presenting research findings for dissemination

DEAN WHITEHEAD, DOUG ELLIOTT AND ZEVIA SCHNEIDER

Learning outcomes

By the end of this chapter, you should be able to:

- identify the importance and relationship of research dissemination as part of the research process
- understand the nature of and dilemmas associated with publishing research findings
- understand how to avoid many of the pitfalls associated with publishing research findings
- identify different avenues, other than publication, by which research findings can also be disseminated

Introduction

'Reading maketh a full man; conference a ready man; and writing an exact man.'

Francis Bacon (1561–1626)

An increasing expectation of nurses and midwives, as professional groups, is that they contribute to the development of quality service provision, through the sharing or dissemination of their research findings — thus actively reporting the results of clinical innovation and best practice (Albarran & Scholes 2005). Walsh and Downe (2006), as midwives, state that this trend is driven further by an increasing complexity of healthcare interventions, an increasing emphasis on client-based experiences, and a specific focus on changing clinicians' practice. Today, these facts are as true as they have ever been. Much of the space in this book has been devoted to the importance of understanding, using and applying research in practice as a means of proving an evidence base for our actions and strategies. This said there is little in the nursing and midwifery literature that explores or describes the reporting of research findings — namely presenting, publishing and publication. This chapter discusses the dissemination of research findings through such media — although the main focus lies with the major format of the formal processes of academic journal-related publication.

There is an expectation that those who do research can automatically formulate their findings into a written format suitable for coverage or publication in the public domain. Those who have experienced this phenomenon, however, often tell of a different story. Even beginning to write for publication, for some, proves to be a daunting and formidable task. Actually getting published can prove a step too far for others. As early as 1995, Hicks (1995) identified that a significant shortfall in nursing-related research publications existed. There is no more recent evidence to suggest that this situation has changed that much today. In the absence of a concerted body of literature, this chapter aims to provide a guide for leading potential or novice authors towards the final step of the research process — dissemination and, ultimately, publication of findings. While it is acknowledged that publication of research findings, in academic journals, is one of several forums for disseminating this information it is, by far, the most recognised and practised means. Therefore, the majority of this chapter's content is devoted to the nature, mechanism and structure of such published accounts.

TT Tutorial trigger 1

Why do you think it is that there remains a significant shortfall in nursing and midwifery-related research publications when compared to many other health disciplines?

The importance of disseminating research findings

Undertaking research, in itself, presents a huge challenge for many nurses and midwives on the basis of historical challenges, such as limited training, understanding, resources, support and medical hegemony issues. Many researchers, at an individual level, undertake research purely as a means of fulfilling the requirements of higher degrees, in the anticipation that successful completion may result in a career promotion or a change in direction of career. Those then who do complete higher degrees often breathe a 'sigh of relief' and equate completion with closure. Perhaps for some, with the intention of eventually writing for publication, the moment escapes the individual and the research is never disseminated at a wider level other than the thesis archives of a university library — as is always the requirement of submission for higher degrees. Individuals who are viewed as being in the best position to undertake research — academics — are reported to be equally disadvantaged, in that they too often lack the time, confidence and resources (Crookes & Bradshaw 2002).

The previous paragraph talks only of the requirement of higher degrees and intentionally neglects to mention undergraduate studies. The reason for this is that it is not usually a requirement of undergraduate programs to ask students to conduct research. Instead, the program outcomes are usually related to developing research awareness and an introduction to research consumerism. If undergraduate students are asked to participate in the processes of research it is usually to raise awareness of part of the design process; for example, collecting blood pressure measurements of peers to demonstrate how certain data can be analysed, rather than the whole design. This does not, however, preclude undergraduate students from publishing. In the absence of conducting primary research work, undergraduate students are still at liberty and are encouraged to publish anecdotal accounts of their activities; that is, letters to journals, perform literature reviews or develop theoretical/conceptual papers, using the best available research literature to support these.

Crookes and Bradshaw (2002) have stated that, within both Australasia and the UK, hallmarks of professional individual development and success are underpinned by the ability to conduct and publish research. Against such terms as academia, scholarship and scholarly integrity, success is closely associated with the degree, range and quality of an individual's publication portfolio. The popular term 'publish or perish' has subsequently been attributed to this phenomenon. Rhoads (2006) offers an account of what comprises the process of scholarly publication. The attributes of the terms used here, so far, are often only associated with successful academics. This view may well have been the case a long time ago but certainly does not hold true today. Beyond academia, many clinical practitioners are now contractually bound to contribute

to the development of theory and practice through research and publication (Albarran & Scholes 2005). Therefore, where the mantra of 'publish or perish' used to apply just to those in academic positions, it applies equally today to those who hold middle and senior clinical positions. Alongside this though, there often exists an expectation that more junior staff will still engage in at least aspects of research process and design.

Another advantage of disseminating research findings is not just at the individual level, but at the institutional and professional level. Often, health organisations (i.e. hospital division or university faculty) are presented in a good light according to their research profile. Where this profile is a concerted and visible one many benefits for the individual can be observed, such as recruitment and retention of high profile research-active staff, excellent higher degree supervision, research-based teaching, evidence-based practice, consumer confidence and sustainable research funding. Accompanying this, with a high research profile, health organisations ably demonstrate that 'success breeds more success'. Of course this does hinge on the organisations actively disseminating and promoting their research findings and outcomes. An organisation may conduct a great deal of research but, in the absence of actively highlighting outcomes and benefits for the community at large, may enjoy less of a research profile than it otherwise could.

At the professional level, nursing and midwifery often find themselves competing against more established and more successful health professional disciplines. Their research standing, both within the health-related academic and clinical community, is often found wanting. Nursing and midwifery, therefore, have a vested interest in increasing their research profile, standing and capacity. Crookes and Bradshaw (2002) have identified that there is no overall source of central data that identifies nursing research capacity in both Australasia and the UK and, subsequently, no clear picture of nursing research skills or expertise in these countries. In the absence of similar data, a similar picture is assumed for midwifery research. Subjective evidence would suggest that the same is so for most other countries, as well as Australasia and the UK.

Point to ponder

▶ If undertaking a postgraduate qualification, seek out programs and supervisors that actively encourage and support the writing up of findings for publication. Beware of unscrupulous supervisors and co-ordinators, however, who may take more credit for the publication than they are due.

A problem for many potential research writers is that they find it difficult to formally translate the findings and outputs of their research into an understandable and publishable format (Albarran & Scholes 2005). If researchers find it difficult to effectively promote their findings in the written form, then it is most likely that those that read them will have difficulty too. Oermann et al. (2006) report that researchers limit the dissemination of their findings if they publish only in traditional nursing or midwifery research journals where many subscribers may not understand the context of the research or how to apply it to their practice. Supporting this notion, there is much evidence which supports the fact that the eventual consumer of published research does find it difficult to translate findings into practice (Edwards et al. 2002; Olade 2003, 2004; Veeramah 2004). The fault here though, according to some authors, lies with the way that findings are presented in their published form. French (2005) subsequently reports that the quality, context, and nature of presented evidence influence the extent to which research findings are subsumed into practice. Hutchinson and Johnston (2004), for instance, report that nearly 65% of their study respondents were unable to understand the statistical analyses of research results, thus could not be confident of applying results to practice. Furthermore, Holland (2004) (a journal editor) states that many authors, writing for international

publications, do not consider the international audience. She argues that writers often use terminology and language that is specific to their own cultural/organisational contexts and fail to consider the value and application of their practice to (or against) that elsewhere in the world.

Leeman et al. (2006) identify the specific barriers that prevent nursing practitioners adopting and utilising published research findings in their practice environments. Walsh and Downe (2006) identify similar issues for midwives when appraising qualitative research studies, by means of a meta-synthesis, for practice. Their findings conclude that most of the critically reviewed studies failed to provide a clear map of criteria used, were theoretically dense and excessively detailed. Those wishing to disseminate their research findings, in such a way as to make them accessible and relevant to practice, are advised to formulate their publications in a manner that avoids the pitfalls that Leeman et al. (and to some extent, Walsh & Downe) identify. They are:

- an absence of information on 'how to' implement finding interventions
- too much emphasis on persuading the reader of the internal validity of findings
- lack of information on the complexity of an intervention or to guide the implementation in practice
- lack of information on cost and cost-effectiveness of intervention
- lack of exploration of underlying theory
- minimal guidance on process applied to the population or setting
- lack of fidelity of the implementation.

Oermann et al. (2006) help to counter the above-identified pitfalls by suggesting ways that they can be overcome. These include:

- collaborating with other practitioners (sound-boarding and proofreading)
- selecting a title that attracts clinical attention
- writing 'catchy' abstracts that convince nurses to read the research throughout
- writing introductions that are aimed at clinicians
- presenting the clinical purpose of papers early on
- writing methods sections with clinicians in mind

Research in brief

Leeman et al. (2006) report on their study into how well reports on research findings facilitate the use of findings in practice. They conducted a content analysis (using a coding scheme based on Roger's theory of the diffusion of innovations) of 46 published research reports into diabetes self-management interventions and matched their findings against Roger's stages of adopting a clinical intervention and implementing it in practice. They concluded that research publications often neglected to provide adequate information to convince practitioners of the benefits in implementing intervention findings.

- presenting the results clearly and concisely — avoiding technical language
- focusing the discussion and recommendations on clinical implications.

TT Tutorial trigger 2

Before reading on, what perceived barriers would prevent you from publishing in a peer-reviewed health professional journal? Do they fit with the points under the following discussion: 'Barriers to publishing'? To what extent are these perceived barriers real or imagined?

Barriers to publishing

It might appear a negative stance to begin a section on successful publication with the potential barriers to publication. However, it is argued here that, in identifying and avoiding the pitfalls of the publication process early on, half of the battle is already won. Lessons and skills learned, at this stage, will help the writer to avoid potential problems and enhance the eventual written outcome. This, in turn, is more likely to result in a successful publication. Potential barriers to publishing therefore include those discussed below.

Lack of confidence and experience

For many authors, their first publication may often be the most testing and demanding. It's often a 'catch-22' situation. When an author is at their most vulnerable or least confident and would most benefit from possessing skills, that are more likely to convert to the currency of successful publication, they tend to lack such skills. Accompanying this, many novice researchers do not put forward their findings for publication because of a lack of confidence and experience. This can be referred to as the 'glass ceiling' effect, whereby the notion exists that the researcher can only climb a developmental ladder so far before they encounter an unseen yet perceivably impenetrable barrier. For some, this barrier may be at the level of the first rung. This unseen barrier is not an actual physical barrier, but more an internally constructed emotional, cognitive or psychological one. For the tentative first-time publisher this perception may ensure that the individual

never gets started. As potential authors might appreciate though, if they do not at least try to publish they will never gain the required experience.

Fear of failure or rejection

For many beginning authors they too are novice researchers. These things combined may have the potential author feeling that their findings are either not relevant or significant enough to warrant publication. This situation could manifest itself in such a way that potential authors feel certain that their publishing attempts will be subject to 'automatic' rejection or, worse still, being discredited. This very rarely happens though, even with poor quality research. Authors may well have their work rejected but, usually, there is feedback and indication as to why and how to possibly rectify it. It is often obvious to reviewers and editors who the beginning researchers and publishers are and, in most cases, they will extend a helping hand, rather than knock confidence.

Fear of scrutiny — peer reviewers and editors

Often there is a perception that journal peer reviewers and editors are an elite gathering of gate-keepers, there to maintain an impeccable standard for research. This is simply not the case. These people are essentially volunteers who juggle their normal working commitments with a desire to share their experiences in the form of a published format. Busy people are fallible too. This means that some editors and reviewers will be seen as 'poor' compared to others — but this should be tempered against the fact that they also normally hold full-time positions for which they get no compensatory time for reviewing or editing (Davidhizar et al. 2006). Experienced authors, instead, learn to differentiate between those journals they have had undesirable experiences with or avoid those that have a poor word-of-mouth reputation.

The notion that all published research must be good quality research because it has passed through the peer-review and editorial process is highly flawed. Reviewers and editors cannot know everything. In the pages of even the most highly regarded nursing and midwifery journals, there is as much poor to moderate research as there is good-to-excellent quality research. The research consumer for this reason should always be vigilant when reviewing the research literature. To assist in this process, Chapter 16 devotes its pages to the critical review of research articles.

TT Tutorial trigger 3

Again, before reading on, if you were to write for publication in a health professional journal, what actions would most help you overcome the potential barriers? Are your notes/thoughts reflected in the points discussed below, under 'Overcoming the barriers towards publication'?

Overcoming the barriers towards publication

Now that the potential barriers to publication have been identified and, hopefully, from hereon avoided, it is prudent to identify what factors assist the process of successful publication and dissemination of research findings. They include those discussed below.

Publishing research is part of the research process

Many, including the authors here, would argue that research is not complete until it is appropriately disseminated for scrutiny in the public domain. Disseminating study results is part of research design and process, and not something separate from it. Therefore, within the planning of all research, it is useful to have in mind the type of dissemination format and potential audience that would best suit when the outcomes are known. A useful exercise is to write up research, as it progresses, in such a way that it requires minimal amendment to conform with a range of academic journal house styles. For those undertaking research for higher degrees, who present their work in the form of a thesis, writing two versions (one for publication and one for a university requirement) is a labour-saving technique. In the case of completing a higher degree, it is a good idea to prepare and submit an article for publication while still engaged in the study and then include it in the reference list.

Be confident of your ability to publish and the quality of your research

If you have invested the time, personal resources and effort into conducting successful research, following the systematic processes highlighted in the preceding pages of this book, the chances of successful publication-related outcome are very high. Getting published is just part of the overall 'research game'. Be confident in the fact that, if the right medium for publication has been chosen in the first instance and that the conducted research is sound and original (or, if not original, a good quality replication study), the chances of eventual success are very much in the researcher's favour. It is recognised that well-structured, designed and conducted research has a much higher chance of being published (Cleary & Freeman 2005).

Many researchers view the peer-review process as something to be wary of and intimidating. Better, instead, to realise that reviewers are mostly researchers who enjoy offering the benefit of their experience to help others and, along the way, to help generate higher quality nursing research publications for professional consumption. The reviewing forum is not a forum to undermine research. Viewed this way, the publication process route should seem less daunting to the would-be author.

● **Evidence-based practice tip**

Replicating nursing and midwifery research studies is important, particularly if the findings of a study are of topical interest and have the potential to be implemented, because all findings provide a level of evidence.

Begin small and work your way up

Good quality research is good quality research and this usually shows. Good research is also usually original and creative — further making it desirable to the potential reader and editor. There is no need to think that a first publication could not be in the pages of the *Journal of Clinical Nursing, Journal of Advanced Nursing, Midwifery, Journal of Nursing Scholarship* or *Advances in Nursing Science*, but caution is advised. Rejection from journals, such as those mentioned, may not simply reflect the fact that a submission lacks quality, but that much higher levels of competition and experience can dictate quality thresholds. For some, their first setback is often their last, whereby any chance of further setback is avoided by not submitting again. If potential rejection poses no problem for the author though, then submission to higher-end journals can be attempted. The expertise of reviewers and quality of review are usually high with these types of journals and so, even with rejection, useful commentary can be obtained to improve the manuscript for submission elsewhere.

Chances are higher of getting first-time acceptance within more specialised discipline-focused journals, but this is usually tempered against smaller readerships and impact factors (see later in this chapter, under 'Journal impact factors'). An important point to remember with peer-reviewed journals, however, is that it is very rare for original manuscript submissions to be accepted on first draft. Reviewers, even if advocating acceptance of a first-draft submission, will nearly always recommend amendments to be made before final editorial acceptance is confirmed.

Starting small can also refer to the point that writing a full research article is not always the only option available. Many journals now offer the scope to submit a summary of research (e.g. *Journal of Clinical Nursing* and *Journal of Advanced Nursing*). Here, a précis of research findings (usually a page or two) is presented. It is, however, suggested that this option best serves research that is ongoing — and so promotes the fact the research is ongoing and that the final results will not be too far away. Similarly, Johnson (2003) states that journal editors are very keen to publish letters that are responses to existing research. While this is not reporting a researcher's own primary research, it allows researchers to discuss how the results of other research may compare to, or differ, from their own.

Work with others

Much as it is recommended that beginning researchers work initially with more experienced researchers, the same is so for beginning authors. In any professional endeavour it is better to learn from those with experience than to tentatively engage solo in the unknown. Experienced authors and researchers are often looking to engage with others in good quality research and cannot come up with all the ideas themselves. Approaching experts with a sound proposal can often result in a positive response and possible collaboration. Another consideration here is that, in securing research funding (see Chapter 19), agencies will usually look to the publication record of the lead researcher for credibility before releasing funds. More often than not, experienced authors are as approachable as the next person and actually value the opportunity to 'share their wares'. The right approach and a positive outlook can open many doors for the novice researcher and publisher.

Of further help is being aware of what research is being contemplated or conducted where you either study or work. There may be an area where you can actively seek to get a foothold and contribute, no matter how limited, to ongoing research and the publication of its findings. It is sometimes more realistic as a beginning author, and yet still very useful, to be named the third, fourth or even fifth author in a publication.

Know your medium

In most cases this will be academic nursing and midwifery journals. Be aware though that some of the more 'popular' magazine-style journals do not publish primary study findings. Those that do publish primary research in their pages will have a clearly identified structure for presentation of manuscripts. General guidelines for authors on manuscript style and submission will usually be found, if online, on journal homepages or located somewhere within the pages of the hard copy. Some journals occasionally run special editorials or commentary on how to ensure the best possible outcome for publication in their journals (Webb 2001, 2002). Some journals might favour or only call for certain types of articles. *Qualitative Health Research*, for instance, would obviously not be a useful forum for those conducting quantitative research. Some journals will present a generic range of papers from all nursing disciplines and settings (e.g. *Australian Journal of Advanced Nursing*) while others are far more specific (e.g. *International Journal of Mental Health Nursing*). Quite commonly, journals will put out a timely call for 'special' theme editions. Recently for instance, after such a call, the *Journal of Clinical Nursing* (July 2006, vol. 15, issue 7) devoted the contents of an entire volume to spirituality-related nursing issues.

> ● **Evidence-based practice tip**
>
> Most academic journals are international in their scope but others have a more national scope; for example, *Nursing Praxis in New Zealand*. There would be an expectation, within such journals, that a national, regional or local perspective, at least, is presented.

Most journal editors, while often very busy people, welcome the opportunity to discuss manuscript proposals. This said, very few authors take advantage of this service. Editors are usually best placed to know what they want in their journals and when they want it. Initial consultation, either way if your submission is acceptable or not, can save a lot of time and frustration.

Keep it simple, keep it brief

Most journals will specify a certain word limit for submitted research articles — usually up to 7000 words, but more usually around 4000–5000 words. A lot of work goes into conducting research and this means there is usually a lot to tell and write about. Five thousand words or so is not a lot to achieve this task. Stages of the research process, therefore, can only be summarised in terms of the main activities. For instance, researchers can only include 'snippets' of information on their collected data. To include all the data would, in many cases alone, take up 20 000 words or elements. One skill that is essential for effective presentation of research for publication then is that of summarising.

Many novice authors are under the illusion that, to get an article accepted in a top-rated nursing journal, they must write either very eloquently or technically or both. This is a complete fallacy. Most journal editors will insist that submissions are written in a clear, understandable, uncomplicated and approachable manner (Webb 2002). Webb (2001) has stated that, while nurses have advanced in terms of conducting research,

they do not seem to have advanced in relation to writing up research. She also denotes the tensions that arise from authors being unsure how to write in either the first-person or third-person (personalised or distant stance) perspective.

Where a researched area is highly technical, a good deal of supporting explanatory discussion is usually required. As a less research 'savvy' profession than others, nursing and midwifery research is often published with high levels of description of the whole process from beginning to end — especially in the methodology sections. This is based on the fact that many target readers of this research may not yet be active research consumers or overly-familiar with research terminology. In many medical journals, these levels of description are omitted in the expectation that the readership is more conversant with research processes.

Be patient

For those who do submit manuscripts for publication, the initial experience of getting published is necessarily one of patience and perseverance — getting published is never a quick process. A few rejections and subsequent modifications later can see a publication in print several years after the research was completed. This is another good reason to write up research for publication as research progresses, rather than at some point after completion. Writing up research findings, as the research process progresses, effectively ensures that a manuscript is ready to send off soon after completion. Even with first-time acceptance, the initial peer-review process can be time-consuming (anywhere between 3 and 6 months), while recommended amendments may take further months to complete and final confirmation several months later. With major amendment recommendations, the revised manuscript may go back to the original peer reviewers for further review. All manuscripts, therefore, are best viewed as 'works in progress'. Even with confirmation, time from acceptance to publication can take up to a year or more. Davidhizar et al. (2006), in offering publishing advice in the form of six steps, identify 'don't give up' as their last step. The other steps, in sequence, are 'read the potential journals', 'communicate with the editor', 'choose your journals', 'follow your manuscript' and 'keep track of journals and editors'.

The process and structure of writing for peer-reviewed publication

As noted earlier, the final step in the primary research process is to disseminate the findings of the study to the community. From a professional community perspective, the favoured approach is to publish in a scholarly peer-reviewed journal. Now that the potential barriers and the means to overcome these have been explored, it is useful to begin thinking how an author can set out to plan and complete the writing process — through to the submission phase and beyond. The information presented below acts as both a summary of points made earlier in this chapter and as a further elaboration on process and structure.

Academic writing spans a range of purposes, from developing research review committees, ethics committee proposals and grant applications (see Chapter 19), abstract writing for conference presentations, dissemination at conferences by poster or verbal presentations (see later in this chapter), through to full-text papers in peer-reviewed journals or books. Writing for publication in a refereed journal can also take a number of forms — a review paper (as outlined in Chapter 4), a clinical paper describing a practice or a series of clinical cases, a scholarly or theoretical paper discussing a concept or phenomenon of disciplinary interest, or a report of a research project. In line with the intent of this book, however, the focus of discussion here will be on the latter form — a research paper.

Selecting a journal

Selecting a set of journals to target for submission is an important process for the writing team to consider early in the writing process. A range of issues needs to be considered in this process, including:

- matching the manuscript topic, approach and target audience to the journal's scope, intent and readership

- identifying the submission process, including the journal's timelines for peer review and publishing accepted manuscripts
- determining whether the impact factor of the journal is important in this instance (see later in this chapter, under 'Journal impact factors').

While you can submit your manuscript to only one journal at a time (due to copyright laws), it is important to have other options if the first journal rejects your paper. This will generally mean targeting other journals of similar scope and house style, so that a resubmission will not require a radical rewrite.

Identifying an appropriate journal to target (van Teijlingen & Hundley 2002) can be facilitated by asking experienced colleagues and reviewing previous issues of the journal for the style and scope of papers published. Journal readership is important for authors to consider, in terms of focus (national versus international application), scope (general disciplinary versus specialty knowledge) and orientation (clinician and/or academic readers). Most journals provide information for potential authors, which notes the range of manuscripts considered, the requirements for the manuscript (e.g. word length, paper structure, reference list format), and submission processes. This information is usually now available on the website of the journal or publisher. If undecided, it is advisable to contact the journal's editor to gauge their interest in your manuscript.

Manuscript submission processes vary considerably between journals and publishers, ranging from mailing a set of printed copies of the manuscript, mailing a disc or CD, emailing the manuscript (as an attachment) to the editorial office, through to complete online submission through the journal's website. More so recently, many of the main publishing houses, such as Blackwell Science and Elsevier, have moved to online submission, review and article proofing (usually available as a 'pdf' (portable document format), on the publisher's article database) — prior to publication. The type of process used by different publishers will also influence the time for peer review and feedback to the authors. This varies widely so, if the author has a particular publication deadline, they are advised to consult on 'average' processing times for various journals.

Increasingly, it is important for nursing and midwifery researchers (particularly academics and senior clinicians) to develop and maintain an ongoing publication track record. The aim therefore is to have a number of writing projects in various stages of development and submission (see Figure 21.1).

FIGURE 21.1 Schema of publication pipeline

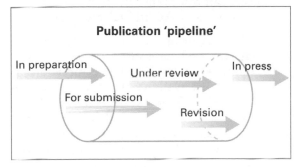

Journal impact factors

The Research Quality Framework (RQF) in Australia, and the Performance-Based Research Funding (PBRF) exercise in New Zealand, have asserted the prominence of measures of impact in relation to research outcomes. One disputed measure of 'impact' and 'quality' of research publications is the use of journal citation rates and impact factors. Citation indexes were first developed in the 1950s (Garfield 1955), as a means to measure the average citations of articles in journals (Bloch & Walter 2001). Contemporary 'bibliometrics' are sourced from a US-based company, Thomson Scientific's Institute of Scientific Information (ISI), via annual Journal Citation Reports (JCR). The most common citation index is the 'impact factor' (IF). The JCR have both 'science' and 'social science' editions, which provide discipline-specific lists of journals, detailing the IF and other information, such as an 'immediacy index' (how quickly an average article in a journal is cited), and 'cited half-life' (the rate of continuing citations to a journal's articles). University libraries commonly subscribe to JCR. At the time of writing, the nursing and midwifery journals (29 journals are listed) with the highest impact factors were (Institute of Scientific Information 2005):

1. *Birth — issues in perinatal care:* IF = 1.84
2. *Nursing Research:* IF = 1.53
3. *Research in Nursing and Health:* IF = 1.08
4. *Journal of Clinical Nursing:* IF = 1.03
5. *Nursing Science Quarterly:* IF = 0.98

Midwives might find it interesting that, currently ranked first, is the well-subscribed to and well-respected US-based *Birth* journal. Unfortunately, no Australasian-based journals feature in the ISI rankings at this time — but it should be noted, instead, that many Australasian-based research studies figure prominently in these mainly European or US-based journals.

There are numerous critiques demonstrating conceptual and technical reasons why the impact factor is not necessarily an ideal indicator for evaluating research (Seglen 1997; Bloch & Walter 2001; Bevan 2004; Cheek et al. 2006). For example:

- less than 5% of all journals are actually included in the database and indexes
- English-language, and in particular US-based journals, are favoured
- factors are usually based on levels of readership rather than the quality of published research.

As an example, Cheek et al. (2006) provide an insight into citation metrics from a qualitative perspective within the Australian context of impending change in measuring research outcomes.

> **Point to ponder**
> ▶ Impact factor is the number of citations of a journal's articles, as a proportion of all articles published in the journal over the preceding two years.

Developing and refining a manuscript

Box 21.1 outlines a range of issues to address when developing a manuscript (article/paper) for publication. It is important to consider both aspects of content and format when developing the work. Writing the content is relatively straightforward, as it is documentation of the research completed, with some of the early material (background, literature review, methods used) already developed for other purposes (such as an HREC proposal). The format includes the overall structure and sections of material flow, which may be guided by the journal's requirements (e.g. in-text reference format and reference list style).

The two common types of reference style (each with numerous variants) are:
1. author–date style ('Harvard'; also 'APA'; favoured by humanities and social science journals, including many nursing and midwifery journals; this style is used in this book)
2. numbered style ('Vancouver'; favoured by biomedical and numerous nursing journals — see 'Additional resources').

These styles dictate the in-text referencing style (author and date cited in parentheses, or a number often as superscript is used, respectively) as well as the format of the reference lists (references are listed in alphabetical order, or in numerical order as cited in-text, respectively). There are benefits and limitations of each style. It is best to note how these are presented in the house style of a targeted journal (especially in reference lists) as subtle variations exist between journals.

Another aspect to consider during development of the background and discussion material is 'author orientation' in sentence structure. Allocation of author prominence (style) is influenced by conventions of the discipline and the reference style, the degree of importance ascribed to an author as a sentinel figure or 'guru' in the field, and for variety in writing. The types of author orientation are 'strong', 'weak' and 'no' orientation (see Table 21.1). Another factor to consider here is the preference for writing in the first-person (personalised), third-person (distant)

BOX 21.1 Developing a manuscript for publication

- Title is a concise and descriptive statement reflective of the manuscript.
- Draft an outline of the manuscript for direction, including the structure of sections.
- When writing as a team, assign sections, tasks or roles in writing for members, but maintain a 'single' voice during editing.
- Develop a timeline for completion of stages, drafts, and the target date for submission.
- Attract and maintain a reader's interest by stating the purpose and aims early.
- Provide a comprehensive but concise background to the topic, including a justification for the study.
- Use a simple sentence structure to maintain reading clarity.
- Provide content linkages between sentences and between paragraphs to maintain flow.
- Maintain the original intent throughout the paper, with logical linkage between the title, purpose, approach, findings and discussion.
- An abstract or summary is a self-contained précis of the manuscript, using appropriate keywords, and is often written (or at least completed) last. Sometimes journals ask for a bulleted list of 'key points' to summarise.

TABLE 21.1 Comparison of author orientation in sentence structure

Type	Description	Example*
Strong	Primary focus is on what the authors said or did; the author therefore takes a prominent position in the sentence.	'Elsevier (2006) concluded that a comparison of previous studies was problematic because of varying study methodologies.'
Weak	Information is again presented as the author doing it or writing about it, although the author details are placed outside the grammatical structure of the sentence.	'A comparison of previous studies was shown to be problematic because of varying study methodologies' (Elsevier 2006).
None	Information is presented as fact, and author details located outside the grammatical structure of the sentence.	'A comparison of previous studies was problematic because of varying study methodologies' (Elsevier 2006).

* using an author–date reference style.

or passive-voice (assumed) perspective (Webb 2001).

Progressive refinement occurs through multiple drafts of the manuscript. This may include using functions in the word-processing software, such as 'track changes' and 'insert comments' to facilitate editing and communicating in a writing team. Self-editing is an important experiential skill to develop and refine as a writer. Some time is required between completion of a draft, and the next edit, so that you can review with a fresh set of critical eyes. Once you (an individual writer or a team) are satisfied with the development of the manuscript to almost-completion, it is important to then engage a 'critical friend' to review and improve the quality of the manuscript. This aspect of 'informal review' can also be achieved through the use of a 'publication syndicate' (Sadler 1994; McVeigh et al. 2002) — a small group of colleagues who review each other's work-in-progress on a regular basis in a safe and collegial context. The aim of these refinement and editing processes is to produce a manuscript that reflects clarity and eloquence.

Submitting the manuscript

When you are satisfied that the manuscript is complete and satisfies the journal's submission requirements, then follow the processes outlined by the journal including the submission format, need for a cover letter, or assignment of copyright of the material to the journal's publisher. The journal's editorial office may send an acknowledgment of receipt. Waiting for feedback can be difficult, so check for the statement timeframe for peer review, and follow up with the editor after that time has lapsed. They may do the same with you if they require feedback; that is, between several reviews. This 'transition time' may also be a good time to commence another writing project.

Receiving and responding to peer-review feedback

The common decisions for a manuscript from a journal editor are: acceptance (+/- minor revisions); revisions (requiring response to substantive comments by the reviewers); and rejection, with variations on these processes evident. Acceptance to peer review or rejection can also occur at the initial submission stage to the editor. Depending on the editor and journal, you may receive a compilation of the reviewers' comments, or the original review from each of the peer reviewers (Morse 2004). Remember that reviewer comments (should) relate to the manuscript, not you as a person, and so attempt to be dispassionate when receiving the feedback and crafting your response. The majority of manuscripts require some form of revision prior to acceptance by the journal, so consider this aspect as part of the usual process for academic writing. Respond to each issue raised by the peer reviewer(s) in a systematic way — either defend your position in an objective, justifiable way, or comply with the suggestion by modifying the text. Follow the editor's instructions, and resubmit in a timely fashion.

There may be a further review by the peer reviewers, requiring some response from the author. At some point, a final decision will be made by the editor to accept or reject the manuscript. If the former, the editor will detail the publication process, including the possible timeframe for publication, and whether the author will be involved in copy editing of the page proofs. This process usually has a tight timeframe, often requiring the author to respond within 48 hours by faxing the annotated page proofs to the editorial office.

Other forums for research dissemination

It can potentially take years for an academic research-based article to find its way into print. This is from conception, through submission, then peer review, possible rejection, then re-submission to another journal, more peer review revisions, final acceptance, journal panel editing, proofing and then placement in the volume 'queue' of a popular journal for eventual publication. This is not always the case but, in such an eventuality, the use of other dissemination forums, either in place of or in conjunction with journal publication, is desirable.

Publishing in academic journals, while generally regarded as the most effective way to reach a broad audience, is not the only way that researchers can disseminate their study findings. Other means can be oral dissemination at local clinical forums, local, national and international conferences and poster presentations at conferences. Those applying for oral presentations at national and international conferences, where unsuccessful, may be offered poster presentations instead. Others may apply for this type of forum as first choice. Either way, poster presentations can be a very useful means of disseminating findings — with the added benefit that the posters can be displayed elsewhere later on.

Although potentially reaching much smaller audiences, the above-stated presentation avenues are still very important for disseminating research findings — especially if used in conjunction with presenting findings in academic journals too. They generally allow the extra dimension of personal interaction, networking and problem-solving. For some, acceptance of an abstract submission for a conference and subsequent publication in conference proceedings marks the beginning of their publication career. This said, we are at pains here to point out that as much effort, patience and diligence that is required for publishing in academic journals, can also be required for oral and poster presentation formats.

There is little nursing- or midwifery-related literature that relates to the writing of abstracts and presenting for oral forums and conferences. Cleary et al. (2003) and Cleary and Walter (2004) are the exception to the rule. They offer sound advice in relation to oral and poster presentation, both in terms of avoiding pitfalls and effective presentation. To avoid the pitfalls, they advise:

- reviewing proposed presentation with experienced colleagues
- ensuring that the content does not marginalise or discriminate and avoids offensive humour
- reviewing for potential legal or ethical issues; that is, sensitive or confidential information
- ensuring that content complies with professional and organisational codes and standards
- that due acknowledgment is given to all contributors to research projects — not just presenters

- that both benefits and limitations to research findings are presented
- ensuring that departmental heads are informed of forum and have copy of presentation (Cleary et al. 2003).

For effective presentation, they advise:
- a wide range of presentation material; that is, graphics, photos, videos etc
- while enhancing presented information with visuals, colour and sound, ensure that this does not 'swamp' or take place of the intended information
- ask departmental audio-visual services to offer their expertise
- the use of concise and relevant information alongside catchy titles and headings.

Summary

Disseminating research findings, whatever medium is used, is an integral part of the research process. It is understandable perhaps why some researchers do not promote their findings to a wider audience, such as time constraints, lack of confidence in findings etc. These, however, are not really true justifications. The effective researcher will have in mind, from the beginning stages of their research, a well-planned strategy for how, when and where they will disseminate and promote their research efforts and endeavours even if, at a minimum, this is at a local level for peers and colleagues. Better still, however, is representation at several levels (local, national and international) and using a variety of dissemination media. Good quality research should be celebrated and wide-ranging audiences should have the opportunity to embrace it through responsible and effective reporting. It is through such reporting that research is converted to publication which, in turn, leads to readership and, hopefully, to implementation in practice (see Chapters 17 and 18). Research dissemination is usually seen as the final stage of the research process and hence this book closes with this chapter. This said, and as for many structured processes in nursing and midwifery, the process is often viewed as cyclical. Dissemination of research findings does not always represent closure of research projects — but rebirth or new birth of the next.

K EY POINTS

- The dissemination of research findings is an integral part of the research process — and needs to be planned and structured early on in any research study. Dissemination of findings is often viewed as, at least, a moral obligation of the nurse or midwife researcher — so as to open up their research for critical scrutiny and to benefit peers and colleagues.

- Disseminating research findings is necessarily a rigorous process, whereby expectation of authors may be high but success does not always follow (at least immediately). Careful planning and perseverance, however, are essential to eventual success.

- Authors do not have to restrict themselves to a narrow range of mediums to promote their research. There exist many different formats and at many different discipline/setting-specific or generic levels.

- Disseminating research findings adds to the overall database for supporting nursing/midwifery-based knowledge.

Learning activities

1. The final stage of the research process is:
   (a) reading as many research articles as possible
   (b) conducting research
   (c) disseminating research findings
   (d) talking to fellow clinicians.

2. Many potential nurse and midwife researchers appear reluctant to write up their research for publication, mostly because:
   (a) they do not write well
   (b) they have already presented their findings at a clinical forum
   (c) they can contribute to the clinical area in other ways
   (d) they fear rejection of their article.

3. Other reasons why researchers may be reluctant to write up their research findings are:
   (a) they fear that their results may be incorrect, or incomplete
   (b) they lack confidence and fear public scrutiny
   (c) they worry that they might not have chosen the correct research method
   (d) they do not see how their findings will benefit others.

4. All published nursing and midwifery research findings are important because:
   (a) it is important to implement them in the practice area
   (b) they encourage all nurses to conduct research
   (c) they add to the sum of nursing knowledge
   (d) they provide an outlet for good writing skills.

5. The Research Quality Framework (RQF) in Australia, and the Performance-Based Research Funding (PBRF) exercise in New Zealand, have:
   (a) made it easier to publish research
   (b) highlighted the importance of nursing and midwifery research
   (c) made research findings more credible
   (d) asserted the prominence of measures of impact in relation to research outcomes.

6. The most common styles of referencing are:
   (a) Harvard, APA and Vancouver
   (b) Yale, APA and Ottawa
   (c) West Point, APA and Toronto
   (d) UCLA, APA and Ontario.

7. Undergraduate nursing and midwifery students should welcome the opportunity to participate in a research study because:
   (a) they can then write their own research proposal
   (b) they can meet other nurses and midwives doing research
   (c) they can learn, at first-hand, aspects of the research process
   (d) they can tell their colleagues about it.

8. It is helpful to consult colleagues who have research publication experience when you have started writing an article because:
   (a) you can tell them all about your research
   (b) they will probably enjoy the opportunity to share their knowledge and experience with you
   (c) they can point out the weaknesses in your article
   (d) because the journal editor wants to know that you have had help with your article.

9. Which of the following points are not pitfalls or barriers that prevent health practitioners using research findings:
   (a) becoming involved in the research process
   (b) an absence of information on 'how to' implement the findings
   (c) lack of fidelity of the implementation
   (d) minimal guidance on process.

10. Disseminating your research findings is important because:
   (a) you will be well known
   (b) you need to feel how good it is to publish your research findings
   (c) your research would enhance your faculty's research profile
   (d) you will have professional recognition.

Additional resources

Clare J, Hamilton H (eds) 2003 *Writing research: transforming data into text*. Churchill Livingstone, Edinburgh

El-Masri M M, Fox-Wasylyshyn S M 2006 Scholarship in nursing: what really counts? *Nurse Researcher* 13:79–80

International Committee of Medical Journal Editors [ICMJE] *Uniform requirements for manuscripts submitted to biomedical journals*. Online. Available: http://www.icmje.org [accessed 9 October 2006]

Lambert V A, Lambert C E, Tsukahara M 2003 Basic tips about writing a scholarly manuscript. *Nursing and Health Sciences* 5:1–2

Thody A 2006 *Writing and Presenting Research*. Sage Publications Limited, London

van Manen M 2006 Writing qualitatively, or the demands of writing. *Qualitative Health Research* 16:713–22

Wager E 2005 *Getting research published: an A to Z of publication strategy*. Radcliffe Publishing, Oxford, UK

References

Albarran J W, Scholes J 2005 How to get published: seven easy steps. *Nursing in Critical Care* 10:72–7

Bevan D 2004 Impact 2002: too much impact? [editorial]. *Clinical Investigations in Medicine* 27:65–6

Bloch S, Walter G 2001 The impact factor: time for change. *Australian and New Zealand Journal of Psychiatry* 35:563–8

Cheek J, Garnham B, Quan J 2006 What's in a number? Issues in providing evidence of impact and quality of research(ers). *Qualitative Health Research* 16:423–35

Cleary M, Freeman A 2005 Facilitating research within clinical settings: the development of a beginner's guide. *International Journal of Mental Health* 14:202–8

Cleary M, Hunt G, Walter G, et al. 2003 Guidelines for presentations and publications. *International Journal of Mental Health Nursing* 12:158–9

Cleary M, Walter G 2004 Apportioning our time and energy: oral presentation, poster, journal article or other? *International Journal of Mental Health Nursing* 13:204–7

Crookes P A, Bradshaw P L 2002 Developing scholarship in nursing — steps within a strategy. *Journal of Nursing Management* 10:177–81

Davidhizar R, Bowd S D, Harris A 2006 Evaluating and choosing journals and editors. *Nurse Author & Editor* 16 Online. Available: http//:www.nurseauthoreditor.com/article.asp?id=48 [accessed 9 October 2006]

Edwards H, Chapman H, Davis L M 2002 Utilization of research evidence by nurses. *Nursing and Health Sciences* 4:89–95

French B 2005 Evaluating research for use in practice: what criteria do specialist nurses use? *Journal of Advanced Nursing* 50:235–43

Garfield E 1955 Citation indexes to science: a new dimension in documentation through association of ideas. *Science* 122:108–11

Hicks C 1995 The shortfall in published research: a study of nurses' research and publication activities. *Journal of Advanced Nursing* 21:594–604

Holland K 2004 Writing for an international readership [editorial]. *Nurse Education in Practice* 5:1–2

Hutchinson A M, Johnston L 2004 Bridging the divide: a survey of nurses' opinions regarding barriers to, and facilitators of, research utilization in the practice setting. *Journal of Clinical Nursing* 13:304–15

Institute of Scientific Information (ISI) 2005 *Journal Citation Reports Social Science Edition*. Thompson Corporation, Stamford, Connecticut

Johnson S H 2003 The Outcome-orientated Publishing Work Group. *Nurse Educator* 28:284–6

Leeman J, Jackson B, Sandelowski M 2006 An evaluation of how well research reports facilitate the use of findings in practice. *Journal of Nursing Scholarship* 38:171–7

McVeigh C, Moyle K, Forrester K, et al. 2002 Publication syndicates: in support of nursing scholarship. *Journal of Continuing Education in Nursing* 33:63–6

Morse J M 2004 How to revise an article [editorial]. *Qualitative Health Research* 14:447–8

Oermann M H, Galvin E A, Floyd J A, et al. 2006 Presenting research to clinicians: strategies for writing about research findings. *Nurse Researcher* 13:66–74

Olade R A 2003 Attitudes and factors affecting research utilization. *Nursing Forum* 38:5–15

—— 2004 Evidence-based practice and research utilization activities among rural nurses. *Journal of Nursing Scholarship* 36:220–5

Rhoads J 2006 Scholarly publication. *Nurse Author & Editor* 16 Online. Available: http//:www.nurseauthoreditor.com/article.asp?id=49 [accessed 9 October 2006]

Sadler R 1994. Publication Syndicates. In: Conrad L (ed.) *Developing as researchers*. Griffith Institute of Higher Education, Brisbane

Seglen P O 1997 Why the impact factor of journals should not be used for evaluating research. *British Medical Journal* 314:498–502

van Teijlingen E, Hundley V 2002 Getting your paper to the right journal: a case study of an academic paper. *Journal of Advanced Nursing* 37:506–11

Veeramah V 2004 Utilization of research findings by graduate nurses and midwives. *Journal of Advanced Nursing* 47:183–91

Walsh D, Downe S 2006 Appraising the quality of qualitative research. *Midwifery* 22:108–19

Webb C 2001 Editorial. *Journal of Clinical Nursing* 10:417–18

—— 2002 How to make your article more readable. *Journal of Advanced Nursing* 38:1–2

Answers

TT Tutorial trigger 1

There remains a significant shortfall in nursing and midwifery-related research publications when compared to many other health disciplines because of:

- being unsure about publication process
- a lack of time, resources and support
- a belief that findings of conducted research are insignificant
- being unsure where to publish or what format to use
- a belief that publishing is only done by academics
- a lack of interest in conducting and presenting research
- a belief that research findings should be 'protected' and kept at the local level.

TT Tutorial trigger 2

Personal observation/experience exercise, not requiring suggested answers.

TT Tutorial trigger 3

Personal observation/experience exercise, not requiring suggested answers.

Learning activities

1. c	2. d	3. b	4. c
5. d	6. a	7. c	8. b
9. a	10. c		

Index